Essentials of
Radiology

Essentials of Radiology

Fred A. Mettler, Jr., M.D., M.P.H.
Chairman, Department of Radiology,
University of New Mexico
School of Medicine,
Health Sciences Center,
Albuquerque, New Mexico

W.B. SAUNDERS COMPANY
A Division of Harcourt Brace & Company
Philadelphia   London   Toronto   Montreal   Sydney   Tokyo

W.B. SAUNDERS COMPANY
A Division of Harcourt Brace & Company

The Curtis Center
Independence Square West
Philadelphia, Pennsylvania 19106

Library of Congress Cataloging-in-Publication Data

Mettler, Fred A., Jr.

Essentials of radiology / Fred A. Mettler, Jr.—1st ed.

p.   cm.

ISBN 0–7216–6744–9

1. Radiography, Medical.   I. Title
   [DNLM: 1. Radiography.   WN 445 M595eb 1996]

RC78.M397 1996

616.07′572—dc20
DNLM/DLC   95–17721

Essentials of Radiology   ISBN 0–7216–6744–9

Printed in the United States of America.

Last digit is the print number: 9   8   7   6   5   4   3   2   1

Preface

Writing a basic textbook on medical imaging is a daunting task. There are, of course, many radiologists who have walked down this path before. Some have been much more successful than others.

The challenge comes from a basic question: "What should be included in such a book?" The answer depends upon the intended audience. I have spent many hours interviewing medical students and entry-level residents in departments other than radiology about what they did and did not like about the many radiology textbooks currently available. The most common complaint was that most books written by radiologists address what radiologists think is important, rather than answering the questions faced by non-radiologists engaged in daily patient care.

After many hours of deliberation, three criteria were chosen to govern what should be included here. The first criterion was the inclusion of normal images and common variants. A clinician needs to be able to recognize and differentiate abnormal from normal on frequently done examinations. The second criterion was that clinicians be able to identify abnormalities that are common in day-to-day practice. The third criterion was that life-threatening abnormalities, even if somewhat rare, be included.

A large number of excellent images were collected and then put aside, because the pathology was quite rare, easily visible, or not immediately important to patient care. For such cases the clinician will seek out a radiologist for consultation. I have included selected examples of techniques (such as angioplasty, magnetic resonance imaging, and so on) to indicate what the radiologist's armamentarium has to offer clinicians.

Educators, medical students, and residents have encouraged me to include more images, tables, and differential diagnoses and at the same time to make the text relatively brief. They have also asked that common terminology (such as *chest x-ray* instead of *chest radiograph*) be used. Whether all these aims have been met successfully, only time will tell.

Fred A. Mettler, Jr.

Acknowledgments

As with any book, some of the credit must go to persons other than the author. I would like to thank Dr. Scott Obenshain for his hours spent reviewing the illustrations and his helpful comments regarding medical student teaching philosophy. I would also like to thank my family for their patience. In addition, I am grateful for the editorial and logistical help of Jonathan Briggs, Percy Bryant, Gabriela Miranda, Adriana Blake, Floyd Willard, and John Stroupe. My radiology residents were wonderful in terms of helping to collect cases for inclusion. The idea for the book and continued support have come from Lisette Bralow of the W.B. Saunders Company.

Fred A. Mettler, Jr.

Contents

Chapter 1

Introduction

AN APPROACH TO IMAGE INTERPRETATION

The first step in medical imaging is to examine the patient and determine the possible cause of his or her problem. Only after this is done can you decide which imaging study is the most appropriate. A vast number of algorithms or guidelines have been developed, but there is no consensus on the "right" one for a given symptom or disease. This is because a number of imaging modalities have similar sensitivities and specificities. In this text, I have chosen to give you my opinion on the initial study to order in a specific clinical setting.

What should you expect from an imaging examination? Typically, one expects to find the exact location of a problem and hopes to make the diagnosis. This is often easier said than done. Although some diseases present a very characteristic picture, most can appear in a variety of forms depending upon the stage. As a result, image interpretation will yield a differential diagnosis that must be placed in the context of the clinical findings.

Examination of images requires a logical approach. First you must understand the type of image, the orientation, and the limitations of the technique used. For example, I begin by mentally stating, "I am looking at a coronal CT scan of the head done with intravenous contrast." This is important, since intravenous contrast can be confused with fresh blood in the brain.

Next I look at the name and age on the film label. This keeps you from mixing up patients, and it allows you to make a differential diagnosis that applies to a patient of that particular age and sex. You would not believe the number of times that this seemingly minor step will keep you from making very dumb mistakes.

The next step is to determine what the abnormal findings on the image are. This means that you need to know the normal anatomy and variants of that particular part of the body as well as their appearance on the imaging technique used. After this you should describe the abnormal areas. This needs to be done because it will mentally help you order a differential diagnosis. The most common mistake is to look at an abnormal image and immediately name a disease. When you do this, you will find your mind locked on that diagnosis (often the wrong one). It is better to say to yourself something like, "I am going to give a differential diagnosis of generalized cardiac enlargement with normal pulmonary vasculature in a 40-year-old male," rather than to blurt out "viral cardiomyopathy" in a patient who really has a malignant pericardial effusion.

After practicing for 20 years or so, a radiologist knows the spots where pathology most commonly is visualized. Throughout this text, I will point out the high-yield areas for the different examinations. Although there are no absolute rules, knowing the pathology and natural history of different diseases will help you. For example, if you are interested in hyperparathyroidism, a film of the hands may be all that is needed, since bone resorption is likely to occur there first. When you have the hand film, the place to look is on the radial aspect of the middle phalanges.

After reviewing the common causes of the x-ray findings that you have observed, you should reorder the etiologies in light of the clinical findings. At this point you probably think that you are done. Not so. Often there is a plethora of information contained in the patient's film jacket. This comes in the form of previous findings and histories supplied for the patient's other imaging examinations. Reviewing the old reports has directed me to areas of pathology on the current film that I would have missed if I had not looked into the folder. A simple example is a pneumonia that has almost but not completely resolved or a pulmonary nodule that, because of inspiratory difference, is hiding behind a rib on the current examination.

You probably think that you are done now. Wrong again. There are a certain number of entities that could cause the findings on the image, but you just have not thought of them all. After I have finished looking at a case, I try to go through a set sequence of categories in search of other differential possibilities. The categories that I use are congenital, physical/chemical, infectious, neoplastic, metabolic, circulatory, and miscellaneous.

X-RAY

Regular x-rays (plain radiographs) account for over 80 per cent of imaging examinations. X-ray examinations, or plain radiographs, are made by an x-ray beam passing through the patient. The x-rays are absorbed in different amounts by the various tissues or materials in the body. Most of the beam is absorbed or scattered. This represents deposition of energy in the tissue but does not cause the patient to become radioactive or to emit radiation. A small percentage of the incident radiation beam exits the patient and strikes a fluorescent screen, which produces light that exposes the film.

There are four basic densities, or shades, visible on plain films. These are air, fat, water (blood and soft tissue), and bone. Obviously, air does not absorb much radiation, so that in the area of the lungs on a chest x-ray, more of the beam passes through the patient, striking the fluorescent screen, exposing the film more and causing it to be dark. On radiographs, fat is generally gray and darker than muscle or blood (Fig. 1–1). Bone and calcium appear almost white. Items that contain metal (such as prosthetic hips) and contrast agents also appear white. The contrast agents generally used are barium for most gastrointestinal studies and iodine for most intravenously administered agents.

It should be remembered that standard or plain radiographs are a two-dimensional presentation of three-dimensional information. That is why frontal and lateral views are often needed. Without these, mistakes can easily be made. You must remember that an object visualized on one view is somewhere in the path of the x-ray beam (not necessarily in the patient) (Fig. 1–2). Each

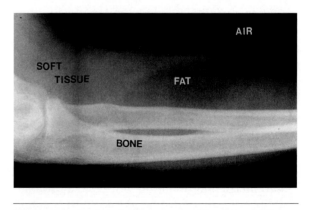

FIGURE 1–1. **The four basic densities on an x-ray.** A lateral view of the forearm shows that the bones are the densest, or white; soft tissue is gray; fat is somewhat dark; and air is very dark. The abnormality in this case is the fat in the soft tissue of the forearm, which is due to a lipoma.

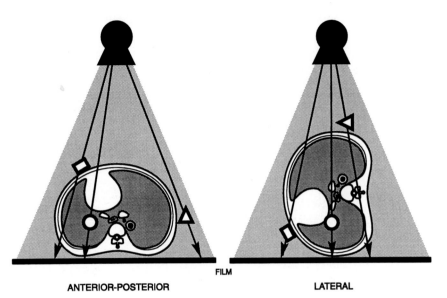

FIGURE 1–2. Spatial localization on an x-ray. On both AP and lateral projections, the square and round objects will be seen projecting within the view of the chest, even though the square object is, in fact, located outside the chest wall. If you can see an object projecting outside the chest wall on at least one view (the triangle), it is, in fact, outside the chest. If, however, an object looks as though it is inside the chest on both views, it may be either inside or outside.

ANTERIOR-POSTERIOR　　FILM　　LATERAL

additional view needed to make a diagnosis requires an additional x-ray exposure and therefore adds to the patient's radiation dose.

The terminology used to describe plain films is usually quite straightforward. Chest and abdominal films are referred to as upright or supine depending upon the position of the patient. In addition, chest x-rays are usually described as PA or AP (Fig. 1–3). These terms indicate the direction in which the x-ray beam traversed the

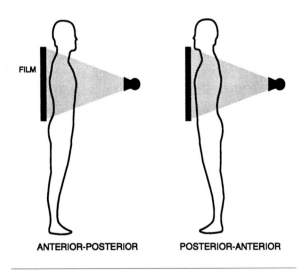

FILM

ANTERIOR-POSTERIOR　　POSTERIOR-ANTERIOR

FIGURE 1–3. Typical x-ray projections. X-ray projections are typically listed as AP or PA. This depends on whether the x-ray beam passed to the patient from anterior to posterior (AP) or the reverse. Lateral (LAT) and oblique (OBL) views are also commonly obtained.

patient on its way to the film. PA means that the x-ray beam entered the posterior aspect of the patient and exited anteriorly. AP means that the beam direction through the patient was anterior to posterior. A left lateral decubitus view is one taken with the patient's left side down.

Position is important to note, since it can affect magnification, organ position, and blood flow and therefore significantly affect image interpretation. For example, the heart appears larger on AP than on PA films. This is because on an AP film the heart is farther from the film and is magnified more by the diverging x-ray beam. It also appears larger on supine than on upright films because the hemidiaphragms are pushed up, making the heart appear wider. A portable film is taken with the tube closer to the patient than on upright films, and this also magnifies the heart.

Use of contrast agents permits visualization of anatomic structures that are not normally seen. For example, intravenous or intra-arterially injected agents allow visualization of blood vessels (Fig. 1–4). If imaging is done with standard format, the blood vessels appear white. Newer imaging technology uses computers. Digital imaging allows subtraction or removal of unwanted structures, such as the bones, from an image (Fig. 1–4B). Often the computer manipulation is done in such a way that the arteries may appear black instead of white, although this

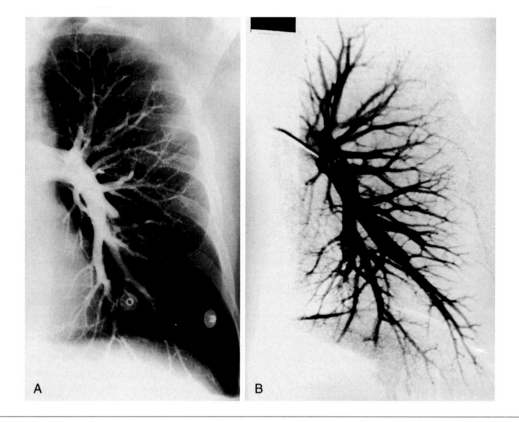

FIGURE 1–4. Pulmonary angiogram. A conventional view of blood vessels can be obtained by injecting iodinated contrast material into the vessels *(A)*. On these images, the vessels will appear white, and the bones will be seen as you would normally expect (white). A digital subtraction technique utilizing computers may show the vessels either as black *(B)* or as white, but the bones will have been subtracted from the image.

usually does not present a problem in interpretation.

Contrast agents are used to fill either a hollow viscus (such as the stomach) or anatomic tubular structures that can be accessed in some way (such as blood vessels, ureter, and common bile duct). When you see an abnormality on one of these studies, you need to determine whether the location is intraluminal, mural, or extrinsic. This usually requires seeing the abnormality in perpendicular views (Fig. 1–5). Unless you are careful about this determination you will make errors in diagnosis.

Contrast agents instilled orally, rectally, or retrograde into the ureter or bladder have little or no risk unless there is aspiration or perforation. With the intravenously or intra-arterially administered agents there is a small but real risk of contrast reaction. This is something that you should definitely consider before ordering an intravenous pyelogram or a contrast-enhanced

CT scan. About 5 per cent of patients will experience an immediate mild reaction, such as a metallic taste or a feeling of warmth; some experience nausea and vomiting or wheeze or get hives as a result of these contrast agents. Some of these mild reactions can be treated with 50 mg of intramuscular diphenhydramine (Benadryl). Because contrast agents also reduce renal function, they should not be used in patients with compromised renal function or multiple myeloma.

A small number (about 1 in 1000) patients have a severe reaction to the contrast. This may be a vasovagal reaction, laryngeal edema, severe hypotension, an anaphylactic type reaction, or cardiac arrest. A vasovagal reaction can be treated with 0.5 to 1.0 mg of atropine intravenously. The most important initial therapeutic measures in these severe reactions are to establish an airway, ensure breathing and circulation, and give intravenous fluids. Other drugs obvi-

FIGURE 1–5. Appearances of different lesions depending upon their location when utilizing contrast. Contrast medium is used to visualize tubular structures, including the spinal canal, blood vessels, gastrointestinal tract, ureters, and bladder. Intraluminal lesions *(A)*, such as stones or blood clots within the lumen of the given structure, produce a central defect on both AP and lateral projections. On AP and lateral views, the contrast will show acute angles on both sides and in both projections. Intramural lesions *(B)* will produce a defect that indents the column of contrast. When seen tangentially, there will be an acute angle between the normal wall and the beginning of the indentation. Extramural lesions *(C)* can also indent the wall, but at the point of indentation the angle will be somewhat blunted as compared with the intramural lesion.

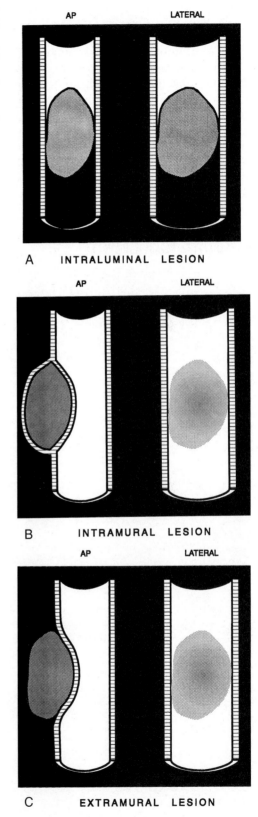

ously may also may be necessary. The risk of death from a study using intravenously administered ionic contrast agents is about 1 in 40,000.

There are newer and very expensive (about $100 per injection) nonionic contrast agents that reduce the risk of severe, but not of less severe, reactions. Most hospitals now use nonionic agents on patients under the age of 6 and over the age of 60 years and in those with a history of asthma or previous severe reactions. As expected, some hospitals use the expensive nonionic contrast agents on everybody in order to avoid lawsuits.

COMPUTED TOMOGRAPHY

Computed tomography (CT) is accomplished by passing a rotating fan beam of x-rays through the patient and measuring the transmission at thousands of points. The data are handled by a computer that calculates exactly what the x-ray absorption was at any given spot. The data can be manipulated in a number of ways, displayed on a screen, and photographed. Since the data points are in the computer memory, it is possible to "window" the image and obtain a number of filmed pictures without additional radiation exposure (Fig. 1–6). The computers can even display the data as a three-dimensional rotating image, although this is rarely necessary for diagnosis. Compared with plain x-rays, CT uses about 10 to 100 times more radiation.

The basic four densities on CT images are the same as for plain radiographs. The advantage of CT is that actual absorption of a specific tissue can be displayed. The units used are

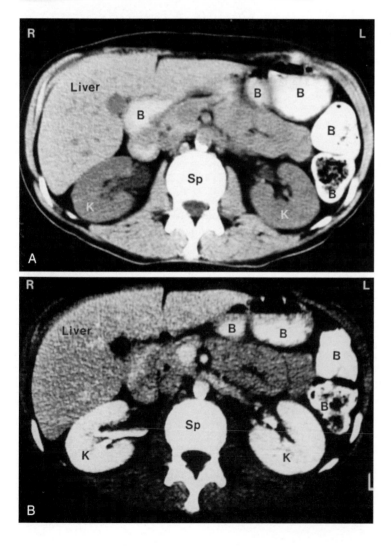

FIGURE 1–6. Computed tomography (CT). Images of the abdomen are presented here. A, The image was done utilizing relatively wide windows during filming, and no intravenous contrast was used. B, The windows have been narrowed, producing a rather grainy image, and intravenous contrast has been administered so that you can see enhancement of the aorta, abdominal vessels, and both kidneys (K). In both images, contrast has been put in the bowel (B) in order to differentiate bowel from solid organs and structures.

Hounsfield units, and the density of water is zero. The greater sensitivity of the computer compared with plain radiographs allows differentiation of acute hemorrhage from old blood and often shows areas of minor calcification that cannot be seen on routine radiographs.

CT scans are presented as a series of slices of tissue. The method is similar in principle to slicing a loaf of bread and pulling up one slice at a time to examine it. Thus, CT is a two-dimensional display of two-dimensional information, and objects appear where they really are in space. The scans or slices are shown as if you are viewing the patient from the foot of the patient's bed. Thus, the individual's right side is on your left (Fig. 1–7). This is also the convention used for the transverse images of ultrasound and magnetic resonance imaging.

Contrast agents, frequently employed in CT scans, are usually the same water-soluble oral, rectal, or intravenous iodinated agents used in other imaging studies. Intravenous contrast agents are common, being used in probably 50 to 75 per cent of all CT studies, and obviously carry the risk of contrast reactions discussed previously.

The appeal of CT is that a large number of structures are visualized simultaneously. In a patient with abdominal pain, one CT examination shows the liver, adrenal glands, kidneys, spleen, aorta, pancreas, and other structures. This allows the clinician to quickly identify macroscopic pathology.

ULTRASOUND

Ultrasound utilizes high-frequency sound waves to make images. The technology is that of sonar or a glorified fish-finder used by fisherman. The image is made by sending high-frequency sound into the patient and assessing the magnitude and time of returning echoes. Echoes are the result of interfaces or changes in density. Typically, a cyst has few if any echoes, since it is mostly water. Tissues such as liver and spleen give a picture with rather homogeneous small echoes due to the fibrous interstitial tissue (Fig. 1–8). High-intensity echoes are caused by calcification, fat, and air.

The technology of ultrasound is attractive

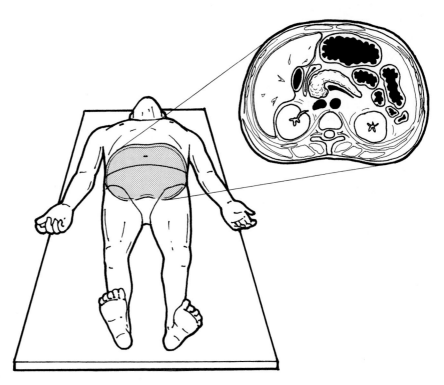

FIGURE 1–7. Orientation of CT and MR images. CT and MR usually present images as transverse (axial) slices of the body. If, as you stand and look at the patient from the foot of the bed, you think of these images as slices lifted out of the body, you will have the orientation correct.

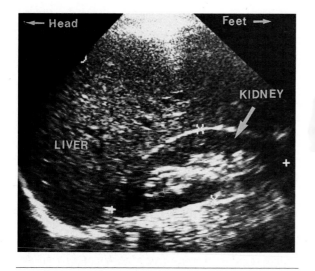

FIGURE 1–8. Ultrasound of the liver and kidney. This is a longitudinal image, and you are essentially looking at the patient from the side. The patient's head is to your left. The liver has rather homogeneous echoes, and the kidney is easily seen as a bean-shaped object posterior to the right lobe of the liver.

because it does not use ionizing radiation and the machines are relatively inexpensive. For these reasons ultrasound has found widespread use in obstetrics. The use of so-called real-time ultrasound allows the images to be seen in sequential frames just like a movie. This capability has proved popular for imaging rapidly moving structures, such as the heart. Unfortunately, ultrasound images can be quite dependent upon operator-set parameters, and the field of view within the patient is limited. Thus, unless there are clear labels relative to orientation the images can be difficult or impossible for the novice to interpret. Another confusing point is that ultrasound images are usually presented as white echoes on a black background but occasionally as black echoes on a white background.

In addition to using echoes to generate images, you can analyze the returning echo frequencies. This Doppler analysis allows identification of moving blood as well as its direction and magnitude. One example of its use is to identify and quantitate stenoses of the carotid arteries.

NUCLEAR MEDICINE

Nuclear medicine images are made by giving the patient a short-lived radioactive material. The most commonly used radionuclides decay rapidly and have half-lives of only hours. Most materials administered are not detectable within a day or so after administration. By attaching a radionuclide (such as technetium-99m) to specific carrier compounds, there can be concentration of the radioactivity in a chosen organ or tissue, such as the thyroid, bone, lung, heart, abscess, or tumor. There are essentially no significant patient reactions to radiopharmaceuticals used for diagnosis.

Nuclear medicine images are made by a gamma camera that records radiation emanating from the patient and makes an image of the distribution of the radioactive material (Fig. 1–9). The radiation dose to the patient is determined by the amount of radioactive material initially injected into the body. Therefore, once the dose has been given, additional images can be obtained without increasing the radiation. Images are usually obtained as planar images which, like plain radiographs, display three-dimensional data in two dimensions. These images are labeled as anterior, lateral, and so forth. Computer technology (similar to CT) has been

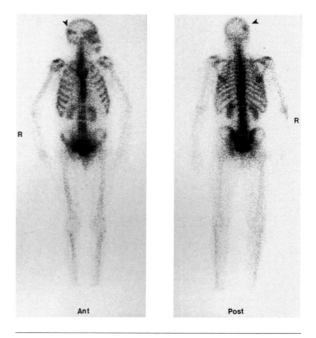

FIGURE 1–9. Nuclear medicine bone scan. Radioactivity has been introduced intravenously and localizes in specific organs. In this case, a tracer has been given that makes the radioactivity localize in the bone and the kidneys. Nuclear medicine can obtain images of a number of organs, including lungs, heart, and liver. An abnormality can be seen here in the posterior aspect of the skull.

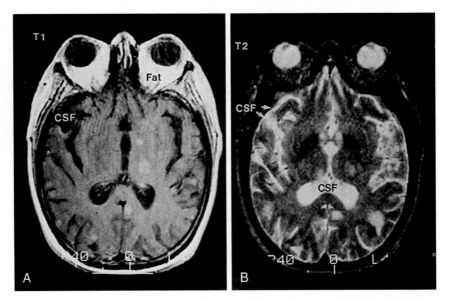

FIGURE 1–10. Magnetic resonance imaging of the brain. There are a wide variety of imaging parameters that can make tissues appear very different. The two most common presentations are T1 images *(A)*, in which fat appears white, water or cerebrospinal fluid appears black, and brain and muscle appear gray. In almost all MR images, bone gives off no signal and will appear black. With T2 imaging *(B)*, fat is dark, and water and cerebrospinal fluid have a high signal and will appear bright or white. The brain and soft tissues still appear gray.

applied to nuclear medicine and allows images to be displayed as slices of the tissue of interest. This single-photon emission computed tomography (SPECT) technology is usually applied to brain, cardiac, and bone imaging.

The major advantage of nuclear medicine is in its ability to obtain an image of physiologic function. For example, there is virtually no other imaging technique that can assess regional pulmonary ventilation or hepatic function.

MAGNETIC RESONANCE IMAGING

Magnetic resonance imaging (MRI) generates images by applying a varying magnetic field to the body. The magnetic field aligns atoms. When the field is released, radio waves are generated. The frequency of the emitted radio waves is related to the chemical environment of the atoms as well as to their location. With computer analysis of these data, MR images (which are essentially hydrogen maps) can be generated.

Although there are many MR techniques, there are two basic types of images, T1 and T2. T1 images show fat as a white or bright signal, whereas water (or cerebrospinal fluid {CSF}) is dark. On a T2 image, fat is dark and blood, edema, and CSF appear white (Fig. 1–10). Un-

fortunately, calcium and bone are difficult to see on MR images. What people think are the (white) bones is really visualization of fat in the marrow. Computer manipulation of MR images allows slices similar to CT orientation to be used. An intravenous contrast agent (gadolinium) is often used in conjunction with brain

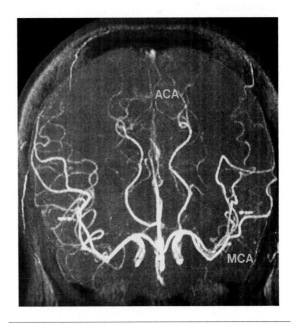

FIGURE 1–11. MR angiogram. An anterior view of the head showing intracerebral vessels, including the anterior cerebral artery (ACA) and the middle cerebral artery (MCA). These images were obtained without injection of any contrast agent.

imaging. This contrast is very expensive, adding about $100 to $200 to the cost of the examination. There are not many significant patient reactions to this agent.

The primary advantages of MR are that it obtains exquisite images of the central nervous system and stationary soft tissues (such as the knee joint). It also does not use ionizing radiation. Recent developments have allowed images of blood vessels to be generated without the need to inject anything into the patient (Fig. 1–11).

Disadvantages have been artifacts due to patient motion, the inability to bring ferrous objects near the magnet, and high cost. The major safety problems with these magnets is that they are so strong that if you bring a ferromagnetic object (such as a wrench) into the room it can accelerate to 150 miles per hour as it is ripped out of your hand and flies into the bore of the magnet. Large floor polishers have been sucked into magnets (Fig. 1–12). If a patient is

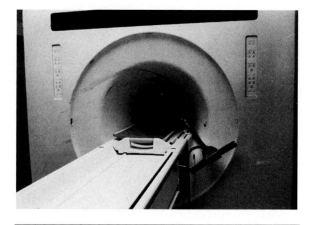

FIGURE 1–12. Floor polisher in a magnet. The high magnetic field strength of an MR machine is shown by a heavy floor polisher sucked into the scanner. The polisher was inadvertently brought into the room by cleaning personnel. (Courtesy of T. Haygood, M.D.)

in the machine at the time, there will be lethal consequences. You should be aware that some "sandbags" used for neck stabilization actually contain small BBs and can destroy magnets.

General Suggested Readings

General Radiology

Juhl J, Crummy A: Paul and Juhl's Essentials of Radiologic Imaging, 6th ed. Philadelphia, JB Lippincott, 1993.
Keats T, Lusted L: Atlas of Roentgenographic Measurements, 5th ed. Chicago, Year Book Medical Publishers, 1985.
Keats T: Atlas of Normal Roentgen Variants That May Simulate Disease, 4th ed. Chicago, Year Book Medical Publishers, 1988.

Nuclear Medicine

Mettler F, Guiberteau M: Essentials of Nuclear Medicine Imaging. Philadelphia, WB Saunders, 1991.

Ultrasound

Mittlestaedt C: General Ultrasound. New York, Churchill Livingstone,1992.
Rumack C, Wilson S, Charboneau J: Diagnostic Ultrasound. St. Louis, CV Mosby, 1991.

Computed Tomography and Magnetic Resonance

Haaga J, Lanzieri C, et al: Computed Tomography and Magnetic Resonance Imaging of the Whole Body, 3rd ed. St. Louis, CV Mosby, 1994.
Lee J, Sagel S, Stanley R: Computed Body Tomography, 2nd ed. New York, Raven Press, 1989.

Chapter 2

Head and Soft Tissues of the Neck

SKULL AND BRAIN

The Normal Skull and Variants

The skull consists of a large number of overlapping bones in the face and the cranial vault. In this text the face will be treated later. Normal anatomy of the standard x-ray projections is shown in Figure 2–1. The most common differential problem on plain skull films is distinguishing cranial sutures from vascular grooves and fractures. The main sutures are coronal, sagittal, and lambdoid. There is also a suture that runs in a rainbow shape over the ear. In the adult, sutures are symmetric and very wiggly and have sclerotic (very white) edges.

Vascular grooves are usually seen on the lateral view and extend posteriorly and superiorly from just in front of the ear. They do not have sclerotic edges and are not perfectly straight. Fractures are dark lines that have very sharp edges and tend to be very straight (Fig. 2–2). Clinical examination of the patient and a search for overlying scalp swelling on the film can be helpful in locating a fracture. If there is a fracture over the middle meningeal area there may be an associated epidural hematoma. If there is a depressed fracture, the lucent fracture lines can be stellate or semicircular Fig. 2–3). In either of these cases there can also be substantial brain injury, and a CT scan including bone windows is indicated.

Skull films are ordered much too frequently. A skull fracture without loss of consciousness is very rare. There also may be significant brain injury without a skull fracture. You should examine the patient clinically and decide whether physical findings and the history indicate moderate to severe head injury or mild head injury. If there is moderate or severe injury and the

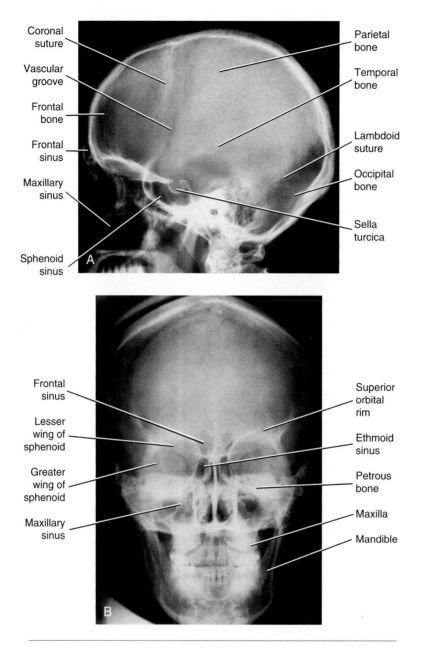

Coronal suture

Vascular groove

Frontal bone

Frontal sinus

Maxillary sinus

Sphenoid sinus

Parietal bone

Temporal bone

Lambdoid suture

Occipital bone

Sella turcica

Frontal sinus

Lesser wing of sphenoid

Greater wing of sphenoid

Maxillary sinus

Superior orbital rim

Ethmoid sinus

Petrous bone

Maxilla

Mandible

FIGURE 2–1. Normal skull. Lateral *(A)*, AP *(B)*, AP Towne's projection *(C)*, and the AP Waters' view *(D)*.

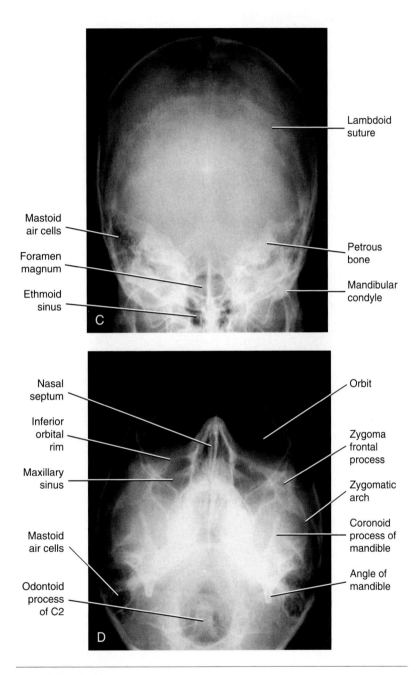

FIGURE 2-1 *Continued*

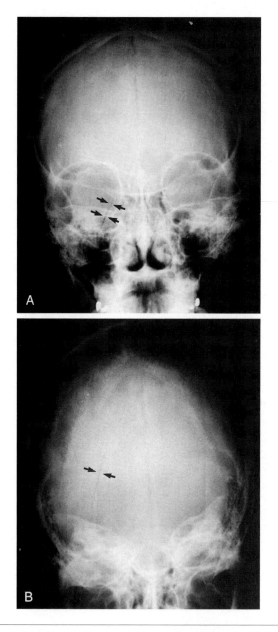

can be observed. If there is a persistent headache, CT scanning should be performed. The appropriate initial imaging studies for various clinical problems are shown in Table 2–1.

There are a few common variants on skull films. Hyperostosis frontalis interna is a benign condition of females in which sclerosis or increased density is seen in the frontal region. It

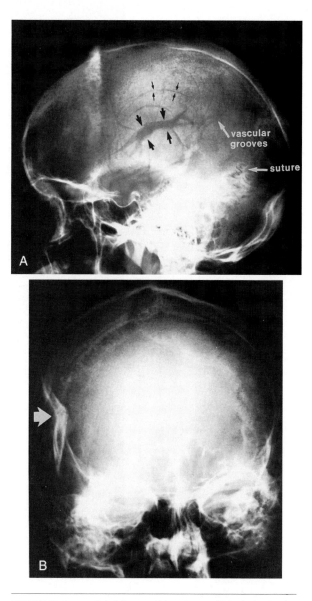

FIGURE 2–2. Linear skull fracture. Skull fractures *(arrows)* are usually dark lines that are very sharply defined and do not have white margins. On the AP view *(A)*, you cannot tell whether the fracture is in the front or the back of the skull. With a Towne's view, however, in which the neck is flexed and the occiput is raised *(B)*, the fracture can clearly be localized to the occipital bone.

patient is neurologically unstable, a CT scan should be done to exclude a hematoma. If the patient is neurologically stable, an MR scan is preferable to look for parenchymal shearing injuries. In mild head injury (with no loss of consciousness or neurologic deficit) the patient

FIGURE 2–3. Depressed skull fracture. This patient was hit in the head with a hammer. The lateral view *(A)* shows the central portion of the fracture, which is stellate *(large arrows)*, and the surrounding concentric fracture line *(small arrows)*. Note the very wiggly posterior suture lines and the normally radiating vascular grooves. The AP view *(B)* shows the amount of depression of the fracture, although this is usually much better seen on a CT scan.

TABLE 2-1. Imaging Modalities for Neurologic Problems

Suspected Cranial Problem	Initial Imaging Study
Skull fracture (depressed)	CT brain scan and with bone windows
Major head trauma	CT (neurologically unstable)
	MRI (neurologically stable)
Mild head trauma	Observe
	CT (if persistent headache)
Acute hemorrhage	Noncontrasted CT
Hydrocephalus	Noncontrasted CT
Acute stroke	Noncontrasted CT (to exclude hemorrhage)
Multiple sclerosis	MRI
Tumor or metastases	MRI or contrasted CT
Aneurysm (chronic history)	MR angiogram or contrasted CT
Abscess	CT with contrast or MRI
Meningitis	Lumbar tap
	CT (to exlude complications of stroke or abscess)
New seizures (idiopathic)	Nothing
(neurologic deficit or known primary tumor elsewhere)	MRI
Dementia	Nothing, or MRI
Alzheimer's disease	Nuclear medicine SPECT scan

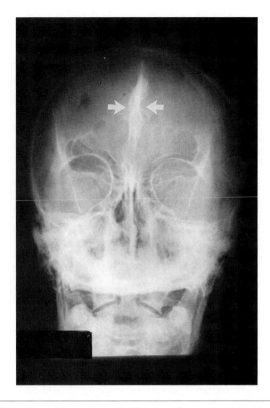

FIGURE 2–5. Calcification of the falx. A normal variant that appears as a flame-shaped or linear vertical calcification (usually seen on the AP projection).

typically spares the midline (Fig. 2–4). A number of benign intracranial calcifications can be seen on skull films. A vertical linear calcification seen in the midline on the frontal film is almost always due to calcification of the falx (Fig. 2–5). A punctate central calcification can be due to benign pineal calcification, and occasionally symmetric bilateral calcification of the choroid plexus can be seen. None of these conditions is of clinical importance. Large, asymmetric, or amorphous focal intracranial calcifications should always raise the suspicion of a benign or malignant neoplasm (Fig. 2–6).

There are occasionally areas of lucency (dark areas) where the bone is thinned. The most common normal variants that cause this are vascular lakes or biparietal foramen (Fig. 2–7). Asymmetric round or ill-defined "holes" should raise the suspicion of metastatic disease (Fig. 2–8).

Paget's disease can affect the bone of the skull. In early stages there may be very large lytic or destroyed areas, but the late stage is more commonly seen. With this there is softening, increased density (sclerosis), and marked overgrowth of the bone causing a "cotton-wool" appearance of the skull (Fig. 2–9). Bone overgrowth can cause impingement of the cranial nerves as they exit the skull. You should always

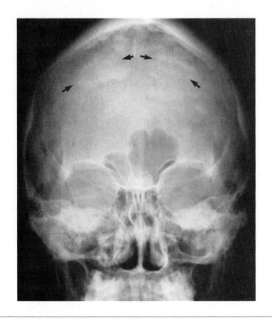

FIGURE 2–4. Hyperostosis frontalis interna. A normal variant, most common in women, in which there is increased density of the skull in the frontal regions. Notice that there is sparing of the midline.

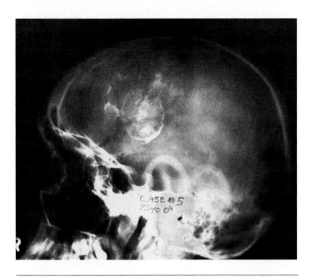

FIGURE 2–6. Calcification in an arteriovenous malformation. The amorphous, as well as rounded, calcification in an asymmetric distribution is suggestive of a vascular malformation or a neoplasm.

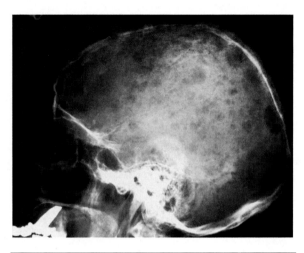

FIGURE 2–8. Multiple myeloma. Multiple asymmetric holes in the skull are really seen only with metastatic disease. Metastatic lung or breast carcinoma can look exactly the same as this case of multiple myeloma.

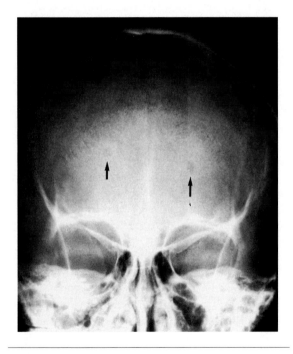

FIGURE 2–7. Biparietal foramen. This is a normal variant in which two lucent or dark areas are seen in the parietal region. Typically, these are 1 to 2 cm in diameter; they should always be symmetric.

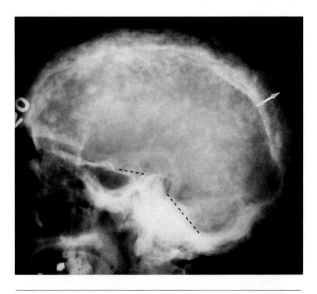

FIGURE 2–9. Paget's disease. The fluffy cotton-wool densities overlying the skull are caused by bone expansion. Note also that the calvarium is very thick. The base of the skull has become softened; the cervical spine and foramen magnum look as though they are pushed up, but in reality the skull is sagging around them.

be aware that both prostate and breast cancer can cause multiple dense metastases in the skull and that both diseases are more common than Paget's disease.

BRAIN

Normal Anatomy

Both CT and MRI are capable of displaying anatomic "slices" in a number of different planes. Usually the study that you are looking at will show a "scout view," which is an image with numbered lines drawn across it. This view can be helpful in orienting yourself with regard to a particular slice (Fig. 2–10). The normal anatomy of the brain on CT and MR images is shown in Figure 2–11. Coronal and sagittal images are much more common with MR than CT (owing to differences in technology that you don't care about). However, you should be able to identify some anatomy on these images (Fig. 2–12). Table

---

TABLE 2–2. Examination of a CT Brain Scan

Look for:

- focally decreased density (darker than normal) due to stroke, edema, tumor, surgery, or radiation

- increased focal density (whiter than normal) on a noncontrasted scan
  - in ventricles (hemorrhage)
  - in parenchyma (hemorrhage, calcium, or metal)
  - in dural, subdural, or subarachnoid spaces (hemorrhage)

- increased focal density on contrasted scan
  - all items above
  - tumor
  - stroke
  - abscess or cerebritis
  - aneurysm or AVM

- asymmetric gyral pattern
  - mass or edema (causing effacement of sulci)
  - atrophy (seen as very prominent sulci)

- midline shift

- ventricular size and position (look at all ventricles)

- sella for masses or erosion

- sinuses for fluid or masses

- soft tissue swelling over skull

- bone windows for possible fracture

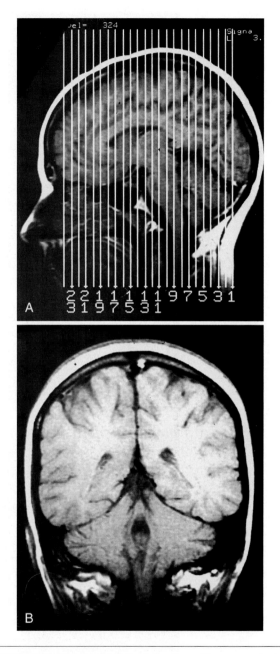

FIGURE 2–10. Scout view image. Scout view images (A) are commonly obtained during CT and MR imaging. Lines are seen across the image; they have numbers at one end, which help you localize the slice. In this particular case, slice # 8 has been pulled out and turned sideways, showing a coronal view of the brain (B).

2–2 gives a methodology or checklist of items that you should look for on a CT scan.

Intracranial Calcifications. As mentioned, intracranial calcifications can be seen occasionally
Text continued on page 23

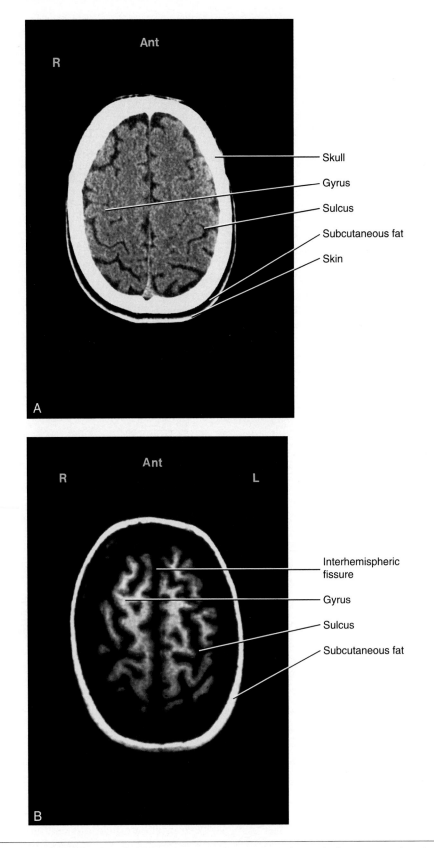

FIGURE 2–11. Normal anatomy of the brain in transverse (axial) images. *A* to *H,* Noncontrasted CT and T1 weighted MR images are shown for the same levels.

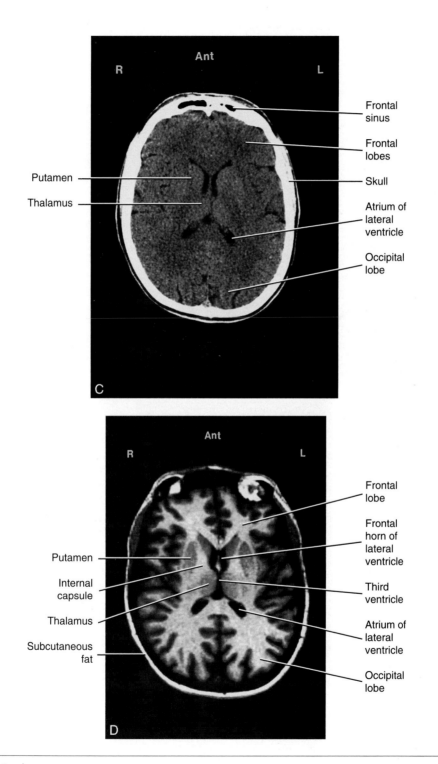

FIGURE 2–11 *Continued*

Illustration continued on following page

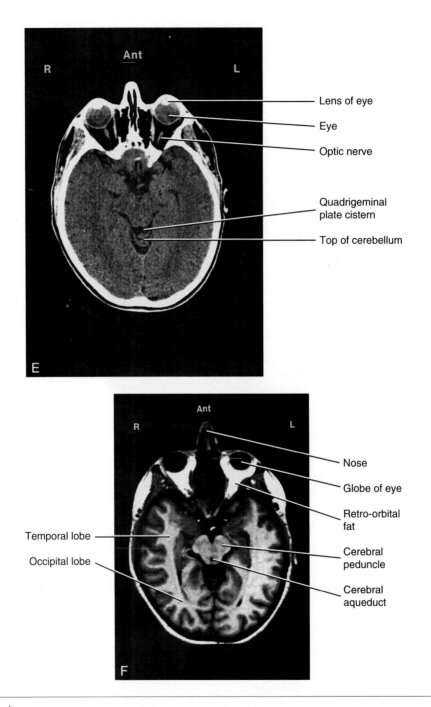

FIGURE 2–11 *Continued*

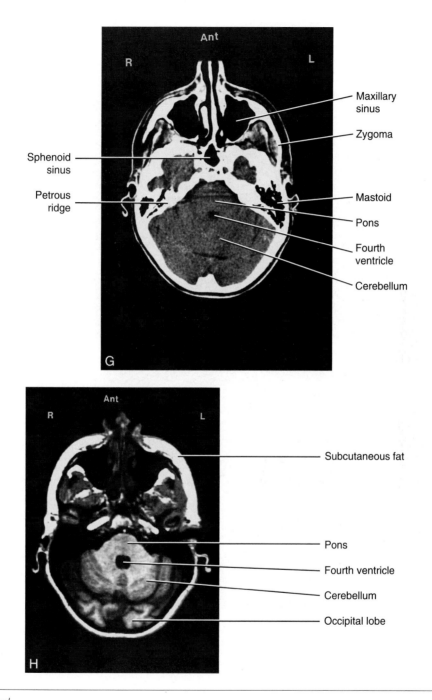

FIGURE 2–11 *Continued*

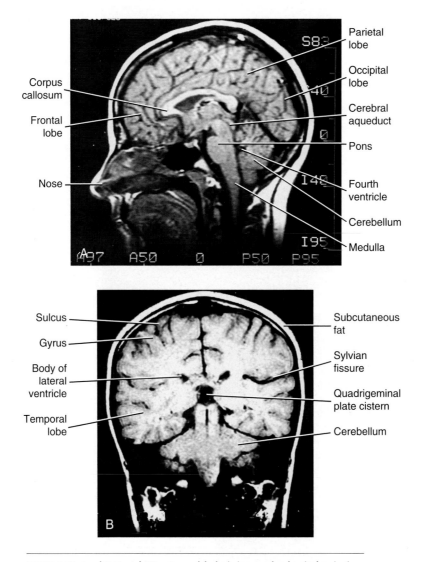

FIGURE 2–12. *A* and *B*, Normal MR anatomy of the brain in coronal and sagittal projections.

on a skull film, but they are seen much more often on CT. There are myriad causes for intracranial calcifications. There can be normal pineal as well as ependymal calcifications. Scattered calcifications can occur from toxoplasmosis, cysticercosis, tuberous sclerosis (Fig. 2–13), and granulomatous disease. Unilateral calcifications are very worrisome, sincethey can occur in arteriovenous malformations, gliomas, and meningiomas (Fig. 2–14).

Intracranial Hemorrhage. If you suspect that there may be acute intracranial hemorrhage, the study of choice is a CT scan done without intravenous contrast. The reason for doing the scan without contrast is that acute hemorrhage appears to be white on a CT scan (Fig. 2–15) and so does contrast . Hemorrhage into the ventricles is usually seen in the posterior horns of the lateral ventricles. Blood is denser than CSF and therefore settles dependently. This settling process is not seen with subarachnoid or intraparenchymal blood. The presence of hemorrhage is a contraindication to anticoagulation.

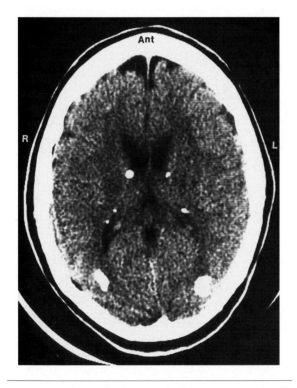

FIGURE 2–13. Tuberous sclerosis. Scattered calcifications are seen about the ventricles in the posterior parietal regions. Other diseases that could present with this appearance include intrauterine TORCH infections (toxoplasmosis, rubella, CMV, herpes).

Intraparenchymal bleeds can result from a ruptured aneurysm, stroke, trauma, or tumor. They are a common complication of hypertension. Grave prognostic factors are large size or brainstem location. Most (80 per cent) hypertensive bleeds occur in the basal ganglia. Ten per cent occur in the pons and 10 per cent in the cerebellum. There can be an associated mass effect with compression of the ventricles or midline shift. The findings of acute hemorrhage on a noncontrasted CT scan are increased density in the parenchyma (Fig. 2–16). Differentiation from calcification usually is easily made by clinical history and, if necessary, by having the area of interest measured on the scan in terms of density (Hounsfield units).

Subdural hematomas are seen as crescent-shaped abnormalities between the brain and the skull. They can cross suture lines, but they do not cross the tentorium or falx. In some cases subdural hematomas can be quite difficult to see. The reason for this is that acute blood in a subdural hematoma appears denser or whiter than brain tissue (Fig. 2–17A). As the blood ages (over several weeks) it becomes less dense than brain (Fig. 2–17B). Obviously, it follows that there is a subacute phase during which the blood is the same density as the brain (isodense). In this stage sometimes the only clue that a subdural hematoma is present is effacement of the gyral pattern on the affected side, a midline shift away from the affected side, or ventricular compression on the affected side.

Epidural hematomas follow the same changing pattern of density as subdural hematomas. The major differential point from an imaging viewpoint is that they are lenticular rather than crescentic (Fig. 2–18) and tend not to cross suture lines of the skull. Epidural hematomas are associated with temporal bone fractures that have resulted in a tear of the middle meningeal artery.

Subarachnoid hemorrhage is usually the result of trauma or a ruptured aneurysm. It is most often accompanied by a very severe sudden-onset headache. Subarachnoid hemorrhage can really be visualized only in the acute stage, when the blood is radiographically denser (whiter) than the cerebrospinal fluid (CSF). The most common appearance is increased density in the region around the brainstem, in a pattern

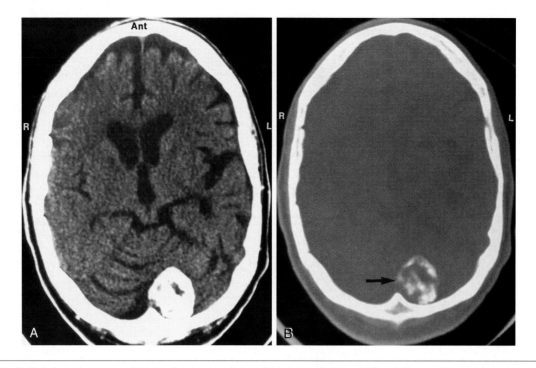

FIGURE 2–14. Meningioma. A noncontrasted CT scan *(A)* shows a very dense, peripherally based lesion in the left cerebellar area. A bone window image *(B)* obtained at the same level shows that the density is due to calcification within this lesion.

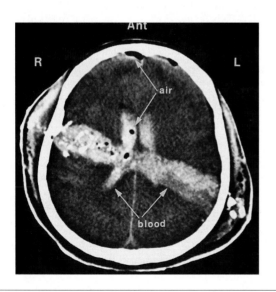

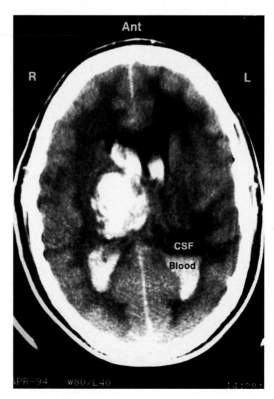

FIGURE 2–15. Gunshot wound of the head. A noncontrasted CT scan shows bilateral soft tissue swelling and a hemorrhagic track across the brain. Blood appears white, and it is also seen within the lateral ventricles. Several small air bubbles are seen in the lateral ventricles along the track and along the anterior surface of the brain.

FIGURE 2–16. Intracerebral hemorrhage. In this hypertensive patient with an acute severe headache, the noncontrasted CT scan shows a large area of fresh blood in the region of the right thalamus. Blood is also seen in the anterior and posterior horns of the lateral ventricles. Since blood is denser than CSF, it is layered dependently.

FIGURE 2–17. Subdural hematomas. A noncontrasted CT scan of an acute subdural hematoma *(A)* shows a crescentic area of increased density in the right posterior parietal region between the brain and the skull. An area of intraparenchymal hemorrhage (H) is also seen; in addition, there is mass effect causing a midline shift to the left *(open arrows)*. A chronic subdural hematoma is seen in a different patient *(B)*. There is an area of decreased density in the left frontoparietal region effacing the sulci, compressing the anterior horn of the left lateral ventricle, and shifting the midline somewhat to the right.

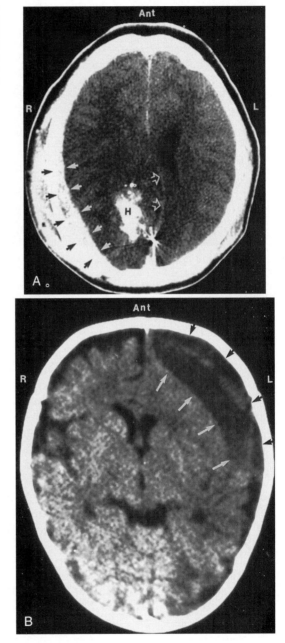

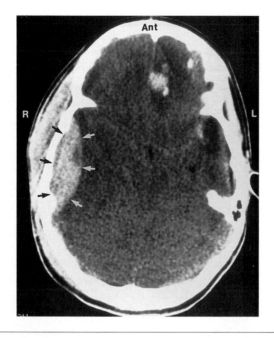

FIGURE 2–18. Epidural hematoma. In this patient who was in a motor vehicle accident, a lenticular area of increased density is seen on a noncontrasted axial CT scan in the right parietal region. These typically occur over the groove of the middle meningeal artery. Areas of hemorrhage are also seen in the left frontal lobe.

sometimes referred to as a Texaco star (Fig. 2–19). Increased density due to blood can also be seen as a white line in the sylvian fissures, in the anterior interhemispheric fissure, or in the region of the tentorium. In the absence of trauma, a ruptured aneurysm should be suspected, and an angiogram may be useful.

As will be discussed in Chapter 9, in infants both intraventricular and intraparenchymal hemorrhage can be visualized and followed using ultrasound. This can be done only if the fontanelles have not closed.

Pneumocephalus. Air within the cranial vault is almost always the result of trauma. Even tiny amounts are easily seen on CT as decreased density (blackness) (see Fig. 2–15). It is preferable to do a CT scan instead of an MRI examination because of the superior ability of CT to localize skull fractures and fresh hemorrhage. It is also easier to manage an unstable patient in a CT scanner than in an MRI machine. The intense magnetic fields associated with the latter can make ferrometallic objects (such as hemostats and oxygen tanks) into lethal flying objects.

Hydrocephalus. Dilatation of the ventricles can be either obstructive or nonobstructive. The ventricles are easily seen on a noncontrasted CT or MRI study. If the cause is obstructive, both modalities have a good chance of finding the site of obstruction.

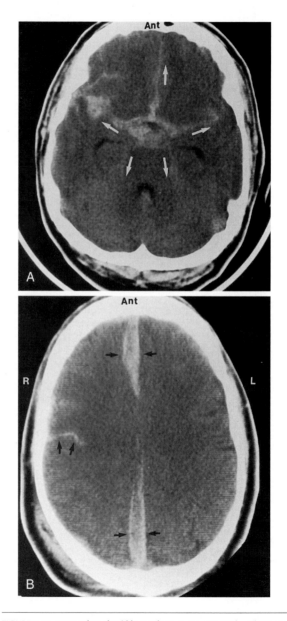

FIGURE 2–19. Acute subarachnoid hemorrhage. A noncontrasted axial CT scan shows the blood as areas of increased density. A transverse view (A) near the base of the brain shows blood in the "Texaco star" pattern, formed by blood radiating from the suprasellar cistern into the sylvian fissures and the anterior interhemispheric fissure. A higher cut (B) shows blood as an area of increased density in the anterior and posterior interhemispheric fissures as well as in the sulci on the right.

Stroke. A stroke may be ischemic or associated with hemorrhage. An acute hemorrhagic stroke is most easily visualized on a noncontrasted CT scan, since the fresh blood will be quite dense (white). A diagnosis of stroke cannot be excluded even with normal results on a CT scan taken within 12 hours of a suspected stroke. A purely ischemic acute stroke is difficult to visualize on a CT scan unless there is mass effect. This is noted as compression of the lateral ventricle, possible midline shift, and effacement of the sulci on the affected side. One key to identification of most strokes is that they are usually confined to one vascular territory (such as the middle cerebral artery). An acute ischemic stroke is very easy to see on an MRI study, since the edema (increased water) can be identified as a bright area on T2 images. In spite of this, an MRI scan is not needed in a patient with an acute stroke. Since anticoagulant therapy is often being contemplated, a noncontrasted CT scan can be obtained to exclude hemorrhage (which would be a contraindication to such therapy).

After about 24 hours, the edema associated with a stroke can be seen on a CT scan as an area of low density (darker than normal brain). If a contrasted CT scan is done one to several days post stroke, there may be enhancement (increased density or whiteness) at the edges of the area (so-called luxury perfusion). During the months after a stroke, there is atrophy of the brain, which can be seen as widened sulci and a focally dilated lateral ventricle on the affected side (Fig. 2–20).

Aneurysm. Intracranial aneurysms occur in about 2 to 4 per cent of the population and are a cause of intracranial hemorrhage. Most aneurysms occur in the anterior communicating artery or near the base of the brain. They can sometimes be seen on plain radiographs if they have eggshell-like calcification. The best initial way to visualize intracranial aneurysms is with CT or MRI.

In a setting of acute headache and suspected acute intracranial bleeding, a noncontrasted CT study should be done; if negative, it is followed by a contrasted CT. The noncontrasted study will show extravascular acute hemorrhage as denser (whiter) than normal brain. If this is

seen, an angiogram is done and the CT scan with contrast is skipped (Fig. 2–21). A completely thrombosed aneurysm is frequently seen as a hypodense region with a surrounding thin ring of calcium. On the contrasted study a large non-thrombosed aneurysm will fill with contrast, although there may be only partial filling because of a thrombus. With MRI, the aneurysm may be seen as an area signal void (black) on the T1 images. If gadolinium contrast is used, the aneurysm may fill and have an increased signal (white) (Fig. 2–22).

In the acute setting, CT or MRI is usually followed by a conventional contrast arteriogram prior to surgery. This is done because of the very high spatial resolution of the conventional arteriogram. Some CT and MR machines can give angiographic images, but many surgeons still demand a regular angiogram. Patients who have an acute bleeding episode as the result of a ruptured aneurysm may have associated spasm (occurring after a day or so and lasting up to a week). This can make the aneurysm hard or impossible to see on an arteriogram. For this reason, if subarachnoid hemorrhage is present and an aneurysm is not seen, the angiogram is often repeated a week or so later. For patients who have a long history of headache, or a familial history of aneurysms, a noninvasive MR arteriogram is probably the procedure of choice.

Tumors. There are a variety of brain tumors. Meningiomas occur along the surface of the brain. They grow quite slowly and often contain calcium. The study of choice is a CT scan with and without intravenous contrast. The noncontrasted scan may show the calcification, while the contrasted scan will show the extent of this typically vascular tumor (see Fig. 2–14).

Astrocytomas can be high or low grade and typically occur within the brain substance. Low-grade tumors may contain some calcium, but they are low density (dark) on a noncontrasted CT scan and have minimal surrounding low-density edema. The more edema that is present and the more enhancement that occurs after administration of intravenous contrast, the more malignant the lesion is likely to be. On MR scans these tumors are usually low signal (dark) in T1 images and bright on T2 images. They can also show enhancement when intravenously

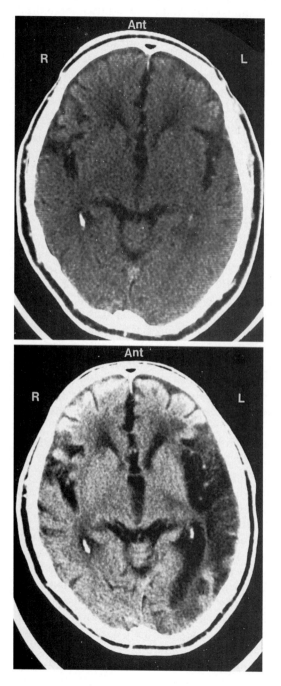

FIGURE 2–20. Acute and chronic stroke. An axial CT scan performed on a patient with an acute stroke *(A)* has little, if any, definable abnormality within the first several hours. Later, there may be some low density and mass effect as a result of edema. Another scan, approximately 2 years later *(B)*, shows an area of atrophy and scarring as low density in the region of the distribution of the left middle cerebral artery.

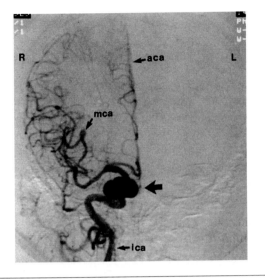

FIGURE 2–21. Intracerebral aneurysm. An AP projection from a digital angiogram shows the right internal carotid artery (ICA), the anterior cerebral artery (ACA), and the middle cerebral artery (MCA). A large rounded density seen in the region of the circle of Willis is an aneurysm *(large arrow).*

administered gadolinium is used as a contrast agent (Fig. 2–23).

Other intracranial tumors, such as pinealomas, papillomas, lipomas, epidermoids, and others, have variable appearances and will not be considered here. A reasonable differential diagnosis can be made from the appearance and location of the lesions on either CT or MR scans.

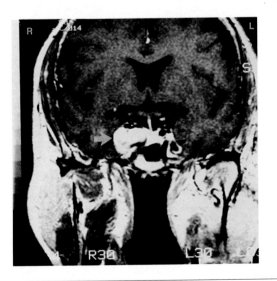

FIGURE 2–22. MR image of intracranial aneurysm. A gadolinium contrast-enhanced scan in the coronal projection shows a large area of enhancement *(arrow)* representing an aneurysm.

There are a wide variety of pituitary tumors ranging from benign microadenomas to malignant craniopharyngiomas. The examination with the best resolution for the pituitary region is MRI, although relatively large lesions can be imaged with thin-cut (1 to 3 mm) CT scans of the sellar region. In either case, the studies are usually done with and without intravenous contrast, since differential enhancement of the tumor and the pituitary allows the margins to be delineated (Fig. 2–24).

Metastases. Metastatic disease is best identified by MRI using intravenous gadolinium (Fig. 2–25). A contrasted CT scan can be used, but it is not as sensitive as MRI. Most metastases enhance with contrast agents. The reason for ordering any study should be carefully considered to determine that the findings will affect the treatment. There is usually little reason to do a cranial MR or CT scan on a patient who has known metastases elsewhere. Almost all metastases to the brain are quite resistant to all forms of therapy.

Multiple Sclerosis. Multiple sclerosis is effectively imaged only by MRI. There are often small high-signal (bright) lesions seen on either T1 or T2 images (Fig. 2–26). These plaques can have contrast enhancement to varying degrees in the same patient. Whether the enhancement is related to activity of disease remains a matter of debate.

Dementia. Imaging of the brain in most patients with dementia is usually an unrewarding exercise. Most of the time a CT scan shows atrophy compatible with age and nothing else. As mentioned, an MR scan can effectively exclude multiple sclerosis, tumor, metastases, and hydrocephalus. Often it is ordered to exclude these rather than to find the true cause of most dementias. It is possible to do a nuclear medicine tomographic brain scan (brain SPECT) using radioactive substances that are extracted on the first pass through the cerebral circulation. It appears that these HMPAO scans show bilateral reduced blood flow to the temporoparietal areas in Alzheimer's disease and scattered areas of reduced perfusion in multi-infarct dementias.

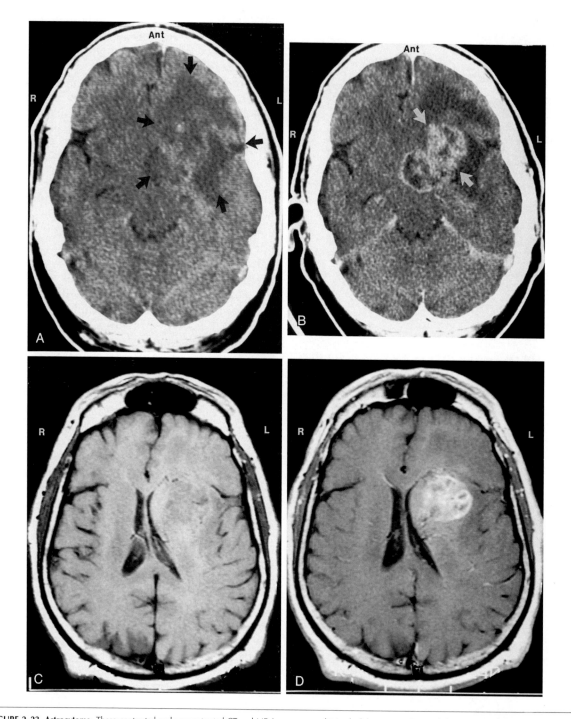

FIGURE 2–23. Astrocytoma. These contrasted and noncontrasted CT and MR images were obtained of the same patient and demonstrate a left astrocytoma with a large amount of surrounding edema. The noncontrasted CT scan *(A)* shows only a large area of low density that represents the tumor and edema. A contrasted CT scan *(B)* shows enhancement of the tumor *(arrows)* surrounded by the dark or low-density area of edema. A noncontrasted T1 weighted MR image (C) clearly shows a mass effect due to impression of the tumor on the left lateral ventricle and some midline shift. A gadolinium-enhanced T1 weighted MR image *(D)* clearly outlines the tumor, but the edema is difficult to see.

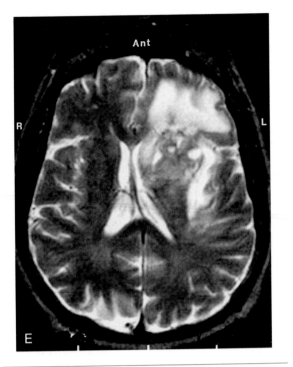

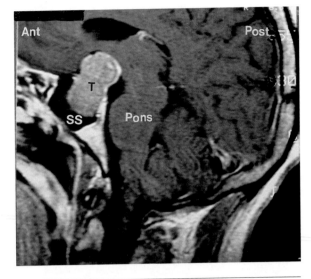

FIGURE 2–24. Pituitary adenoma. A sagittal view of the base of the brain on a T1 weighted MR scan shows the pituitary tumor (T) and its extension down into the sphenoid sinus (SS).

FIGURE 2–23 *Continued* A T2 weighted MR image *(E)* shows the tumor rather poorly, but the surrounding edema is easily seen as an area of increased signal (white).

Such studies may not be cost effective unless you have an effective therapy for these entities.

FACE

Sinuses

The frontal skull film is best used to evaluate the frontal and ethmoid sinuses. The frontal Waters' view (done with the head tipped back) is used to evaluate the maxillary sinuses. The lateral view is used for evaluation of the sphenoid sinus (Fig. 2–27). Sinus series are often inappropriately ordered to rule out sinusitis in children. Sinuses are not developed or well pneumatized until children are about 5 to 6 years old (Fig. 2–28). In adults there is often hypoplasia of the frontal sinuses.

Most patients with suspected sinusitis do not need sinus films for clinical management. Sinusitis is most common in the maxillary sinuses. Acute sinusitis is diagnosed radiographi-

cally if there is an air-fluid level in the sinus (Fig. 2–29) or complete opacification. After trauma, hemorrhage can also cause an air-fluid level. With chronic sinusitis there is thickening and indistinctness of the sinus walls.

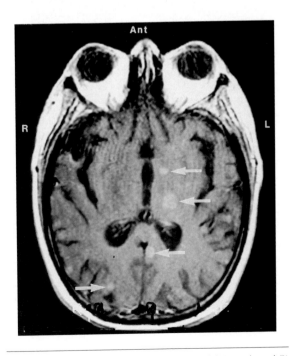

FIGURE 2–25. Metastatic disease to the brain. A gadolinium-enhanced T1 weighted image shows multiple metastases as areas of increased signal *(arrows)*.

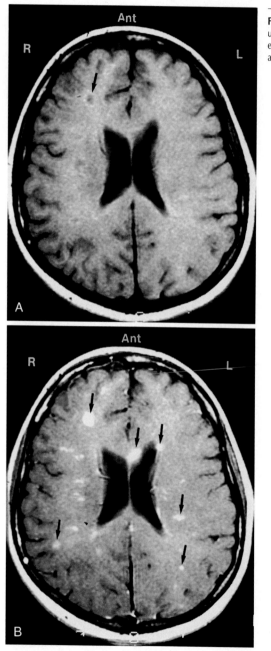

FIGURE 2–26. Multiple sclerosis. The noncontrasted T1 weighted MR scan *(A)* is generally unremarkable with the exception of one lesion in the right frontal lobe. A gadolinium-enhanced scan *(B)* is much better and shows many enhancing lesions, only some of which are indicated by the arrows.

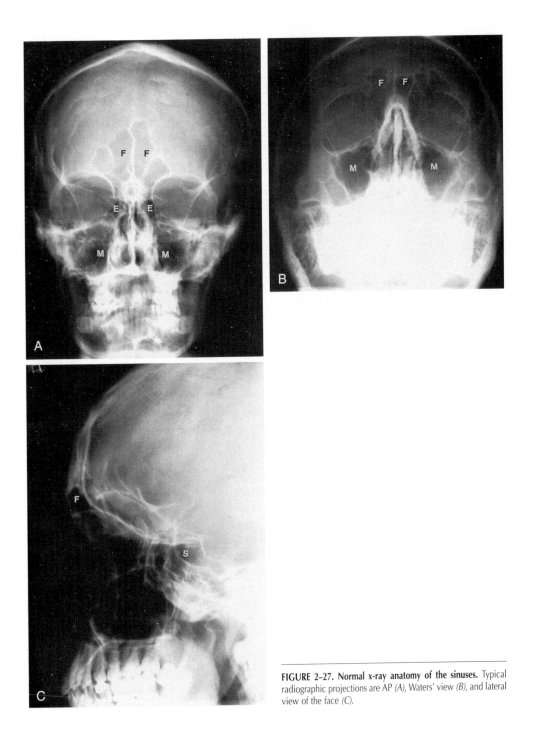

FIGURE 2–27. Normal x-ray anatomy of the sinuses. Typical radiographic projections are AP (A), Waters' view (B), and lateral view of the face (C).

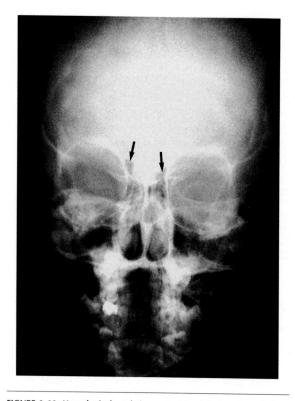

FIGURE 2–28. **Hypoplastic frontal sinuses.** In this adult, there has only been minimal development of both frontal sinuses *(arrows)*. This is a common normal variant.

Facial Fractures

Zygoma. Fractures of the zygoma can result from a direct blow to the arch or to the zygomatic process. The arch and the skull form a rigid bony ring. Just like a pretzel, it cannot be broken in only one place. The view that should be ordered if an arch fracture is suspected is the "jug handle" view (Fig. 2–30). If only one fracture is seen in the arch, then films of the facial bones should be obtained to exclude a so-called tripod fracture.

The tripod fracture results from a direct blow to the zygomatic process. It actually consists of four fractures, not three as the name suggests. The fractures are of the zygomatic arch, lateral orbital rim, inferior orbital rim, and lateral wall of the maxillary sinus (Fig. 2–31).

Nasal. In my view, nasal films are useful only to look for depressed fractures or lateral deviation. The latter is often obvious clinically. On the lateral view, the nasal bone has normal lucent lines that are often mistaken for fractures. If the lines follow along the length of the nose, however, they are not fractures. Fractures are seen as dark lines that are perpendicular or sharply oblique to the length of the nose (Fig. 2–32).

Orbital. Blowout fractures occur from a direct blow to the globe of the eye. Most often this is due to trauma from a small object, such as a racquet ball or fist. The pressure on the eyeball fractures the weak medial or inferior walls of the orbit. The usual blowout fracture is down through the orbital floor. The Waters' view affords the best image to look for this. The findings that may be present are discontinuity of the orbital floor, a soft tissue mass hanging down into the maxillary antrum (Fig. 2–33), fluid in the maxillary antrum, and rarely air in the orbit (coming up from the sinus). Blowout fractures can also occur medially into the ethmoid sinus (Fig. 2–34). You will see this on the frontal skull view only as opacification (whiteness) in the affected ethmoid sinus.

Le Fort Fractures of the Face. These rare injuries are produced by massive facial trauma. They are associated with many other smaller fractures. A Le Fort 1 fracture is a fracture through the maxilla, usually caused by being hit in the upper mouth with something like a baseball bat. A Le Fort 2 fracture involves the maxilla, nose, and inferior and medial orbital walls. A Le Fort 3 fracture is a facial-cranial dissociation or a separation between the face and the skull. Owing to the massive trauma required for the type 3 fracture, there is a high fatality rate from the associated brain injury.

Mandible. Mandibular fractures should be suspected especially if there is malocclusion after trauma. Occasionally there can be temporomandibular joint dislocation. The easiest way to visualize these entities is to order a Panorex view of the mandible. This displays the mandible as if it were flattened out (Fig. 2–35). If a Panorex machine is not available, standard oblique views of the mandible are satisfactory but harder to interpret.

Text continued on page 39

FIGURE 2–29. Sinusitis. A Waters' view taken in the upright position *(A)* may show an air-fluid interface *(arrows)* in acute sinusitis. In another patient who is a child *(B)* there is opacification of the left maxillary antrum *(arrows),* and this may represent either acute or chronic sinusitis.

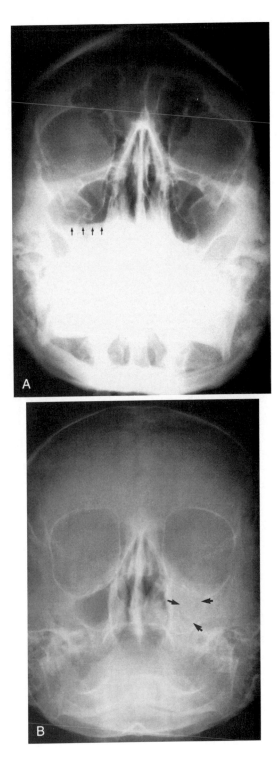

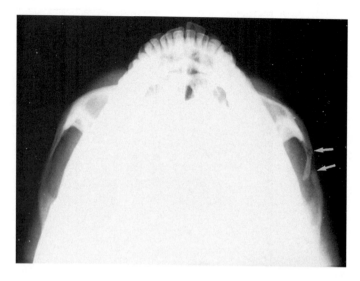

FIGURE 2–30. Depressed zygomatic fracture. A view of the skull from the bottom (jug-handle view) shows the zygomatic arches very well. In this patient, a direct blow to the zygoma has caused a depressed fracture.

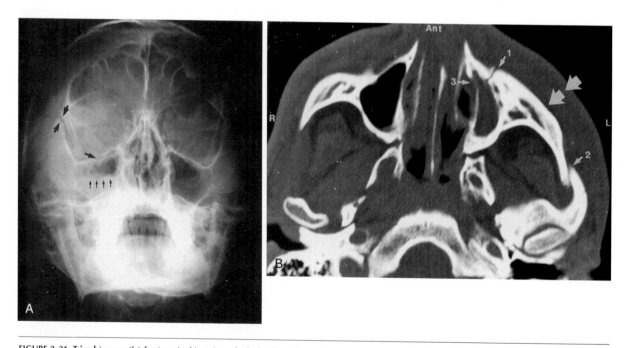

FIGURE 2–31. Tripod (zygomatic) fracture. In this patient who had a direct blow to the zygomatic process, the AP Water's view of the skull obtained in the upright position (A) shows an air-fluid level (as a result of hemorrhage) in the right maxillary antrum. There is also discontinuity of the inferior and right lateral orbital walls, representing a fracture. A transverse CT view in a different patient (B) shows a tripod fracture on the left caused by a direct blow in the direction indicated by the large arrows. Fractures of the anterior (1) and posterior (2) zygoma as well as the medial wall of the left maxillary sinus (3) are seen.

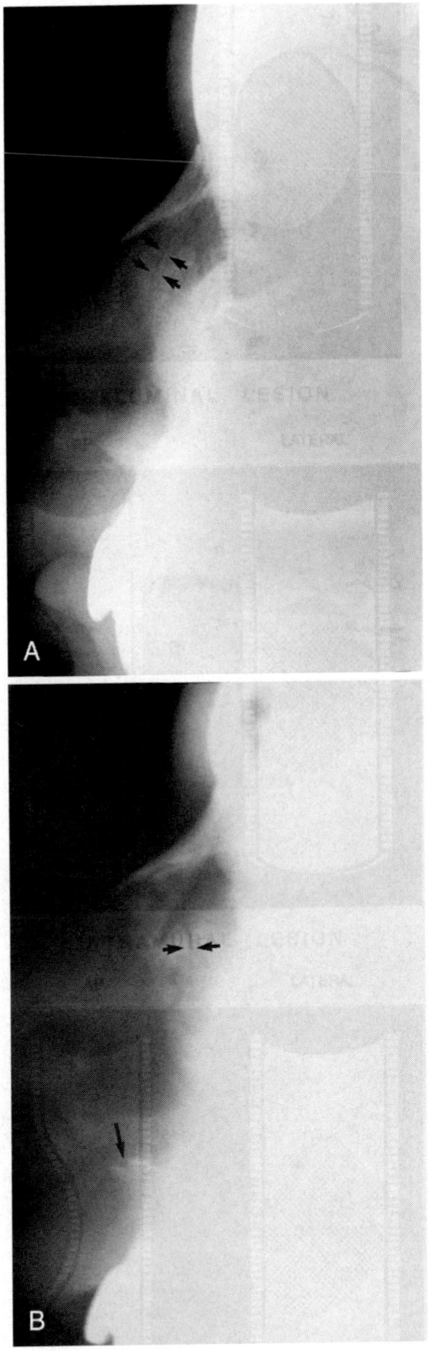

FIGURE 2–32. Normal and fractured nasal bones. A normal lateral view *(A)* of the nose shows normal dark longitudinal lines in the nasal bone. A nasal fracture *(B)* is seen as a lucent line that is not in the long axis of the nose *(arrows)*. A fracture of the anterior maxillary spine is also seen in this patient.

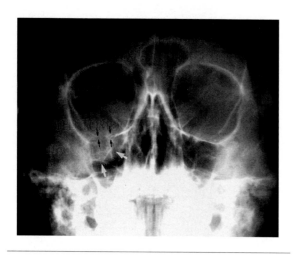

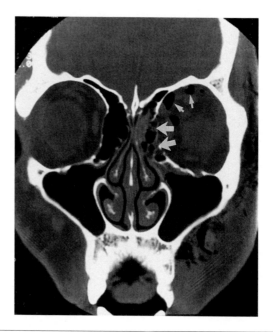

FIGURE 2–33. Inferior blowout fracture of the orbit. An AP view of the face shows air in the orbit, discontinuity of the floor of the right orbit *(black arrows)* as well as a soft tissue mass hanging down from the orbit into the maxillary antrum *(white arrows)* and blood in the dependent part of the sinus.

FIGURE 2–34. Medial blowout fracture. A coronal CT scan shows a fracture of the medial orbital wall with hemorrhage into the left ethmoid sinus *(large arrows).* Air within the orbit *(small white arrows),* is seen in this case.

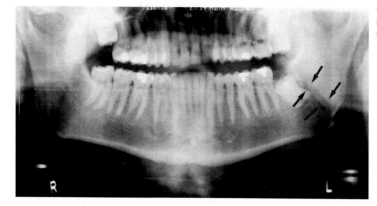

FIGURE 2–35. Mandibular fracture. A panorex view shows a fracture through the left mandibular angle.

FIGURE 2–36. **Normal epiglottis and epiglottitis.** The normal epiglottis is well seen on the lateral soft tissue view of the neck *(A)* as a delicate curved structure. In a patient with epiglottitis *(B)*, the epiglottis is swollen and significantly reduces the diameter of the airway.

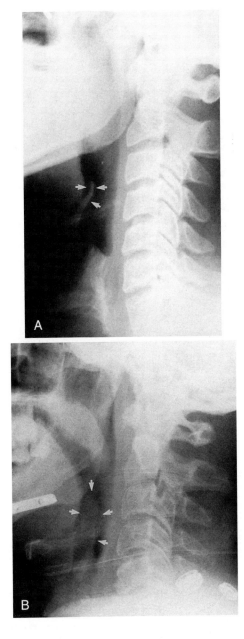

SOFT TISSUES OF THE NECK

For a discussion of cervical fractures and dislocation the reader is referred to Chapter 8.

Epiglottitis

Epiglottitis is usually thought of as a childhood disease, but it can occur in adults as well. The best initial imaging modality for upper airway obstruction or suspected foreign body is a lateral "soft tissue" view of the neck. This is essentially an underexposed lateral cervical spine view, and the airway is usually well seen. With epiglottitis there is swelling of the epiglottis that is seen easily on the lateral view. The epiglottis looks somewhat like a thumbprint rather than a thin delicate curved structure (Fig. 2–36). For a discussion of croup

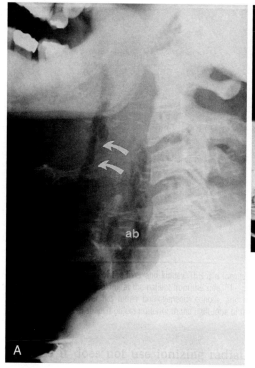

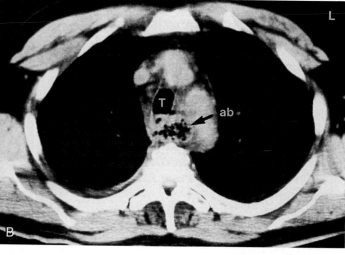

FIGURE 2–37. Retropharyngeal abscess. On a lateral soft tissue view of the neck *(A)*, the normal air column is displaced forward *(curved arrows)*. There is a large amount of soft tissue swelling in front of the cervical spine; gas, which represents an abscess (ab), is seen in the lower portion. A CT scan through the upper thorax in the same patient *(B)* shows extension of the abscess (ab) down into the mediastinum between the trachea (T) and the spine.

and pediatric epiglottitis the reader is referred to Chapter 9.

Retropharyngeal Abscess

This is another cause of upper airway obstruction as well as a cause of dysphagia. The soft tissue lateral radiograph is the initial imaging procedure of choice. There is usually prevertebral soft tissue swelling. There may or may not be air within these swollen soft tissues (Fig. 2–37). An intravenously contrasted CT scan is often of great value to help discern the lateral and inferior margins of the abscess and the location of the great vessels of the neck. Retropharyngeal abscesses can extend interiorly into the mediastinum or laterally into the region of the carotid artery and jugular vein.

Subcutaneous Emphysema

In addition to air within the soft tissues of the retropharynx, you should also be aware of dark vertical lines of air within the anterior and lat-

eral soft tissues of the neck. If you see these you should look at the concurrent chest x-ray, or order one, to exclude either a pneumothorax or mediastinal emphysema. These are both potentially life-threatening abnormalities and the air from these commonly dissects up into the neck. (See Chapter 3 for a full description of these entities.)

Thyroid

The thyroid is a symmetric gland that lies lateral and anterior to the trachea just above the thoracic inlet. Large goiters can compress the trachea in a symmetric fashion, although this is unusual. More commonly, there is asymmetric enlargement and the trachea is deviated to one side or the other. Before diagnosing tracheal deviation you must be sure that the patient is not rotated. On a well-positioned PA or AP film, the medial aspect of the clavicles is equidistant from the posterior spinous processes (Fig. 2–38).

A number of patients will present with hyperthyroidism and a smoothly enlarged gland (Graves' disease) or a lumpy enlarged gland

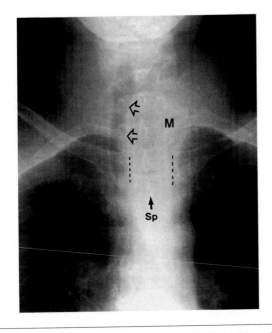

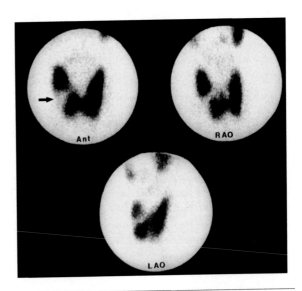

FIGURE 2–38. Thyroid mass. A large thyroid adenoma has displaced the trachea to the right *(open arrows)*. This pattern can be simulated if the patient is rotated slightly when the x-ray is taken. In this case, however, the medial aspects of the clavicles *(dotted lines)* can be seen to be centered over the posterior spinous processes, indicating that, in this case, the patient was not rotated and a mass is truly present.

FIGURE 2–40. Thyroid carcinoma. The right and left lobes of the thyroid are well seen; however, there is a "cold" lesion in the middle of the right lobe *(arrow)*. Lack of uptake of the radioactive tracer can be due to a number of entities, including a cyst or an adenoma, but in this case it was due to thyroid carcinoma.

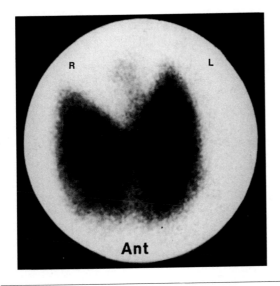

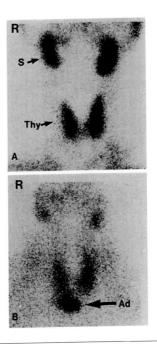

FIGURE 2–39. Graves' disease. An iodine-123 nuclear medicine scan shows a very enlarged right and left lobe of the thyroid. Activity projecting from the upper portion of the left lobe represents a pyramidal lobe commonly seen in Graves' disease patients.

FIGURE 2–41. Parathyroid adenoma. A nuclear medicine scan *(A)* utilizing technetium pertechnetate can show the salivary glands (s) as well as the thyroid (thy). An additional scan done with a cardiac agent, such as thallium *(B)*, will concentrate in and show the aforementioned structures as well as parathyroid adenomas (ad). In cases in which the adenoma is hidden behind the thyroid gland, computer subtraction of the two scans can be done to make it more obvious.

(multinodular goiter). The most appropriate imaging study for these patients is a nuclear medicine thyroid scan done after administration of a radioactive material that concentrates in the thyroid gland (such as technetium-99m pertechnetate or iodine-123) (Fig. 2–39). Radioactive iodine-131 is often given orally to treat both hyperthyroidism and thyroid cancer.

A nuclear medicine scan is the imaging study of choice for patients who have a palpable thyroid nodule. Its purpose is to ascertain whether the nodule has function similar to the normal tissue. If it does, it is not likely to be a cancer. If the nodule has less than normal accumulation of radioactivity it may be a cancer, a necrotic adenoma, or a colloid cyst (Fig. 2–40). Although ultrasound can be performed, it usually does not add much information. Many of these patients will undergo fine needle aspiration of cells for pathologic examination.

Parathyroid

The most common parathyroid problem requiring imaging is hypercalcemia secondary to a parathyroid adenoma (80 per cent) or to hyperplasia (20 per cent). Because adenomas can be very difficult to locate at surgery, a nuclear medicine scan using radioactive compounds that accumulate in the thyroid and parathyroid should be done. The resulting images are very accurate in localizing the adenomas (Fig. 2–41). At this point there is little reason to order CT, MR, or ultrasound for these lesions.

General Suggested Reading

Osborne A: Diagnostic Neuroradiology. St. Louis, CV Mosby, 1994.

Chapter 3
Chest

THE NORMAL CHEST X-RAY

Technical Considerations

Exposure. Making a properly exposed chest x-ray is much more difficult than making radiographs of other parts of the body. This is because the chest contains tissues with a great range of contrast. The range stretches from small vessels in air-filled lungs to dense bony structures located behind the heart. A correctly exposed film should allow visualization of vessels to at least the peripheral one third of the lung and at the same time allow visualization of the paraspinous margins and the left hemidiaphragm behind the heart.

Overexposure causes a film to be dark. Under these circumstances the thoracic spine, mediastinal structures, retrocardiac areas, and nasogastric and endotracheal tubes are well seen, but small nodules and the fine structures in the lung cannot be seen (Fig. 3–1A). Sometimes the interpretation can be salvaged somewhat by using a very bright small light (hot light) to illuminate the film or by copying the film and making it lighter.

Underexposure causes the film to be quite white. This is a major problem for adequate interpretation. It will make the small pulmonary blood vessels appear prominent and may lead you to think that there are generalized infiltrates when none is really present. Underexposure also makes it impossible to see the detail of the mediastinal, retrocardiac, or spinal anatomy (Fig. 3–1B). There is nothing that you can do to an underexposed film to improve interpretation.

Male vs. Female Chest. The major difference between male and female chest x-rays is caused by differences in the amount of breast tissue. This is generally relevant only in interpretation of a PA or an AP film and not of the lateral film. Breast tissue absorbs some of the x-ray beam, essentially causing underexposure of the tissues in the path. This results in the lung behind the breasts appearing whiter and the pulmonary vascular pattern in the same area to appear more prominent. This is not a problem if the inferior aspect of the breasts is above the hemidiaphragms, but if the breasts are pendulous there can appear to be bilateral basilar lung infiltrates.

One common problem is encountered in the

43

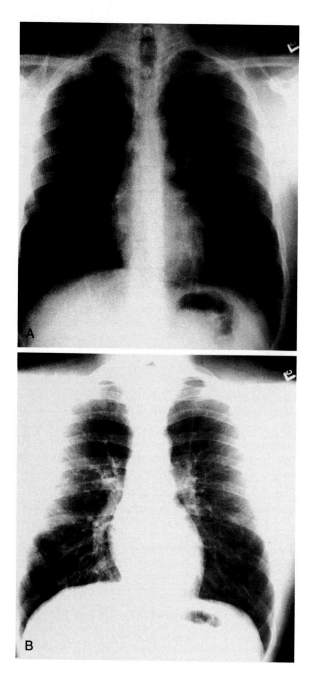

FIGURE 3–1. Effect of over- and underexposure on a chest x-ray. Overexposure *(A)* makes it very easy to see behind the heart and the regions of the clavicles and thoracic spine, but the pulmonary vessels peripherally are impossible to see. Underexposure *(B)* accentuates the pulmonary vascularity, but you cannot see behind the heart or behind the hemidiaphragms.

female who has had a unilateral mastectomy. In this circumstance, the lung density will be asymmetric. The lung on the side of the mastectomy will appear darker than the lung on the normal side. In these circumstances, recognition of the mastectomy will prevent you from making an erroneous diagnosis of an infiltrate or effusion based on the relatively increased density on the side with the remaining breast (Fig. 3–2).

Visualization on a PA or an AP chest radiograph of a single well-defined "nodule" in the lower lung zone should raise the suspicion that you are seeing a nipple shadow and not a real pulmonary nodule. Nipple shadows are common in both men and women. The first thing to do is to look at the opposite lung and see if there is a comparable nodule. If there is, usually you can stop worrying (Fig. 3–3). But before you completely stop worrying, you should also look at the lateral film and make sure that the "nodule" is not seen projecting within the lung. If you can find only one "nodule" projecting over a lung in the PA projection, and no nodule is seen on the lateral view, a small metallic BB

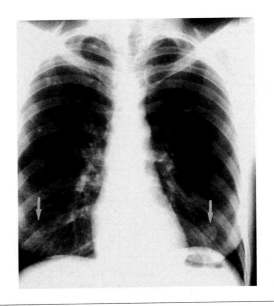

FIGURE 3–3. Nipple shadows. Prominent nipple shadows can be seen in both men and women and are seen in the midclavicular line over the lower half of both the right and the left lung (arrows). These should be bilateral, and sometimes you can see them on the anterior soft tissue of the chest on the lateral view.

can be taped over the nipples and the single PA view repeated to see if you were visualizing the nipple.

PA vs. AP Chest X-rays. Chest x-rays on ambulatory patients are usually done with the subject's chest up against the film holder. The x-ray tube is behind the patient, and the x-ray beam passes in from the back and exits the front of the chest. This is referred to as a PA (posterior to anterior) projection. If the patient is lying down, it is standard practice to take the image with the x-ray beam entering the front of the chest and to have the film cassette behind the patient. This is called an AP (or anterior to posterior) chest x-ray.

For interpretive purposes the main difference is that the heart will be more magnified on the AP projection (Fig. 3–4). This is because in the AP projection the heart is farther from the film and the x-ray beam diverges as it goes farther from the tube. Thus the shadow of the heart appears larger on an AP chest x-ray than on a PA one. All that you have to remember is to make sure that you are looking at a PA view before you interpret a film as showing mild or moderate cardiomegaly. Usually, the technician

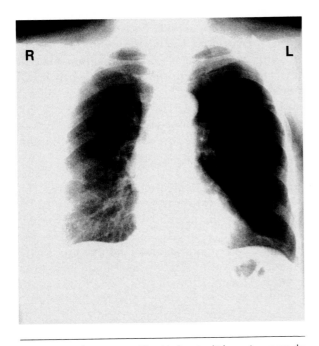

FIGURE 3–2. Left mastectomy. The right breast, which remains, causes the pulmonary vessels at the base of the right lung to be accentuated, and this can be mistaken for a right lower lobe infiltrate. In contrast, the left lung appears darker than the right, and you might mistakenly think there is hyperinflation of the left lung. Notice also that it is easier to see the left lateral ribs and the left axillary region, since the left breast has been removed.

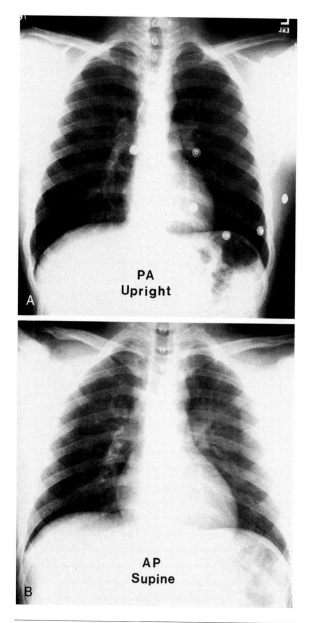

FIGURE 3–4. Effect of position on the chest x-ray. A posterior-anterior upright view *(A)* allows for fuller inspiration than does a supine view. The small round objects over the left lower chest are snaps on the patient's clothing. In an anterior-posterior supine view *(B)*, the abdominal contents are pushing the hemidiaphragms up, and the chest appears hypoinflated. This projection also magnifies the heart relative to a PA view.

will have written the projection on the x-ray requisition, and occasionally it will also be marked on the film.

Upright vs. Supine Chest X-rays. As you can imagine, patients who are able to stand up or sit up usually have their chest x-rays done in that position. There are a number of reasons for this. The amount of inspiration is greater, spreading the pulmonary vessels and allowing clearer visualization. It is obviously easier to see a bird in a tree if the branches can be spread out instead of being all squashed together. Another reason for preferring an upright examination is that small pleural effusions tend to run down into the normally sharp costophrenic angles, allowing relatively small effusions to be identified. Small pneumothoraces tend to go to the lung apex and can be relatively easy to see on an upright chest x-ray.

Now let us think about a patient lying in bed. The typical chest x-ray will be done with a film under the patient. No lateral view is done. Under these circumstances, the patient cannot take a full inspiration; the liver and abdominal contents are pushing up on the lungs and heart, and the result is that the pulmonary vessels are crowded. In the supine position the blood flow to the upper lungs essentially equals that in the lower lobes, and this will mimic congestive failure. On a supine film, the standard AP projection combined with the cephalic push of the abdominal contents will make a normal heart appear large. In addition, with the patient in a supine position, small pleural effusions will layer in the posterior pleural space while small pneumothoraces will go to the anterior pleural surface, and both will probably be missed. For interpretative purposes you must be much more conservative and careful when reading the film of a supine, portable examination.

Inspiration and Expiration Chest X-rays. The degree of inspiration is important not only for assessing the quality and limitations of the examination but also for diagnosing different diseases. When standing, most adults can easily take an inspiration that brings the domes of the hemidiaphragms down to the level of the tenth posterior ribs. When sitting or lying down, often the level is between the eighth and tenth ribs. If the radiograph has the domes of the diaphragms at the seventh posterior ribs, the chest should be considered hypoinflated, and you need to be very careful before diagnosing basilar pneumonia or cardiomegaly (Fig. 3–5). You should be cognizant of the major differences in the appear-

failure in a patient who is, in fact, normal (Fig. 3–6).

Expiration films do have occasional constructive uses. If a small pneumothorax is present, an expiration view makes the lung smaller and denser, and at the same time it makes the pneumothorax relatively larger and easier to see. Thus, if your prime interest is in identification of a small pneumothorax, order an upright expiration film. In the case of a foreign body (such as a peanut) lodged in a major bronchus, an inspiration and expiration film should be ordered. There may be either postobstructive atelectasis or a ball-valve phenomenon. In the latter case, the air can get in past the object during inspiration, but during expiration (as the bronchus gets smaller), the air cannot get out around the object. As a result, on the expiration film there will be air trapping in the affected lung with shift of the mediastinum toward the normal side.

Before hyperinflation is diagnosed on a chest x-ray, the lateral film should be examined. With hyperinflation the diaphragms should be flattened on the lateral view. Many young adults can normally take a very deep inspiration, but on the lateral view they will not have an increased AP diameter or truly flattened hemidiaphragms. In long-standing chronic obstructive pulmonary disease (COPD) there are additional findings, such as an increased AP diameter and an increase in the clear space between the sternum and the ascending aorta.

Chest X-ray vs. Rib Technique. A typical chest x-ray is done utilizing an energy of the x-rays that is a compromise for visualizing lung markings, soft tissues, and bones at the same time. Bones can be well seen by using relatively low voltage x-rays, but then the pulmonary markings are hard to see (Fig. 3–7). If you are interested in rib or spine fractures or other abnormalities of bone, you should order either a "rib" or a "spine" examination rather than a chest x-ray. This will accentuate the detail of the bones.

Normal Anatomy and Variants

Normal anatomy as visualized on a chest x-ray is important to understand, and major structures

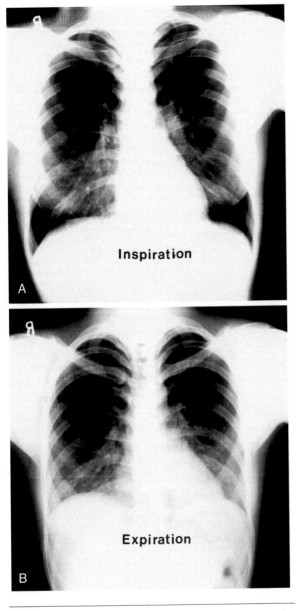

FIGURE 3–5. Effect of respiration. Good inspiration on a chest x-ray *(A)* makes the hemidiaphragms come down to about the level of the posterior tenth or eleventh ribs. The breast shadows are clearly seen on both sides, and this overlying soft tissue accentuates the pulmonary markings behind them. On an expiration view *(B)*, the hemidiaphragms are higher, making the heart appear larger and crowding the basilar pulmonary vessels. The breast shadows overlap the hemidiaphragms, and these findings together may make you think that there are bilateral basilar lung infiltrates when, in fact, this is a normal chest.

ance of a chest x-ray as a result of combining all the factors mentioned above. Unless you are aware of these issues you will diagnosis cardiomegaly, lung infiltrates, and congestive heart

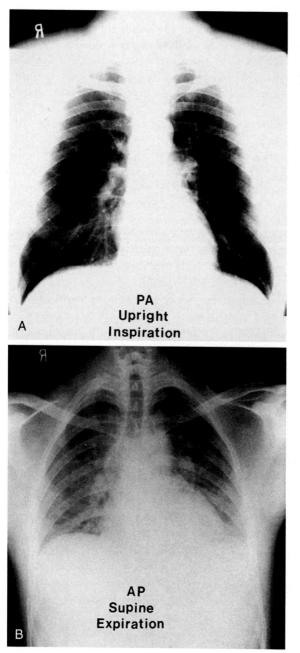

PA
Upright
Inspiration

A

AP
Supine
Expiration

B

FIGURE 3–6. Summation of the effect of position, projection, and respiration. A normal PA upright chest x-ray with full inspiration is shown *(A)*. Another x-ray was taken on this perfectly healthy college student 1 minute later; it was done in an AP projection while he was lying supine and during expiration *(B)*. The wide cardiac shadow and prominent pulmonary vascularity could easily trick you into thinking that this individual was in congestive heart failure.

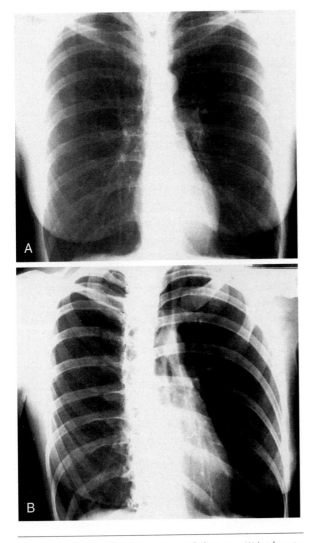

FIGURE 3–7. Chest vs. rib technique. A normal chest x-ray *(A)* is taken at a relatively high voltage, allowing you to see heart, pulmonary vessels, and skeletal structures. By lowering the voltage of the x-ray, the pulmonary vessels become much harder to see and the bones become easier to see *(B)*.

diac chambers mostly overlie each other. As a general rule, if the right side of the heart is enlarged more than the left, there is a right chamber lesion. The same holds true for the left side.

On an upright PA chest x-ray, the greatest width of the heart should be less than half the width of the thoracic cavity at its widest point (Fig. 3–9). This is determined by finding the farthest right and left portions of the cardiac silhouette. These will not be at the same horizontal level, but that is all right. You find the horizontal distance between the two most lateral cardiac margins. Sometimes there are patients with either dextrocardia or situs inversus (Fig. 3–10). Before the latter diagnosis is made, it is important to make sure that the technician did not misplace the right or left marker on the film.

The upper mediastinal structures that are visualized on the right are the brachiocephalic vessels, azygos vein, and ascending aorta. The

---

TABLE 3–1. How To Look at a Chest X-ray

Determine the age, sex, and history of the patient
Identify the projection and technique used:
   AP, PA, lateral, portable, or standard distance
Identify the position of the patient:
     Upright, supine, decubitus, lordotic
Look at the inspiratory effort:
     Adequate, hypoinflated, hyperinflated
Identify the obvious and common abnormalities:
     Heart size, large or normal
     Heart shape, specific chamber enlargement
     Upper mediastinal contours
     Examine airway, tracheal deviation
     Lung symmetry
       Any mediastinal shift?
       Hilar position
     Lung infiltrates, masses, or nodules
     Pulmonary vascularity
       Increased, decreased, or normal
       Lower greater than upper
     Pleural effusions, blunting of costophrenic angles
     Rib, clavicle, and spine fractures or other lesions
     Check tube placement
Recheck what you thought was normal anatomy and look at typical blind
     spots
     Behind the heart
     Behind the hemidiaphragms
     In the lung apices
     Pneumothorax present?
     Costophrenic angles
     Chest wall
     Lytic rib lesions
     Shoulders
Look for old films, not just the last one
Decide what the findings are and their location
Give a common differential diagnosis correlated with the clinical history

---

are shown in Figure 3–8. A method for examining a chest x-ray is given in Table 3–1. The appropriate imaging study to order in various clinical circumstances is shown in Table 3–2.

The heart is the easiest thing to see, so we will begin there. On the PA view of the heart, of course, the left border is much more prominent than the right. It would be nice and simple to say that the left ventricle is on the left and the right ventricle is on the right. Unfortunately, the heart chambers are somewhat twisted in the chest, and on the PA and lateral views the car-

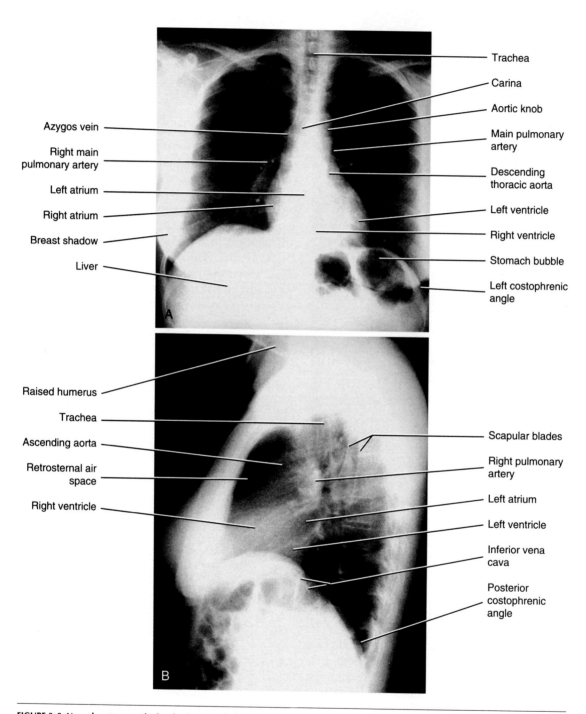

Trachea

Carina

Aortic knob

Main pulmonary artery

Descending thoracic aorta

Left ventricle

Right ventricle

Stomach bubble

Left costophrenic angle

Azygos vein

Right main pulmonary artery

Left atrium

Right atrium

Breast shadow

Liver

Raised humerus

Trachea

Ascending aorta

Retrosternal air space

Right ventricle

Scapular blades

Right pulmonary artery

Left atrium

Left ventricle

Inferior vena cava

Posterior costophrenic angle

FIGURE 3–8. Normal anatomy on the female chest x-ray in the upright PA projection *(A)* and the lateral *(B)* projection.

TABLE 3–2. Suggested Procedures of Various Chest Problems

Clinical Problem	Study
Most chest problems, including	Chest x-ray
Pneumonia	
COPD	
CHF	
Trauma	
Chest pain	
Shortness of breath	
Hemoptysis	
Foreign body	Inspiration/expiration chest x-ray
Mediastinal mass	CT
Lung tumor	CT
Pleural mass or fluid	CT
Localization of pleural effusion for thoracentesis	Stethoscope
	US
	CT
Hemoptysis	Bronchoscopy
Pericardial effusion	Cardiac US
Myocardial thickness	Cardiac US
Cardiac wall motion	Cardiac US
Cardiac ejection fraction	Nuclear medicine (gated blood pool study)
Pulmonary embolism	Nuclear medicine (ventilation/perfusion scan)
	Pulmonary arteriogram
Coronary artery stenosis	Nuclear medicine (myocardial perfusion scan)
	Coronary angiogram
Aortic aneurysm	Contrasted CT
Aortic tear	Angiogram
Aortic dissection	Contrasted CT

The lungs are mostly composed of air, and therefore normally, there is not much to see other than blood vessels. These should be distinct and remain that way as they are traced back to the hila. If you cannot see them clearly near the hila, there may be a perihilar infiltrate or fluid (such as from CHF). Normal hila are sometimes indistinct on portable x-rays because the exposure takes longer and the vessels are blurred by motion.

The blood vessels in the lung are usually clearly seen out to within 2 to 3 cm of the chest wall. Some people say that visualization of vessels in the outer third of the lung is abnormal, but this is not true. It depends on the quality of the film and on how hard you look. Lines located within 2 cm of the chest wall are abnormal and probably represent edema, fibrosis, or metastatic disease. Secondary bronchi usually are not normally visualized except near the hilum, where they can sometimes be seen end-on. The walls of the visualized bronchi normally should not be thicker than a fine pencil point.

A normal variant called an azygous lobe can occasionally be seen in the right upper lung.

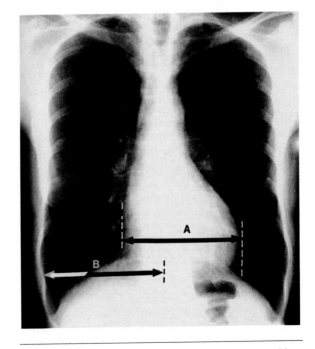

FIGURE 3–9. Measurement of cardiomegaly. The width of the normal heart from its most lateral borders (A) should not exceed the width of half of the hemithorax measured from the middle of the spine to the widest portion of the inner ribs (B).

right border of the ascending aorta can be seen beginning below the right hilum. The aortic arch is most commonly seen to the left of the trachea. The descending thoracic aorta can usually be visualized only along its left lateral border, where it abuts the left lung. The trachea should be midline and can be followed down to the carina. The right and left major bronchi are easily seen. The esophagus is not normally seen on a standard chest x-ray.

HILA AND LUNGS
The hila are made up of the main pulmonary arteries and major bronchi. The right hilum is usually somewhat lower than the left; it should not be at the same level or higher. The pulmonary veins usually are more difficult to see than the arteries. They converge on the atria at a level 1 to 3 inches below the pulmonary arteries. Lymph nodes are not normally seen on a chest x-ray, either in the hilar regions or in the mediastinum.

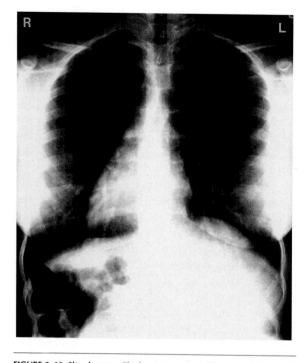

FIGURE 3–10. Situs inversus. The heart, stomach, and liver are all in reversed positions. Before you make this diagnosis, you should make sure that the technician has placed the right and left markers correctly.

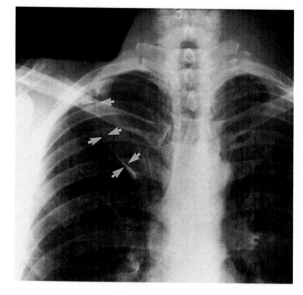

FIGURE 3–11. Azygos pseudolobe. A thin curvilinear line extends from the right lung apex down and medially toward the azygos vein. The line has a teardrop bottom end. This normal variant is seen only on the right side.

This is seen on the PA view as a fine, curved line extending from the right lung apex down toward the mediastinum (Fig. 3–11). It has a teardrop shape at its lower edge. This is caused embryologically by the azygos vein migrating inferiorly from the lung apex while trapping some of the lung medially.

You should remember that on a PA or an AP chest x-ray, the lungs go behind the heart, behind and below the dome of the hemidiaphragms, and behind and in front of mediastinal structures. In fact, 40 per cent of the lung area and 25 per cent of the lung volume will be obscured by these other structures. If you do not look carefully at these regions, you will miss a significant amount of pulmonary pathology.

DIAPHRAGMS

The diaphragms are typically dome-shaped, although there are many people who have polyarcuate diaphragms that look like several domes rather than one. This is an important normal variant and should not be mistaken for a pleural or diaphragmatic tumor (Fig. 3–12). The right hemidiaphragm is usually higher than the left,

and most people believe that this is because the liver is pushing up the right hemidiaphragm. This is nonsense, since the liver, which weighs many pounds, cannot push up into your lungs while you are standing. The diaphragms are at different levels because the heart is pushing the left hemidiaphragm down. The edges of both hemidiaphragms form acute angles with the

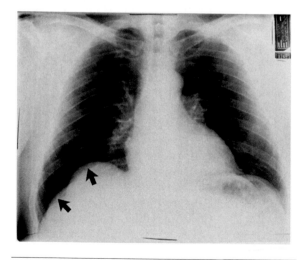

FIGURE 3–12. Polyarcuate diaphragm. This is a common normal variant in which the diaphragm has several small domes instead of one large one.

chest wall, and blunting of these angles should raise the suspicion of pleural fluid.

Most people have trouble telling the right from the left hemidiaphragm on the lateral view, but there are several ways to tell them apart. The right hemidiaphragm is usually higher than the left and can be seen extending from the anterior chest wall to the posterior ribs. The left side usually can be seen only from the posterior aspect of the heart to the posterior ribs. It is the hemidiaphragm most likely to have a gas bubble (stomach or colon) immediately beneath it.

BONY STRUCTURES

Skeletal structures of interest on a chest x-ray include the ribs, sternum, spine, and shoulder girdle. There should be 12 ribs, but only the upper ones are completely seen on a PA chest x-ray. Ribs are very difficult to evaluate on the lateral view owing to superimposition of the right and left ribs and the many soft tissue structures. Evaluation should include searches for cervical ribs (Fig. 3–13), fractures, deformity, missing ribs (from surgery), and lytic (destruc-

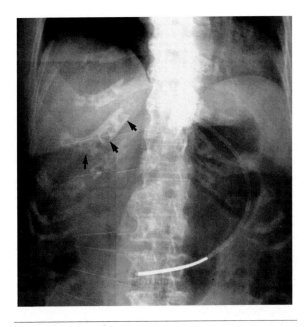

FIGURE 3–14. Costochondral calcification. Calcification between the anterior ends of the ribs and the sternum is quite common, particularly in older persons, and can be quite striking (arrows). A Dobbhoff feeding tube is noted in this patient as well.

tive) lesions. The upper margin of the ribs is usually well seen, since the rib is rounded here. The lower edge of the ribs is usually very thin, and the inferior cortical margin can be difficult to appreciate. What you should do is to look for symmetry between the right and left ribs at the same level. If they are symmetric, they are usually normal. At the anterior ends of the ribs there is cartilage that connects to the sternum. In older individuals there can be significant calcification of this cartilage; this is a normal finding (Fig. 3–14).

The sternum is well seen only on the lateral view of the chest. On this view you can look for pectus deformity, fractures, and lytic lesions. A pectus deformity can cause apparent cardiomegaly. This is because the sternum is depressed and squashes the heart against the spine, making the heart look wider than normal on the PA chest view (Fig. 3–15). Occasionally, overexposed oblique views of the chest can show the sternum well. If this does not work, you may need to resort to a CT scan with bone windows.

The clavicles and shoulders should also be routinely examined. There is often a scalloped

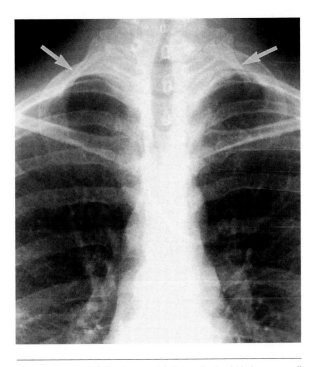

FIGURE 3–13. Cervical ribs. A congenital abnormality in which there are small ribs projecting off the lateral aspect of C7 (arrows). Occasionally, these can be symptomatic.

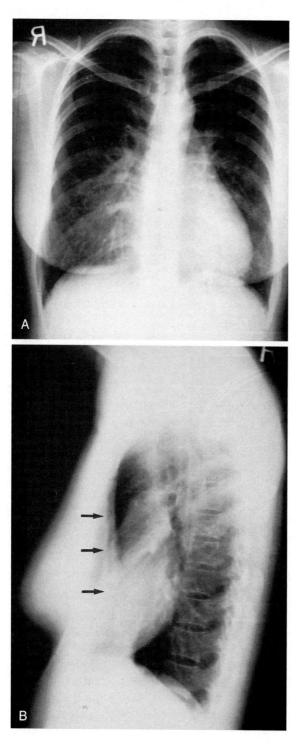

FIGURE 3–15. Pectus excavatum. A congenital abnormality in which the sternum is depressed. Since the heart is squashed between the sternum and spine, it appears big in the frontal view *(A)* of the chest, and the right heart border is indistinct, suggesting a right middle lobe infiltrate. A lateral view *(B)* clearly shows the depressed position of the sternum *(arrows)*.

appearance to the inferior and medial portions of the clavicle. This is called a rhomboid fossa, and it is bilateral. It should not be mistaken for a pathologic bone lesion (Fig. 3–16). The medial aspect of the scapula projects over the upper lateral aspect of the lungs and sometimes can be mistaken for a pathologic line, such as a pneumothorax. When you think that you see a pneumothorax, you should make sure that it is not the scapular border that you are looking at. This is done by noting that the medial scapular border is usually straight rather than curved and by tracing the outline of the scapula.

The thoracic spine is seen only incompletely on a standard chest x-ray. This is because on the frontal view it is obscured by the heart and mediastinal structures. In older people there can be substantial degenerative changes or bone spurs extending laterally from the vertebral bodies. These can often be seen on the PA view (Fig. 3–17), and on the lateral view the spurs can look like pulmonary nodules. A key to differentiating bony spurs from nodules is that spurs project over the vertebral disks on the lateral view and do not look like round nodules on the frontal chest x-ray.

SOFT TISSUES

The soft tissues should also be examined. We have already seen the problems in interpretation

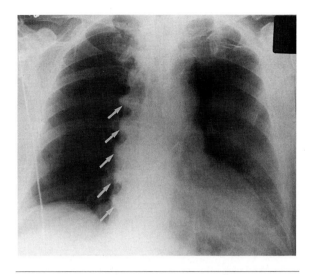

FIGURE 3–17. Degenerative spurs or osteophytes. These projections occur at the level of the disks and can cause an unusual appearance along the lateral aspect of the thoracic spine. On the lateral chest x-ray, these bony spurs can simulate nodules projecting near or over the thoracic spine.

that can arise as a result of a mastectomy or nipple shadows, but other soft tissues are also important. It is important to look for asymmetry of soft tissues or for air or calcium within them. Calcification may be seen in the carotid arteries or great vessels in older persons (Fig. 3–18). A common confusing artifact can be caused by hair (especially braids). If the hair is greasy and braided, very strange artifacts (Fig. 3–19) that may be mistaken for apical lung infiltrates can be seen.

There normally should not be much soft tissue or water density between the peripheral aerated lung and the ribs. The pleura is not normally seen at the lung margins. In some adults there is a collection of fat along the chest wall between the lung and the ribs. This is extrapleural fat, which is usually seen only on the PA view of the chest and almost always in the upper outer portion of the thoracic cavity (Fig. 3–20). The biggest pitfall is mistaking this for bilateral pleural effusions. If there is no other sign of effusion (such as costophrenic angle blunting) and if the finding is bilateral, is seen near the upper lateral lung zones, and does not exceed 3 to 4 mm in thickness, it is almost certainly extrapleural fat rather than pleural fluid.

CT Anatomy. The cross-sectional anatomy of the

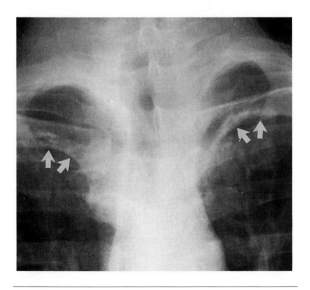

FIGURE 3–16. Rhomboid fossa. A normal finding in which there is an indentation along the medial and inferior aspects of the clavicles. This should be bilateral and is of no clinical significance.

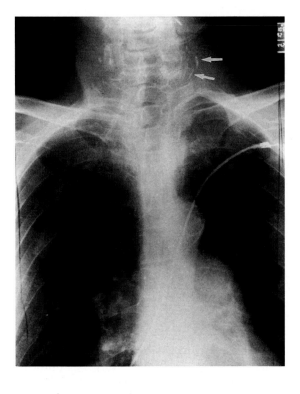

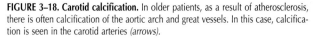

FIGURE 3–18. Carotid calcification. In older patients, as a result of atherosclerosis, there is often calcification of the aortic arch and great vessels. In this case, calcification is seen in the carotid arteries *(arrows).*

FIGURE 3–19. Braid artifacts. Tightly woven or greasy hair can cause streaky artifacts that may resemble an upper lobe infiltrate. A key finding is that these artifacts can be seen extending above the apex of the lung and projecting over the cervical soft tissue region.

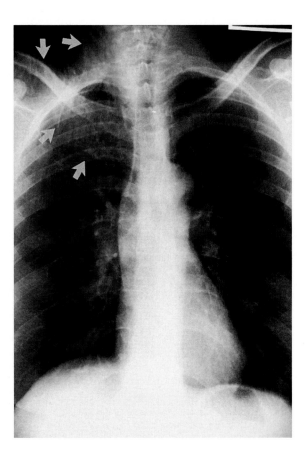

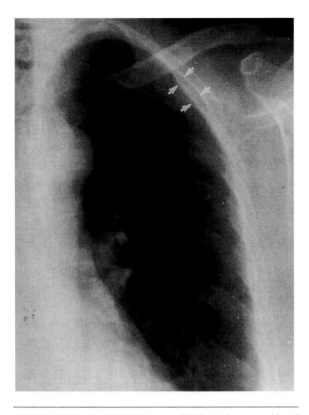

FIGURE 3–20. Extrapleural fat. This is a normal finding in the upper and lateral hemithorax. It is symmetric between right and left and should not be mistaken for a pleural effusion.

chest is very important to understand, since CT is very commonly used for evaluation of thoracic pathology. CT scanning of the chest may be done with or without intravenous contrast. Most standard CT scanning techniques provide you with CT "slice" images that are 1 cm thick. If you are interested in the evaluation of a lung nodule, thinner cuts should be used and intravenous contrast is not needed. For evaluation of a potential dissecting aortic aneurysm, a bolus of intravenous contrast is essential. You should consult a radiologist if you are in doubt about what to order. The radiologist usually will use the correct technique provided you have supplied complete clinical information. If available, spiral CT is often done because the entire chest can be scanned in several seconds while the patient holds his or her breath. After the scan is done, the technologist will film the computer data using both mediastinal windows and pulmonary parenchymal windows. This affords a good look at the pulmonary parenchyma and

still allows differentiation of mediastinal structures (Fig. 3–21A).

There are special circumstances in which you will want to look at the fine detail of the lung. In these circumstances, high-resolution CT (HRCT) can be done. The "slices" that are obtained are 1 to 2 mm thick. This cannot be done for the whole lung, since it would involve too many images and is not necessary to make most diagnoses. For this reason, a regular CT scan is often done with thin cuts at selected levels (Fig. 3–22).

Tubes and Wires

Evaluation of the placement and associated complications of various tubes, wires, and lines is a very common reason for ordering a chest x-ray. On patients who are very sick and in intensive care units, the portable chest x-ray often resembles a plate of spaghetti with tubes, lines, and wires all over the place. Your job is to figure out which parts of the tubes and wires are inside the patient and which are simply lying on the patient. In addition, you need to know if the lines and tubes that are inside the patient are going to the right place or are at the correct level.

The Endotracheal (ET) Tube. This is probably the easiest item to identify, since it is within the air shadow of the trachea. In an adult or child, the ET tip should be at least 1 cm above the carina, and preferably slightly more. A tube in a lower position can obstruct air flow to one side and cause atelectasis (collapse) of a lung or a portion of a lung. An ET tube in low position usually will go into the right mainstem bronchus because it is more vertically oriented than the left mainstem bronchus (Fig. 3–23). The highest that an ET tube tip should be is at the level of the suprasternal notch (which is midway between the proximal clavicles).

Nasogastric (NG) Tubes. A nasogastric tube should follow the course of the esophagus on the frontal chest x-ray and on the lateral view it passes behind the trachea and then along the posterior aspect of the heart (Fig. 3–24). You need to ascertain the position of the tip of an

Text continued on page 62

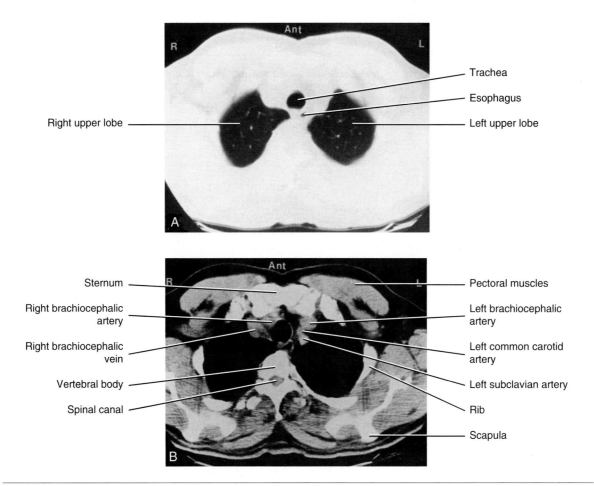

FIGURE 3–21. Normal anatomy of the chest on transverse (axial) CT scans. Identical levels have been filmed using pulmonary parenchymal windows and soft tissue windows.

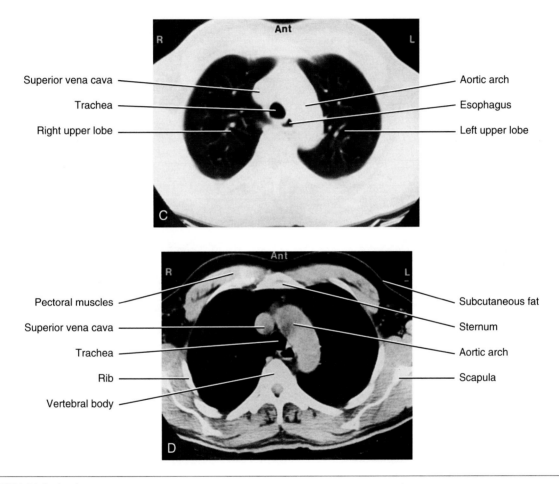

Superior vena cava

Trachea

Right upper lobe

Aortic arch

Esophagus

Left upper lobe

Pectoral muscles

Superior vena cava

Trachea

Rib

Vertebral body

Subcutaneous fat

Sternum

Aortic arch

Scapula

FIGURE 3–21 *Continued*

Illustration continued on following page

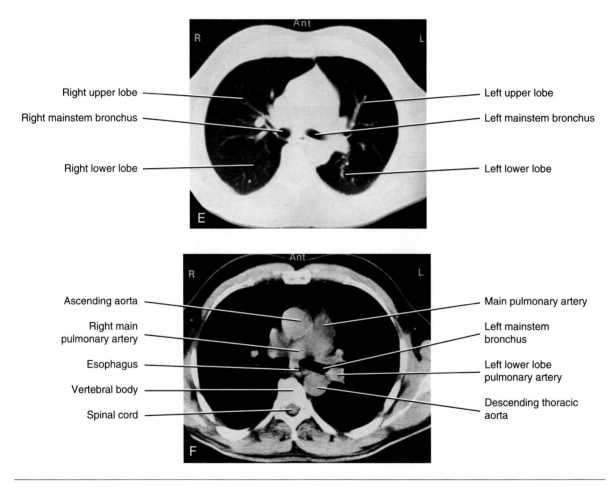

Right upper lobe

Right mainstem bronchus

Right lower lobe

Left upper lobe

Left mainstem bronchus

Left lower lobe

Ascending aorta

Right main pulmonary artery

Esophagus

Vertebral body

Spinal cord

Main pulmonary artery

Left mainstem bronchus

Left lower lobe pulmonary artery

Descending thoracic aorta

FIGURE 3–21 *Continued*

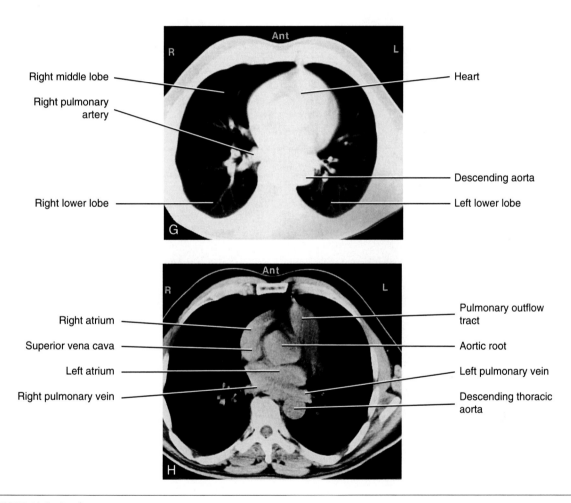

Right middle lobe

Right pulmonary artery

Right lower lobe

Heart

Descending aorta

Left lower lobe

Right atrium

Superior vena cava

Left atrium

Right pulmonary vein

Pulmonary outflow tract

Aortic root

Left pulmonary vein

Descending thoracic aorta

FIGURE 3–21 *Continued*

Illustration continued on following page

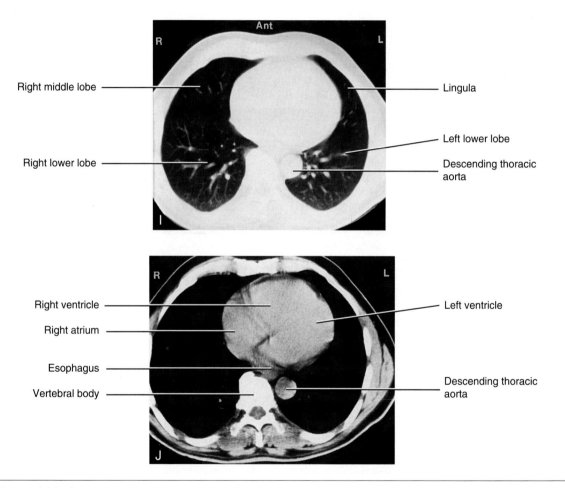

FIGURE 3–21 *Continued*

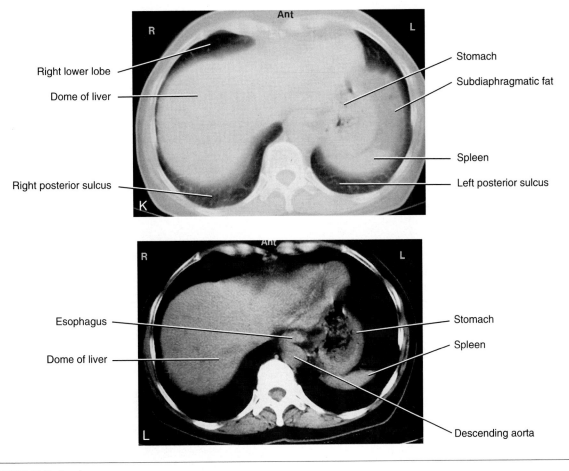

Right lower lobe

Dome of liver

Right posterior sulcus

Stomach

Subdiaphragmatic fat

Spleen

Left posterior sulcus

Esophagus

Dome of liver

Stomach

Spleen

Descending aorta

FIGURE 3–21 *Continued*

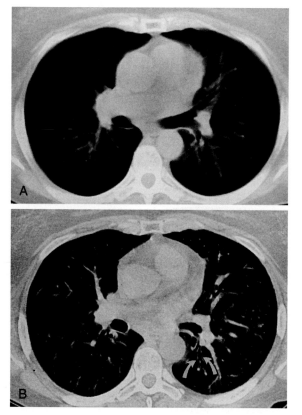

NG tube before putting any liquid through the tube. The position can often be determined by clinical means without resorting to a chest x-ray. The most common method is to put air into the tube and listen over the stomach with a stethoscope.

Nasogastric tubes have two favorite abnor-mal positions. The most common is with the NG tube only partway down the esophagus or coiled in the esophagus. Fluid placed down the tube can reflux and be aspirated into the lungs. Less commonly during insertion the NG tubes can pass into the trachea instead of going into the esophagus. When this happens, they tend to

FIGURE 3–23. Left lung atelectasis. The endotracheal tube is down too far, and the tip is located in the right mainstem bronchus. The left mainstem bronchus has become totally obstructed, the air in the left lung has been resorbed, and there is volume loss of the left lung with shift of the mediastinum to the left.

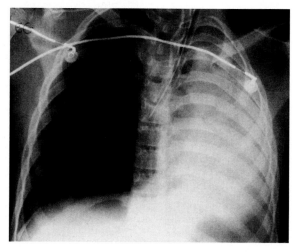

FIGURE 3–24. Normal course of a nasogastric tube. In the PA projection of the chest *(A),* the NG tube passes directly behind the trachea until it gets past the carina and then curves slightly to the left at the gastroesophageal junction. On the lateral view *(B),* the NG tube can be seen behind the trachea (t) and going down behind the heart.

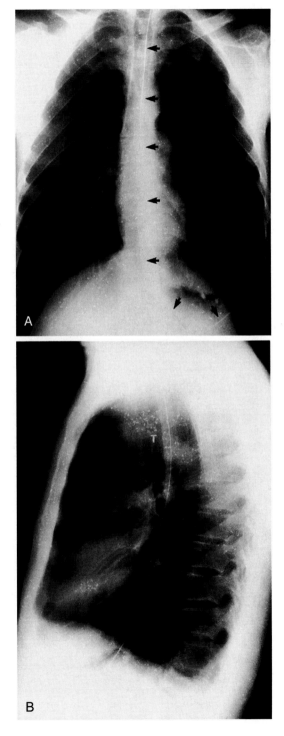

go down the right mainstem bronchus (just like ET tubes that are advanced too far). Since NG tubes can be stiff and have a rigid end, if pushed hard enough they can perforate the lung and go out into the pleural space (Fig. 3–25). Many patients require alimentation via NG tube; this works best if the tube tip is in the distal aspect of the duodenal loop near the ligament of Treitz.

The Short Jugular or Subclavian Venous Line. This is a very common route of venous access. The tip of the catheter should optimally be placed in the superior vena cava (SVC). On the frontal chest x-ray, the catheter tip should be about 1 to 4 cm below the medial aspect of the right clavicle (Fig. 3–26). The favorite abnormal

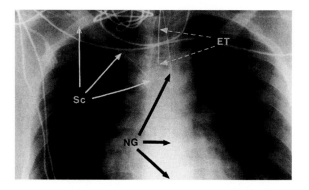

FIGURE 3–26. Normal subclavian catheter course. The subclavian catheter (SC) should progress medially and then inferiorly to the medial clavicle, with the tip being located in the superior vena cava. An endotracheal tube (ET) and nasogastric tube are also present. The remainder of overlying and coiled wires are EKG leads.

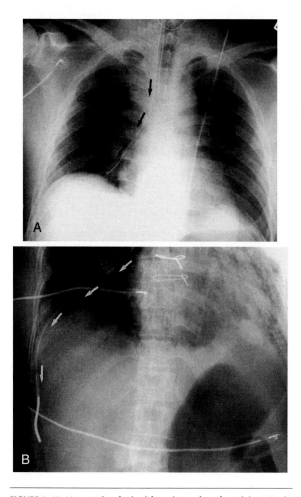

FIGURE 3–25. Nasogastric tube in right mainstem bronchus. If the NG tube gets into the trachea, it will usually go down the right mainstem bronchus (A). These tubes are quite rigid and if pushed, can perforate the lung and go out into the pleural space (B).

positions of subclavian catheter tips are those that have turned up into the jugular vein rather than down into the SVC (Fig. 3–27A) and those that have crossed the midline and extended into the opposite subclavian vein (Fig. 3–27B).

The Swan-Ganz or Pulmonary Arterial Catheter. Central lines are usually placed to monitor cardiac or pulmonary arterial pressures. The normal course is almost circular: down the SVC, through the right atrium and right ventricle, and out into the main pulmonary and peripheral pulmonary arteries. The most common natural course that the catheter likes to follow leads it into the right rather than the left main pulmonary artery (Fig. 3–28). Some venous catheters are placed from the inguinal region. In this case the catheter usually follows a gentle S curve from the IVC into the right atrium and right ventricle and into the pulmonary artery (Fig. 3–29). A central venous catheter placed too far out into a pulmonary artery will obstruct blood flow and can result in pulmonary infarction (Fig. 3–30). The tip of a CVP line should not extend more than halfway between the hilum and the lung periphery or lung infarction can occur. Another problem encountered can be the passage of such a catheter from the SVC into the inferior vena cava (IVC) instead of into the right heart (Fig. 3–31).

Pleural Tubes. Pleural tubes are typically placed to evacuate a pneumothorax or drain a pleural

FIGURE 3–27. Abnormal courses of subclavian catheter. Common abnormal courses include the tip of the catheter going up the jugular vein *(A)* or across the brachioceph- alic vein into the opposite subclavian vein *(B).* Nasogastric tube and EKG leads are also seen. A chest tube is seen on the right. Note the discontinuity in the radiodense line of the pleural tube just outside the ribs. This discontinuity represents a tube port, indicating that the chest tube has not been inserted far enough.

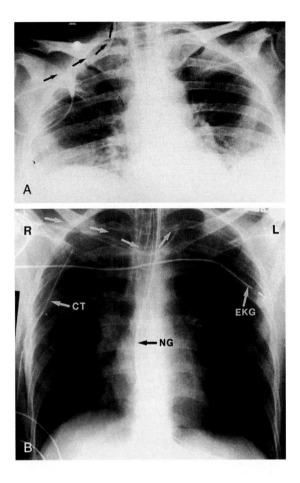

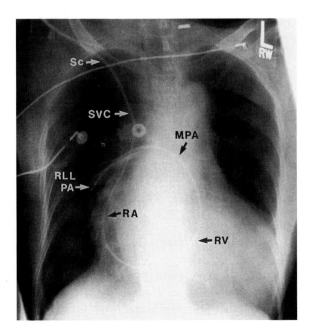

FIGURE 3–28. Normal course of a Swan-Ganz catheter. A Swan-Ganz catheter inserted on the right goes into the subclavian vein (SC), into the superior vena cava, right atrium, right ventricle, main pulmonary artery, and in this case, the right lower lobe pulmonary artery.

fluid collection. They are relatively large bore and are inserted between the ribs in the mid- or lower lateral chest. One common question about these tubes concerns the location of the tip and side port. The tip should not abut the mediastinum. The side port can be seen as a discontinuity in the radiodense marker line, and it should be inside the chest cavity and not out in the soft tissues of the chest (see Fig. 3–27B). Another question relates to whether the tube has kinked and whether it is working to reduce the pneumothorax or fluid collection. Remember, a posteriorly placed tube will have a hard time removing a pneumothorax if the patient is supine and the air collection is located anteriorly.

Cardiac Pacers. Cardiac pacers are wires that extend from a pacing source, down the SVC, through the right atrium, and to the right ventricular apex (Fig. 3–32). Not much that can go wrong with these can be identified on a conventional chest x-ray; however, in the case of pacer failure you should look for a broken wire.

Overlying EKG Wires and Tubes. EKG leads are

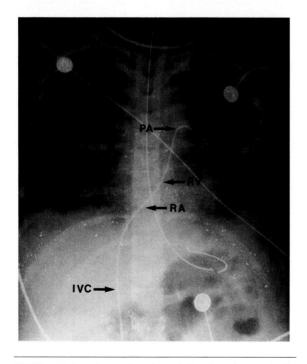

FIGURE 3–29. Swan-Ganz catheter inserted via a femoral approach. This catheter proceeds up the inferior vena cava and follows a gentle S curve through the right atrium, right ventricle, and, in this case, the left main pulmonary artery. The patient also has an NG tube, a left SC catheter and multiple EKG leads.

metallic wires and therefore are denser than most tubes and catheters. They can also be recognized by the fact that they usually have a button or snap on the end, usually are over the upper chest, and do not follow any reasonable internal anatomic pathway (such as venous structures) (see Fig. 3–27B).

Other overlying objects that are often confusing are oxygen supply lines to nasal cannulas and masks. These can look like catheters, but they too do not follow normal vascular or anatomic pathways and are seen mostly over the upper chest and neck. If there is an unsolved issue, you should perform a visual examination of the patient rather than order another x-ray study.

THE AIRWAYS

Issues related to epiglottitis and retropharyngeal abscesses were discussed in Chapter 2. There are several major problems related to airways that you should be able to recognize.

Occlusion. Lung cancer can narrow or totally occlude a bronchus. If the airway is only partially occluded, there will be difficulty clearing mucus and there can be a postobstructive pneumonia. In any older adult who has a focal pneumonia, you should look carefully at the nearby bronchi. In an adult with recurrence of a pneumonia in a particular location you should suspect a lung tumor, and bronchoscopy may be indicated.

If a tumor or mucous plug totally obstructs an airway, there will be resorption of air distally, and this will be accompanied by volume loss. If the obstruction is of a major bronchus, there can be rapid opacification (whiteness) of the lung, accompanied by shift of the trachea and mediastinal structure toward the affected side as a result of volume loss. A major bronchus obstruction can often be identified on the frontal chest x-ray. Additional studies, such as CT, can be useful to determine the extent of tumor, the presence of enlarged lymph nodes, and so forth (Fig. 3–33). In the case of a patient who is young or very sick, a mucous plug is a more likely cause of obstruction and volume loss than a

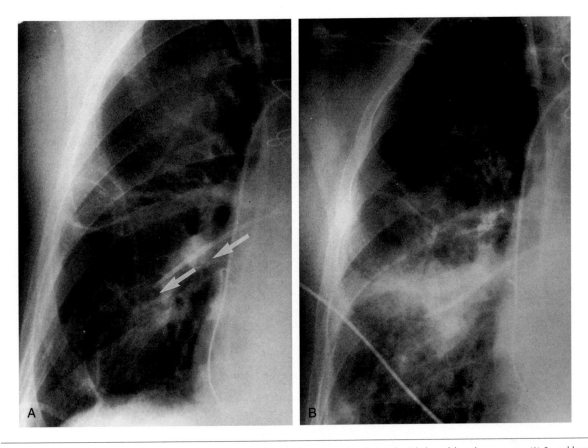

FIGURE 3–30. Swan-Ganz catheter causing infarction. A Swan-Ganz catheter has been inserted too far into the right lower lobe pulmonary artery *(A)*. Several hours later, an infiltrate is present in this region *(B)* as a result of lung infarction, since the catheter obstructed blood flow.

tumor. Bronchoscopy or pulmonary therapy should be suggested rather than a CT scan of the chest.

Foreign bodies are usually the result of aspiration or swallowing an object that was in the mouth. In the case of aspiration, depending on the density of the offending object, it may or may not be seen on a chest x-ray. Metal objects are easily seen (Fig. 3–34), whereas items such as plastic toys and peanuts do not differ in density from soft tissues. The typical location of aspirated foreign bodies is in the right mainstem or right lower lobe bronchus because of the more vertical direction compared with the left side. As mentioned earlier, in cases in which a nonmetallic obstructing foreign body is suspected, you should order inspiration and expiration PA chest views. In uncooperative children, right and left decubitus chest views are sometimes used. The side which does not decrease

in volume during expiration or when placed dependently is abnormal.

Chronic Obstructive Pulmonary Disease (COPD). A chest radiograph can detect only moderate or advanced COPD. In early stages the chest x-ray is normal, and you must rely on pulmonary function tests in order to make this diagnosis. In advanced stages there are obvious signs of hyperinflation. On the PA radiograph the superior portions of the hemidiaphragms may be down to the level of the posterior twelfth ribs, and there is often blunting of the costophrenic angles. Some radiologists use measurements to make the diagnosis. Personally, I do not find them necessary, but here they are. Hyperinflation is diagnosed on the PA chest film if the lungs are longer than 27 cm measured as a horizontal line from the top of the lung apex to the most inferior portion of the lateral costo-

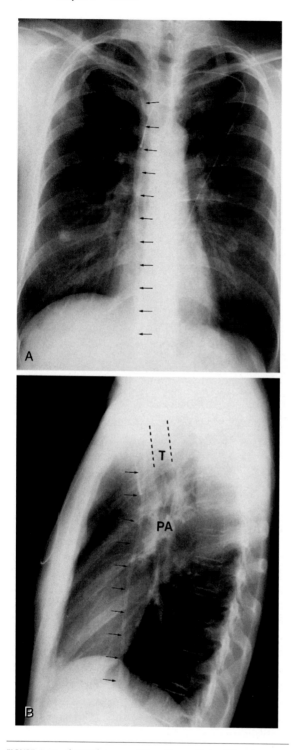

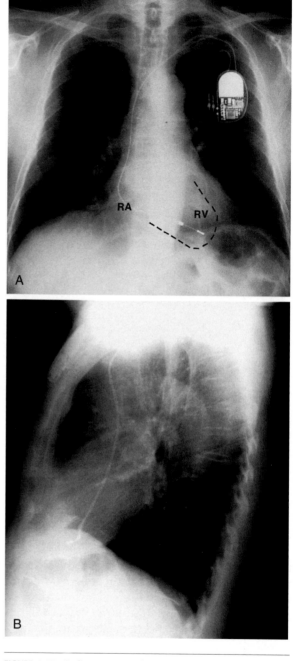

FIGURE 3–32. Cardiac pacer. On the PA view *(A)*, the control portion is underneath the skin and is seen projecting over the right lung apex. It extends into the brachiocephalic vein and down into the right atrium and has the tip in the right ventricle. On the lateral view *(B)*, the course can be clearly identified.

FIGURE 3–31. Abnormal course of Swan-Ganz catheter. This catheter was inserted from a right subclavian approach, and on the PA view of the chest it is seen extending down along the right side of the spine to below the level of the hemidiaphragms *(A)*. On the lateral view *(B)*, it can be seen extending down the inferior vena cava through the heart and down into the inferior vena cava *(arrows)*. The patient also has a left subclavian catheter with tip in the SVC.

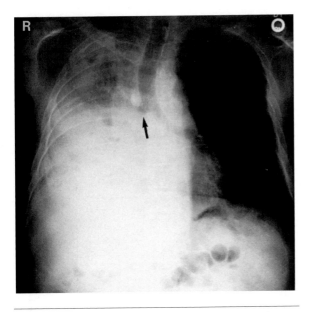

FIGURE 3–33. Tumor obstructing right mainstem bronchus. A sharp cutoff of the air column is clearly identified *(arrow)*. The obstruction has caused a postobstructive infiltrate, with resorption of the air from the right lung, volume loss, and resultant shift of the mediastinum to the right.

phrenic angle. Another quoted measurement for hyperinflation on the PA chest film is the verte-brophrenic angle being less than 1.5 cm above the lateral costophrenic angle on the same side.

With COPD, there is an increase in the AP diameter of the chest on the lateral view, a large anterior clear space between the sternum and ascending aorta, and marked flattening or even inversion of the hemidiaphragms (Fig. 3–35). An associated finding may be the presence of bullae or large air cavities within the lungs as a result of destruction of alveoli. In very advanced COPD there may be what is known as a saber sheath trachea. This refers to a trachea that is compressed from the sides by the lungs, with the trachea appearing narrow on the PA x-ray and wide on the lateral film. Personally, I do not see this very often. Since most COPD is associated with smoking, you should also be looking for an occult lung cancer.

Asthma. Patients with asthma have difficulty with expiration of air as a result of broncho-spasm. The findings on chest x-ray range from a normal appearance (about three quarters of the time) to signs of mild hyperinflation, such as slightly increased AP diameter or hemidi-

aphragms that have their superior aspect level with the posterior tenth to eleventh ribs (Fig. 3–36). With asthma, it is very unusual to have enough hyperinflation to either drive the dia-phragms lower than this or significantly flatten them (as seen on the lateral view). An acute asthma attack can result in a pneumomediasti-num but rarely a pneumothorax. Patients with

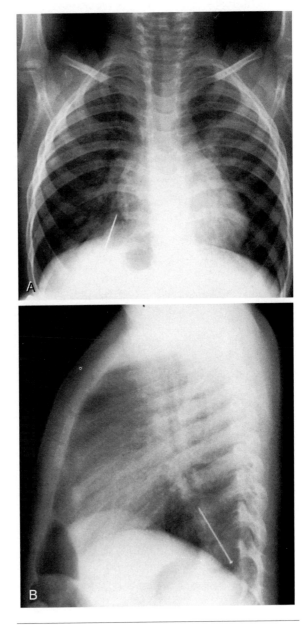

FIGURE 3–34. Aspiration of a nonobstructing foreign body. A metallic straight pin can be seen in the right lower lobe on both the PA *(A)* and the lateral *(B)* chest x-ray.

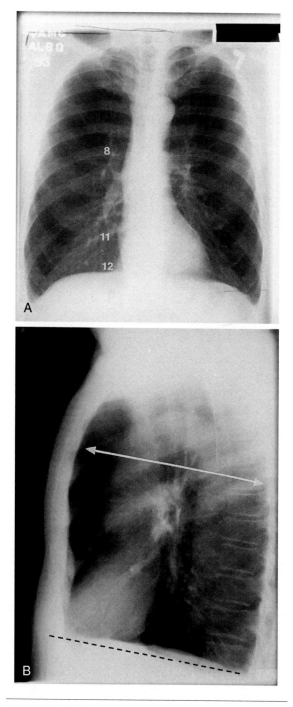

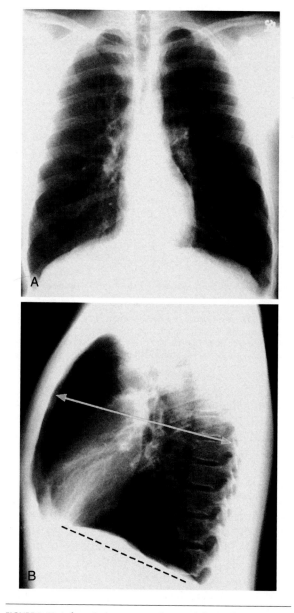

FIGURE 3–36. Asthma. During a severe asthma attack, hyperinflation, similar to that seen in COPD, can be seen. In this case, there is hyperinflation with the superior aspect of the hemidiaphragms located at the level of the posterior eleventh ribs *(A)*; there is a slight increase in the AP diameter and some flattening of the hemidiaphragm *(B)*. The patient does not have the barrel-shaped chest seen in COPD (Fig. 3–35*B*). Most patients with asthma have normal chest x-rays.

FIGURE 3–35. Chronic obstructive pulmonary disease (COPD). The PA view *(A)* shows that the superior aspect of the hemidiaphragms is at the same level as the posterior aspect of the twelfth ribs. Hyperinflation is also seen on the lateral view *(B)* as an increase in the AP diameter and flattening of the hemidiaphragms.

recurrent asthmatic attacks may have a prominent interstitial pattern due to scarring, and they may have slightly thickened bronchial walls. You should also be looking for a focal infiltrate or pneumonia as the precipitating cause of the asthmatic attack.

Bronchiectasis. Bronchiectasis refers to diffuse or focal dilatation of the bronchi. This is usually the result of chronic or childhood infection and subsequent cartilage damage. It is also seen in patients with rare entities such as cystic fibrosis and allergic bronchopulmonary aspergillosis. Symptoms are chronic cough, purulent sputum, and sometimes hemoptysis. Bronchiectasis typically involves the medial aspects of both right and left lower lobes. This is visualized on a plain chest radiograph by the associated bronchial wall thickening, which is the result of infection.

Early bronchiectasis may be associated with a normal chest x-ray, although in later stages the bronchial wall thickening causes the appearance of a stringy or honeycomb (coarse mesh) type infiltrate at both lung bases. In addition, sometimes "tram-tracking" can be seen. This refers to two parallel linear densities seen as white lines that represent the thickened bronchial walls. Usually this is seen for only 2 or 3 cm before it disappears (Fig. 3–37*A* and *B*). Late bronchiectasis is seen as cavities or a honeycomb appearance at the lung bases. Although it is difficult to see bronchiectasis on a plain chest radiograph, it is quite easy to identify utilizing thin-slice or high-resolution CT scanning (Fig. 3–37*C*). You should not order a CT study unless it will make a difference in therapy or outcome.

Atelectasis. Atelectasis refers to collapse of a lung or portion of the lung with resorption of air from the alveoli. This can result from an obstructing bronchial lesion, extrinsic compression (from pleural effusions or bullae), fibrosis, or a loss of surface tension in the alveoli (as in hyaline membrane disease). Atelectasis can involve a small subsegmental region of a lung or the entire lung. Since atelectasis is a very common finding and has clinical implications, you should be familiar with the various appearances and progressions that are associated with focal or generalized volume loss in a lung.

Linear (discoid or platelike) atelectasis is almost always seen in the middle or lower lung zones as a horizontal or near-horizontal line of increased density (whiteness). This minimal form of subsegmental collapse is most commonly seen in patients who have difficulty breathing, such as after recent surgery or rib fractures. The atelectasis may appear very quickly (within hours) and can disappear just as quickly after the patient has been encouraged to breathe deeply or after respiratory therapy (Fig. 3–38).

Atelectasis, or collapse of entire lung segments, occurs typically as a result of a mucous plug, tumor, or malplacement of endotracheal tubes. Early right upper lobe atelectasis is seen on the AP or PA radiograph as a hazy white density in the right upper lung zone. As air is resorbed from the right upper lobe there is increasing density but decreasing right upper lobe volume. During this process, the right minor fissure moves from its normal horizontal position and becomes bowed upward. This looks like an upside-down white triangle at the right lung apex. With complete collapse of the right upper lobe, there may be only a whitish density, which begins at the right hilum and extends up along the right lateral aspect of the superior mediastinum and then curves out over the apex. In this late stage (complete right upper lobe collapse), the diagnosis can be difficult to make. Usually, however, there are other signs of volume loss pointing toward the right upper lobe. These include shift or pulling of the trachea to the right and elevation of the right hilum. Remember that the right hilum should normally be slightly lower than the left; if both right and left hila appear at the same level, you should be thinking about right upper lobe volume loss as one possible cause for this finding.

Atelectasis of the right middle lobe is often difficult to appreciate on an AP radiograph, but it appears as a slightly increased density (whiteness) over the lower portion of the right lung, and there is loss of the normally distinct right cardiac margin. On the lateral chest x-ray there will be a narrow white triangle projecting over the heart, formed by the approximation of the minor fissure and the lower half of the major fissure.

With right lower lobe collapse, there is in-

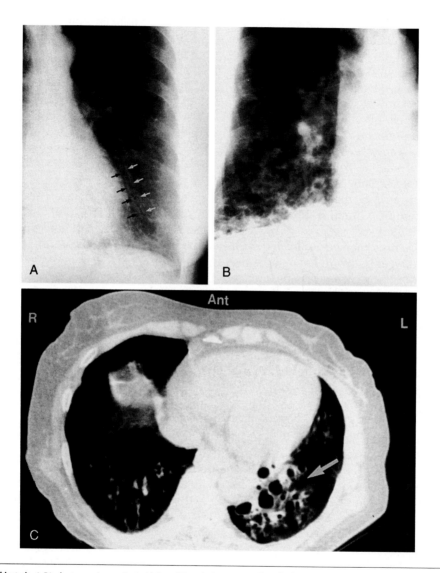

FIGURE 3–37. Bronchiectasis. A PA chest x-ray in a patient with bronchiectasis demonstrates bronchial wall thickening, which is most pronounced at the lung bases *(A)*. This is often referred to as "tram tracking" or linear parallel lines that represent thickened bronchial walls *(arrows)*. In advanced bronchiectasis *(B)*, there are coarse basilar lung infiltrates that may appear cavitary. Bronchiectasis is much better seen on a CT scan *(C)* than on a chest x-ray. The findings are of dilated bronchi with thickened bronchial walls *(arrow)*.

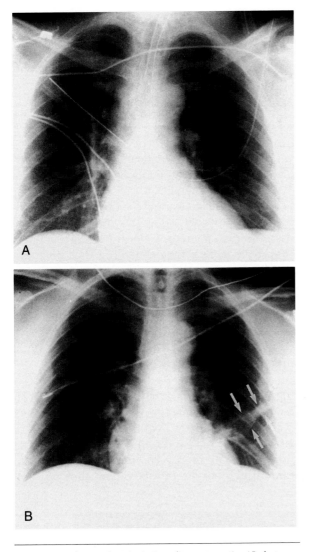

left lower lobe collapse appears as a haziness or increasing density at the left lung base and retrocardiac region. A retrocardiac density is more likely to be atelectasis than a pneumonia, particularly immediately after thoracic surgery. With left lower lobe atelectasis, the left hilum may be pulled down and level with the right one, and the left hemidiaphragm will be hard to see. On the lateral view, there will be posterior and some inferior displacement of the major fissure. As in right lower lobe collapse, there will be increasing density over the lower thoracic spine.

Both right and left lower lobe collapse can mimic or be mimicked by pleural effusions. The way to differentiate the two is to exclude the presence of a pleural effusion. This can be done by looking at the cardiophrenic angles on an upright frontal view of the chest to see if there is blunting or if there is pleural fluid tracking up along the sides of the chest wall. If there is volume loss (indicated by pulling down of the hilum or mediastinal shift toward the affected side), collapse should be suspected. With a large

FIGURE 3–38. Linear atelectasis. An immediate postoperative AP chest x-ray (A) is unremarkable with the exception of an endotracheal tube being present and overlying tubes and EKG leads. A chest x-ray obtained several hours after the patient had been extubated (B) shows an area of linear atelectasis (arrows). This can clear up very quickly if the patient is given appropriate respiratory therapy.

creasing density at the right lung base, loss of the right hemidiaphragm margin, and pulling down of the right hilum. On the lateral chest x-ray, there will be posterior and inferior displacement of the major fissure and increasing density (or whiteness) over the lower thoracic spine (Fig. 3–39).

Lobar atelectasis, or collapse of left lung lobes, can be more difficult to appreciate than you might suspect. On an AP or a PA chest x-ray,

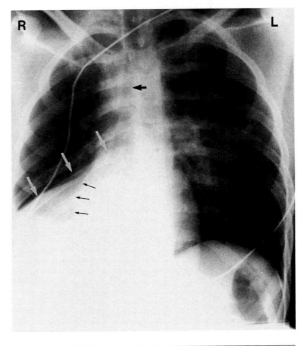

FIGURE 3–39. Right lower lobe atelectasis. Complete collapse of the right lower lobe with volume loss evidenced by shift of the trachea and cardiac border to the right side (black arrows). Air in the right lower lobe has been resorbed, resulting in a diffuse infiltrate (white arrows).

pleural effusion, there often is associated underlying lung atelectasis as a result of direct compression, so you should not be fooled into assuming that only one entity can exist at a given time.

Left upper lobe atelectasis is seen on the frontal chest radiograph as a generalized density in the left upper lung. In the early stages there is increased density anterior to the major fissure on the lateral chest radiograph. As atelectasis of the left upper lobe progresses and becomes complete, the collapsed left upper lobe becomes pancaked along the anterior chest wall and may be visualized only as a dense white line 1 or 2 cm thick in the retrosternal region (Fig. 3–40).

The most severe form of volume loss occurs after surgical removal of one lung. After a pneumonectomy, empty space fills with fluid over several weeks. As this progresses the hemidiaphragm will elevate, the mediastinum will move toward the affected side, and the remaining lung will hyperinflate and often will herniate across the midline. If the mediastinal structures are displaced away from the resected lung, you should be suspicious of a postoperative malignant effusion or an empyema.

Blebs and Bullae. Both these terms refer to a portion of lung in which there is an air space without alveoli. Although I have never known a clear distinction to be made between these two entities, most people consider a bleb to be a relatively small air cavity, usually on the order of 1 cm or less. A bulla is greater than 1 cm and often significantly larger, measuring several inches in diameter. Both a bleb and a bulla should have walls that are very thin and well defined (if they can be seen at all) (Fig. 3–41). If a thick wall is present, you should be thinking in terms of an inflammatory or neoplastic cavitary lesion. Since the walls of blebs and bullae are so thin, the sensitivity of a chest x-ray for detection of these lesions is quite poor, although they are easily seen on a CT scan. The presence of a bulla can sometimes be inferred on a chest x-ray by noting a region of lung that does not seem to have pulmonary vessels.

AIR SPACE PATHOLOGY

Infiltrates

For appropriate diagnosis of a patchy or diffusely increased density in the lungs, you need to characterize the radiographic appearance and correlate this with the clinical history. Most radiologists will report an infiltrate as alveolar, interstitial, nodular, or mixed, and they will tell

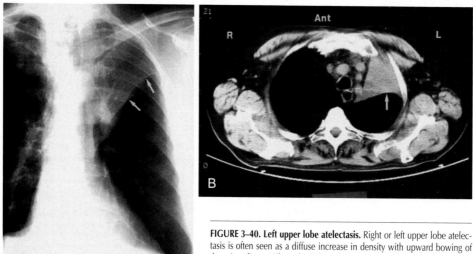

FIGURE 3–40. Left upper lobe atelectasis. Right or left upper lobe atelectasis is often seen as a diffuse increase in density with upward bowing of the minor fissure. The volume loss also elevates the hilum on the affected side (A). A CT scan (B) also shows the atelectasis as a diffuse increase in density of the affected segment or lobe (arrow).

Alveolar simply means that the alveolar spaces are filled with some material. In simple terms, this means that the alveoli are filled with pus, blood, fluid, or cells. Given this, it is not possible radiographically to tell whether an alveolar infiltrate is due to a pneumonia (pus), pulmonary hemorrhage (blood), pulmonary edema (fluid), or alveolar tumor (cells) (Fig. 3–42). Most alveolar infiltrates either are somewhat fluffy or represent areas of complete consolidation. As filling of the alveoli progresses the only things left with air in them are the bronchi, and thus "air bronchograms" can be seen (Fig. 3–43A). If you see a bronchus filled with air and outlined by increased density, you can be certain that you are dealing with an alveolar process.

Interstitial infiltrates are caused by disease processes that affect tissues outside the alveoli. Interstitial processes are usually diffuse and are seen as thin white lines (Fig. 3–43B). Occasionally, they may be somewhat honeycombed in appearance, and the differential diagnosis of these processes often depends on whether the interstitial infiltrate is acute or chronic. Again, the finding of an interstitial infiltrate is nonspecific. Increased fluid in the interstitium and interlobular septa can be seen in congestive heart failure. Interstitial changes can also be seen with

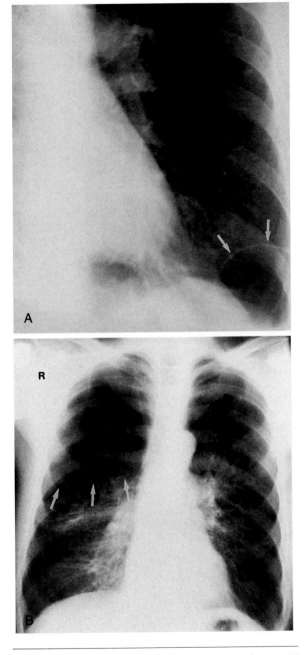

FIGURE 3–41. Bullae. Sometimes small bullae can be seen on a chest x-ray (A) owing to the fact that their thin wall can be visualized. Larger bullae (B) are sometimes identified only by the fact that there is an area on the chest x-ray that does not appear to have any pulmonary vessels (arrows), and at the periphery there may be crowding of the normal lung and vessels.

you whether it is focal (e.g., in the right upper lobe) or diffuse. The terms "alveolar" and "interstitial" are often difficult for the novice and the expert radiologist to differentiate and agree upon.

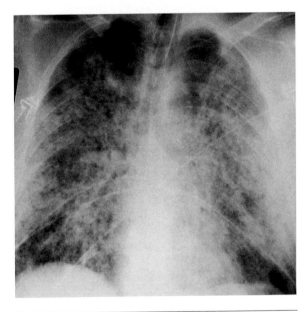

FIGURE 3–42. Pulmonary hemorrhage. The fluffy alveolar pattern is produced by fluid filling the alveoli.

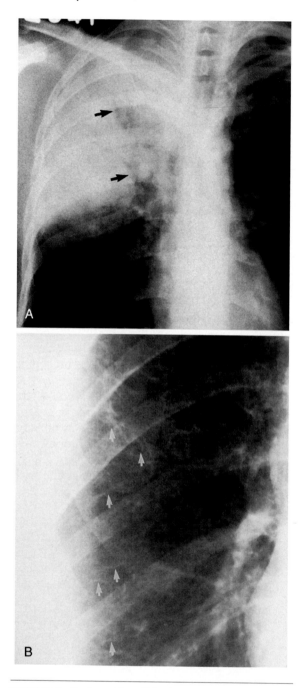

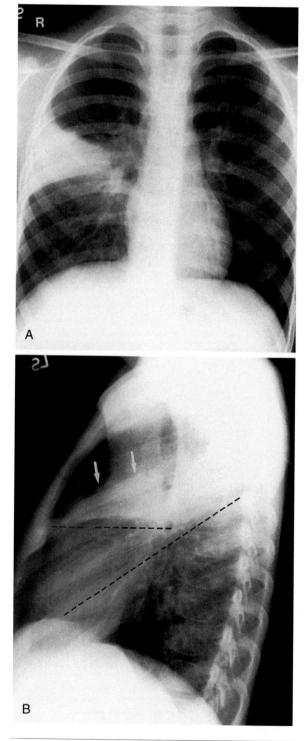

FIGURE 3–43. Alveolar and interstitial pulmonary infiltrates. Alveolar lung infiltrates are seen initially as patchy densities, but as they become more confluent and the process fills the alveolar spaces *(A)* the only air that remains is in the bronchi. This results in what is termed an air bronchogram *(arrows)*. An interstitial infiltrate is seen on the chest x-ray of a different patient as multiple, very white, thin lines *(B)*. Pulmonary vessels are not normally seen at the very periphery of the lung, and, therefore, the lines shown here by the white arrows represent an interstitial process.

FIGURE 3–44. Right upper lobe pneumonia. On the PA chest x-ray *(A)*, note that the right cardiac border is well seen. The alveolar infiltrate is seen in the right midlung. Localization is quite easy on the lateral view *(B)* by noting where the major and minor fissures should be. The infiltrate *(arrows)* can be seen above the minor fissure, indicating that it is in the upper lobe.

what is commonly referred to as lymphangitic spread of tumor as well as idiopathic pulmonary fibrosis, collagen vascular diseases, and other entities. You should not be surprised if you think you see both interstitial and alveolar signs on the same chest x-ray. Many processes, such as congestive heart failure, can cause both findings (i.e., interstitial edema and pulmonary edema with alveolar filling).

Pneumonias. Most bacterial pneumonias produce lobar, segmental, or patchy infiltrates. Although this is an alveolar infiltrate, the alveolar filling and consolidation are usually not enough to be able to see distinct air bronchograms. Accurate localization of a pneumonia to a segment of the lung usually requires both PA and lateral chest radiographs. When the consolidation is fairly dense, the infiltrate is quite easy to localize. A right or left upper lobe infiltrate is usually seen as increased density in the upper portions of the lung on the AP or PA view. The lateral film generally is unnecessary for this diagnosis (Fig. 3–44).

A right middle lobe infiltrate or pneumonia can be in the medial or lateral segment, or both. An infiltrate in the medial segment of the right middle lobe will obscure the right heart border on the frontal view and on the lateral view is seen as a triangular density radiating from the hilum toward the anterior and lower part of the chest (Fig. 3–45).

Right and left lower lobe infiltrates can be visualized by one of three methods. They may obscure the right or left hemidiaphragm on the frontal view. Remember, on an AP or a PA chest x-ray, you should normally be able to see the hemidiaphragms from the lateral costophrenic angles almost all the way to the spine (even behind the heart) (Fig. 3–46A). On the lateral view, lower lobe infiltrates can be identified as being behind the location of the major fissure (Fig. 3–46B); alternatively, they can be identified by utilizing the "spine sign." The vertebral bodies of the thoracic spine usually get darker as you proceed lower in the chest. If the vertebral bodies get darker down to about the midportion of the thoracic spine and then get whiter or lighter inferiorly, you should suspect a lower lobe infiltrate (Fig. 3–36C). Determining whether

this is on the right or left will require correlation with the frontal chest x-ray.

Pneumonias need not always be segmental or lobar; they can be round or diffuse. Round pneumonias can simulate mass lesions, such as a neoplasm, although the clinical presentation is very different, and round pneumonias occur more commonly in children than in adults. These are usually due to streptococcus.

Some characteristics of pneumonias can be used to guess the organism of origin, although none of these is specific or as good as a culture. Lobar pneumonias are associated with streptococcal, staphylococcal, and gram-negative organisms. Lobar enlargement with an infiltrate is characteristically associated with *Klebsiella*. Cavitation in an acute pneumonia is associated with staphylococci and virulent streptococci. Chronic cavitation is associated with tuberculosis, histoplasmosis, and fungal lesions.

Pneumonias that are interstitial and symmetrically diffuse throughout both lungs often are atypical pneumonias. These include pneumonias due to *Mycoplasma*, viruses, and *Pneumocystis*. Viral pneumonias and *Pneumocystis carinii* pneumonia (PCP) are rare in nonimmunocompromised adults; the most likely cause of an interstitial pneumonia in a nonimmunocompromised adult is mycoplasmal infection.

Lobar or segmental infiltrates in immunocompromised adults are most likely bacterial or fungal in origin. A chest radiograph in such a patient may reveal infiltrates (Fig. 3–47A), although a patient who has PCP can have a relatively normal chest radiograph. In these circumstances, a nuclear medicine gallium scan may show increased activity (Fig. 3–47B). Diffuse air space disease in immunocompromised patients is due to *Pneumocystis* with or without cytomegalovirus infection. Early *Pneumocystis* infection can be seen as an interstitial infiltrate, although a more advanced condition may cause diffuse alveolar disease with air bronchograms. This can progress to consolidation within several days. Occasionally there will be upper lobe air-filled cysts that progress to pneumothorax or bronchopleural fistula. These latter findings mimic tuberculosis, but with PCP, adenopathy and pleural effusions are rare. Fungal infections in AIDS patients are uncommon.

In patients with AIDS, there can be diffuse

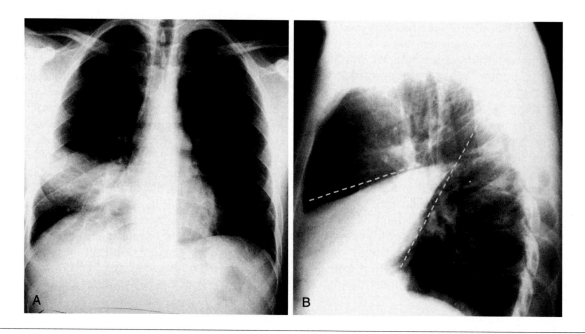

FIGURE 3–45. Right middle lobe pneumonia. On the PA chest x-ray *(A)*, the alveolar infiltrate obscures the right cardiac border. This silhouette sign means that the pathologic process is up against the right cardiac border and, therefore, must be in the middle lobe. This is confirmed on the lateral view *(B)* by noting that the consolidation is anterior to the major fissure but below the minor fissure.

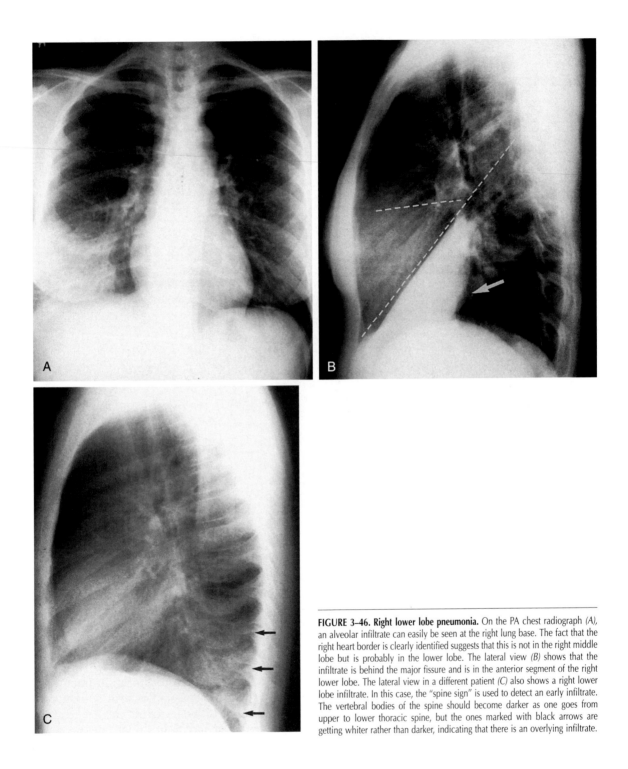

FIGURE 3–46. Right lower lobe pneumonia. On the PA chest radiograph (A), an alveolar infiltrate can easily be seen at the right lung base. The fact that the right heart border is clearly identified suggests that this is not in the right middle lobe but is probably in the lower lobe. The lateral view (B) shows that the infiltrate is behind the major fissure and is in the anterior segment of the right lower lobe. The lateral view in a different patient (C) also shows a right lower lobe infiltrate. In this case, the "spine sign" is used to detect an early infiltrate. The vertebral bodies of the spine should become darker as one goes from upper to lower thoracic spine, but the ones marked with black arrows are getting whiter rather than darker, indicating that there is an overlying infiltrate.

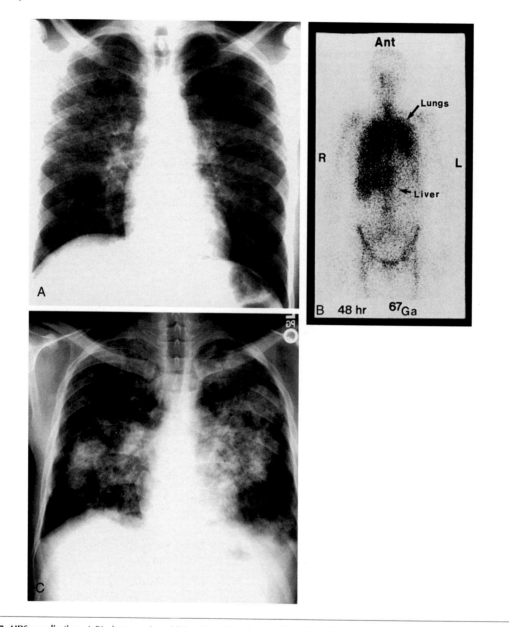

FIGURE 3–47. AIDS complications. A PA chest x-ray in an HIV-positive patient shows a diffuse bilateral perihilar infiltrate due to pneumocystis pneumonia *(A).* In many patients with AIDS, the chest x-ray may be negative when *Pneumocystis* is present. A nuclear medicine gallium scan *(B)* can often show increased activity in the lungs of such patients. A chest x-ray in a different patient with AIDS *(C)* shows bilateral dense patchy alveolar infiltrates, in this case representing Kaposi's sarcoma.

or nodular pulmonary involvement with lymphoma or Kaposi's sarcoma (Fig. 3–47C). A nuclear medicine gallium scan will not be positive in patients with Kaposi's sarcoma but will be positive in PCP, most other infections, and lymphoma. Isolated hilar adenopathy in AIDS patients is more likely due to lymphoma than to mycobacterial infections.

A common indication for ordering a chest radiograph is to exclude aspiration pneumonia. The question of aspirated gastric contents may occur as the result of a seizure, cardiac resuscitation attempt, or alcoholic binge. In the case of aspiration, the chest radiograph is often normal within the first hour or so. If you get a normal chest x-ray interpretation after a recent suspected aspiration, a follow-up film should be obtained in approximately 12 hours. It often takes several hours for the gastric contents to react with the lung to cause fluid exudate and an alveolar infiltrate (Fig. 3–48). A number of other toxic agents, such as water (drowning), hydrocarbons, chlorine, smoke, heroin, and aspirin, as well as radiation therapy can produce alveolar infiltrates. Some drugs, such as busulfan, bleomycin, and cyclophosphamide, produce toxic interstitial disease. Amiodarone can cause a wide variety of pulmonary abnormalities, but the characteristic finding seen on CT scan is increased lung density due to the iodine content of the drug.

Pulmonary infiltrates are common after lung trauma. Pulmonary contusions can occur with-

TABLE 3–3. Abnormalities To Look For on a Postsurgical or Post-traumatic Chest X-ray

Position of the endotracheal tube
           pleural tubes
              venous catheters
Upper mediastinal widening
    Left apical pleural cap
    Ill-defined aortic knob or AP window (signs of aortic tear)
Pneumothorax Apical
               Loculated or basilar
Mediastinal emphysema
Subcutaneous emphysema
Infiltrates (? changing)
Mediastinal shift
Atelectasis Lobar
          Focal
Pleural fluid collection
Rib or sternal fractures
Spine fractures (including paraspinous soft tissue widening)
Shoulder fractures and dislocations
Free air under the diaphragms

out rib fractures and are seen within hours of an accident. About 50 per cent of patients will have hemoptysis. Contusions are seen radiographically as ill-defined pulmonary parenchymal infiltrates due to hemorrhage and edema. If uncomplicated, they normally resolve over 4 to 5 days. Pulmonary hematomas are caused by bleeding as a result of shearing injuries of the lung parenchyma. These can present as nodules or masses, and they may cavitate. They take weeks to resolve. Particular items to look for on a post-traumatic chest study are listed in Table 3–3.

Another post-traumatic abnormality that can produce bilateral ill-defined infiltrates is fat embolism. This is not seen except with fracture of a large bone (such as the femur) that has undergone surgical manipulation. These patients usually present with a clear chest film and have a sudden onset of dyspnea some time afterward. The diagnosis is made by looking for fat globules in the urine.

Tuberculosis. Chest x-rays are often done on patients who have had a positive tuberculin skin test. Of chest x-rays ordered for this reason, 99.9 per cent or more will be normal. It should be pointed out that a normal chest radiograph does not exclude active tuberculosis, since the tuberculosis that results in a positive skin test need not be in the lungs but can be in the kidneys or even in the spine.

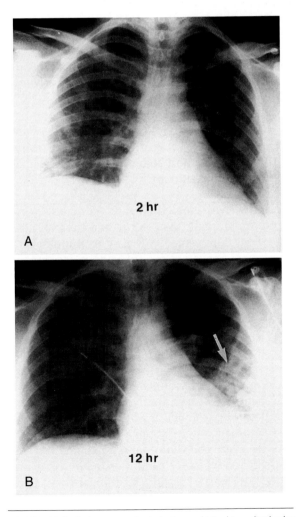

FIGURE 3–48. Aspiration pneumonia. A chest x-ray obtained immediately after aspiration may be quite normal (A). The chemical pneumonia takes 6 or 12 hours (B) to cause an alveolar infiltrate (arrow).

When tuberculosis is visualized on a chest radiograph, the usual sequence of events is as follows. Primary TB is most commonly seen as a focal middle or lower lobe consolidation with lymphadenopathy and sometimes a pleural effusion. Cavitation is rare. Hilar adenopathy is present about 95 per cent of the time and is more commonly seen in children than in adults. A pleural effusion is present about 10 per cent of the time. Reactivation of a primary focus causes infiltrates in the posterior segments of the upper lobes and the superior segment of the lower lobes. Sequelae are miliary tuberculosis, cavitation (40 per cent) (Fig. 3–49), and empy-

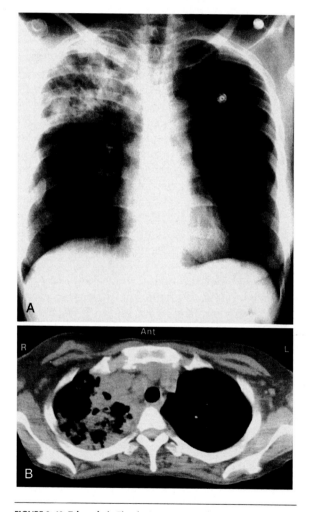

FIGURE 3–49. Tuberculosis. The classic appearance of reactivation tuberculosis is that of an upper lobe infiltrate with cavities (A). Over time, there will be healing and fibrosis, which will pull the hilum up on the affected side. If there is any question about whether the infiltrate is cavitated, a CT scan (B) may be useful.

ema. Adenopathy is rare compared with primary infectious tuberculosis. Healed tuberculosis may present as fibrous changes in the apices or as areas of calcification, either within the lung parenchyma or in the region of the hilar or mediastinal lymph nodes. Most commonly, however, such focal calcifications are due to old histoplasmosis rather than tuberculosis.

Miliary tuberculosis is seen as a diffuse bilateral process with very small nodules scattered throughout both lungs. The nodules are supposed to be the size of a millet seed. Since millet seeds are not very common, it is easier to remember that they are just slightly smaller than sesame seeds. Patients who present with chest x-ray findings of miliary tuberculosis usually are extremely ill. Numerous very small lung nodules can also be seen with histoplasmosis, varicella pneumonia, and metastatic thyroid cancer.

Fungal Lesions. A wide variety of fungal lesions can affect the lung. These may present as focal infiltrates or as discrete lesions. Occasionally, a fungus ball or a mycetoma can be seen within a pulmonary cavitary lesion (Fig. 3–50). Cryptococcus can be seen as a small cavitary lesion within the lung, and sometimes there are small satellite nodules nearby.

Lung Abscess. Inhaled particulate matter or necrotic pneumonias can result in a lung abscess. A typical appearance is that of a lesion several centimeters in diameter that either looks solid (Fig. 3–51) or has a lucent (dark) air-filled center and a shaggy, thick wall. The wall typically is about 5 mm in thickness. The major differential diagnosis of a thick-walled cavitary lesion in the lung is a lung abscess or a cavitating neoplasm (usually squamous cell carcinoma). Lung abscesses may have an air-fluid level in the central portion, but so may infected cavitary neoplasms. CT scanning is commonly utilized to direct a needle biopsy of such lesions to obtain cultures and cytologic studies. Sometimes a lung abscess can be confused with an empyema, but abscesses are typically round, with the lung and blood vessels in normal position; if there is an air-fluid level, it is the same length on PA and lateral films. An empyema is usually elliptical, and the lung and blood vessels are displaced or compressed; if there is an air-fluid level, it often

FIGURE 3–50. Fungal infection. Fungal infections of the lung may initially present as an alveolar infiltrate *(A)*, but several days later *(B)* they may show cavitation *(arrows)* with a central loose mass representing a fungus ball.

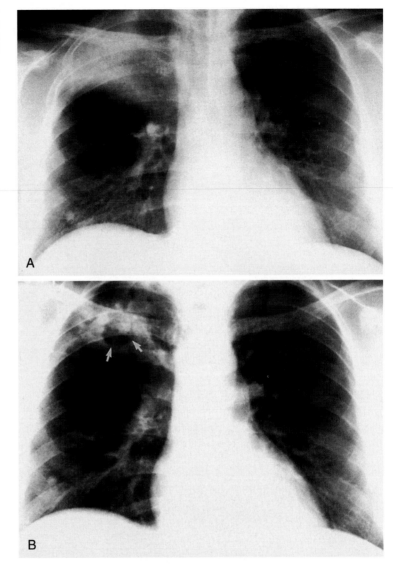

is of a different length on frontal and lateral films.

Adult Respiratory Distress Syndrome (ARDS). ARDS is of uncertain etiology but the damage results from leakage of fluid from the alveolar capillary bed. It is typically seen in patients who have been in an intensive care unit for several days and who have been intubated. ARDS may occur in postoperative patients who have normal pulmonary function in the immediate postoperative period but who then develop tachypnea, anxiety, and breathing fatigue. Systemic nonpulmonary infections can also damage the pulmonary parenchyma and produce ARDS.

The usual pattern is that of diffuse or patchy alveolar infiltrates throughout both lungs (Fig. 3–52). The major difficulty in evaluating these patients is the exclusion of a concurrent bacterial pneumonia or congestive heart failure. The differential diagnosis is probably best made on clinical grounds, although if an alveolar infiltrate changes rapidly (within several hours or within 1 day), the infiltrates most likely represent congestive heart failure or fluid overload. In patients with congestive failure there are usually Kerley B lines, pleural effusions, increased heart size, and infiltrates that are perihilar or basilar. With ARDS, Kerley B lines should not be present, pleural effusions occur only late,

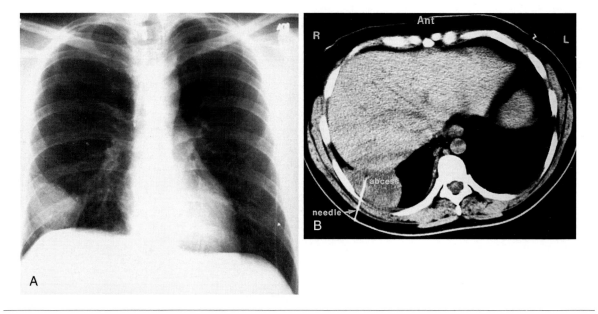

FIGURE 3–51. Lung abscess. On a chest x-ray, a lung abscess may look to be a solid rounded lesion (A), or, if it has a connection with the bronchus, there may be an air-fluid level in a thick-walled cavitary lesion. CT scanning (B) can be used to localize the lesion and to place a needle for drainage and aspiration of contents for culture.

heart size is often normal, and alveolar infiltrates often extend to the lung periphery.

Bacterial pneumonias often take a day or more to change, and patients with ARDS often

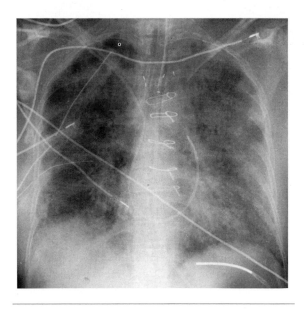

FIGURE 3–52. Adult respiratory distress syndrome (ARDS). The findings of ARDS in this patient who has had a coronary bypass graft are diffuse bilateral alveolar infiltrates. Similar findings may be due to diffuse pneumonia or even pulmonary edema, and the differential diagnosis is ranked on clinical findings.

have a relatively stable appearance over many days. DThe diagnosis of pneumonias is often made on the basis of bacterial cultures. You should be aware that changes in the x-ray technique or in the amount of positive-pressure respiratory therapy may cause significant changes in the appearance of the infiltrates in patients with ARDS.

Chronic Lung Diseases. There are a wide variety of chronic lung abnormalities. Bronchiectasis and chronic obstructive disease have already been described. iseases that preferentially affect the upper lobes are silicosis, sarcoidosis, and eosinophilic granuloma. Silicosis may have "eggshell" calcifications in the hilar nodes in addition to uniformly distributed small (1 to 10 mm) nodules (Fig. 3–53). These small nodules can coalesce to form upper lobe parenchymal masses (progressive massive fibrosis).

Sarcoid is a disease of unknown etiology that most commonly occurs in African-Americans. The manifestations on chest x-ray are hilar and mediastinal adenopathy and pulmonary parenchymal disease. About one third of patients will demonstrate symmetric hilar lymph node enlargement and, occasionally, azygous adenopathy

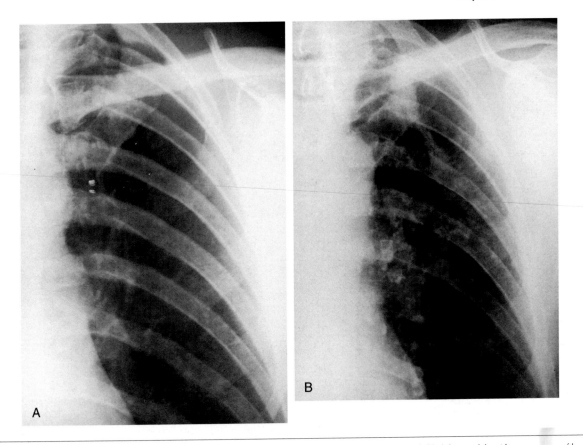

FIGURE 3–53. Silicosis. Chest x-rays on the same person 20 years apart. The initial chest x-ray *(A)* shows an unremarkable left upper lobe. After many years of hard rock mining, rounded calcifications are seen about the left hilum; there is a nodular appearance to the lung parenchyma; and there is fibrosis seen at the left apex *(B)*.

(see Fig. 3–83). About one third will have pulmonaryparenchymal disease manifested as either interstitial or alveolar infiltrates, and one third will demonstrate both adenopathy and pulmonary parenchymal disease (Fig. 3–54). In late stages, a linear interstitial fibrotic pattern develops.

Conditions that preferentially affect the lower lobes are collagen vascular diseases, drug toxicity, asbestosis, interstitial fibrosis, and unusual interstitial pneumonias. My students like mnemonics to help them remember, and they use BADAS for lower lobe diseases. This refers to *b*ronchiectasis, *a*spiration, *d*rugs, *a*sbestosis, and *s*cleroderma (or other collagen vascular diseases). For upper lobe diseases they use CASSET P, which stands for *c*ystic fibrosis, *a*nkylosing spondylitis, *s*ilicosis, *s*arcoid, *e*osinophilic granuloma, *t*uberculosis and *p*neumocystis carinii. For diffuse chronic interstitial disease they use LIFE, which refers to *l*ymphangitic spread of tumor, *i*nflammation (infection),

*f*ibrosis, and *e*dema. For acute interstitial infiltrates they use HEP, referring to *h*ypersensitivity (allergic alveolitis), *e*dema, and *p*neumonia (viral).

Lymphangitic carcinoma and sarcoid can have very small nodules that are concentrated about the bronchi and blood vessels, while most of the other entities have nodules that extend to the periphery of the lung. Most collagen vascular diseases can cause interstitial (fine lines), reticular (meshlike), or honeycombing (coarse mesh–like) pulmonary parenchymal abnormalities. These can be seen with rheumatoid arthritis and systemic lupus erythematosus as well as a number of other entities.

Some chronic lung disease can cause diffuse interstitial changes, honeycombing, or focal patchy infiltrates. Sarcoid has already been mentioned. Other diseases that produce these varied findings include extrinsic allergic alveolitis (caused by a number of antigens such as mold or avian proteins), eosinophilic granu-

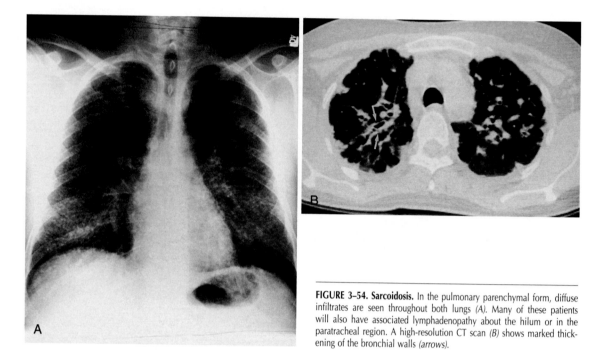

FIGURE 3–54. Sarcoidosis. In the pulmonary parenchymal form, diffuse infiltrates are seen throughout both lungs (A). Many of these patients will also have associated lymphadenopathy about the hilum or in the paratracheal region. A high-resolution CT scan (B) shows marked thickening of the bronchial walls (arrows).

loma, bronchiolitis obliterans, and eosinophilic lung disease. Given the nonspecificity of the radiographic findings and the varied appearance of these diseases, the diagnosis is best made by history and clinical findings. The chest x-ray or high-resolution CT can provide supporting information and be used to monitor progress of a given disease.

Solitary Pulmonary Nodules. A pulmonary nodule is really a small mass. I think of them as being less than 3 cm in diameter, and when there is something in the lung larger than 3 cm, I call it a mass. There are a number of authors who refer to a solitary nodule as a lesion of less than 6 cm in diameter. To me, anything approaching the size of a golf ball is very suspicious for a neoplasm; anything that is only 0.5 cm in diameter that you can see easily and is probably very dense is most likely a granuloma. Age is also a useful discriminating factor. In a patient under 40 years of age a lung cancer may occur, but it is very, very rare.

A solitary pulmonary nodule can represent practically anything. As already mentioned it may be due to a granuloma or lung cancer, but other etiologies include a single metastatic lesion, septic embolus, arteriovenous malforma-

tion, hamartoma, or even a small area of rounded atelectasis (Table 3–4). There are several challenges when you have identified what you think is a solitary pulmonary nodule. The first is to determine that it is, in fact, within the lung and that you are not looking at a nipple shadow or wart that is on the skin surface. A nipple shadow is seen projecting within the lung only on the frontal chest x-ray, is usually in the midclavicular line, and projects over the lower half of the lung. Small nipple markers (BBs) with a repeat chest x-ray may be of some use.

You should locate the "nodule" in a horizontal plane on the frontal chest radiograph (for example, at the level of the aortic arch), and then you should look at the lateral chest x-ray (again at the horizontal plane of the aortic arch) and see whether you can find the nodule at the same level projecting within the chest on both views. If there is any doubt, you can obtain shallow oblique views; if the nodule is truly within the thoracic cavity, it should rotate less than the anterior and posterior ribs.

The second step is to characterize the nodule. If it is well defined and round, it is much more likely to be benign than if it is irregular or indistinct in its margins. Calcification that is very dense (Fig. 3–55) or within a nodule, suggests that it is most likely a granuloma (Fig. 3–56). The calcification, however, should be centrally located in the nodule. If calcification is eccentrically located in a nodule, consider a neoplasm.

The third step of importance is to determine whether the nodule is new or old. A careful review of all available chest x-rays and phone calls to pertinent hospitals should be made before expensive or invasive studies are ordered. A nodule that has remained unchanged in size for 2 years can be considered benign. Stability for a period of 1 year is not enough, since slow-growing tumors may not change appreciably in a 12-month interval. If a 1 cm nodule doubles the number of cells that it contains, its diameter

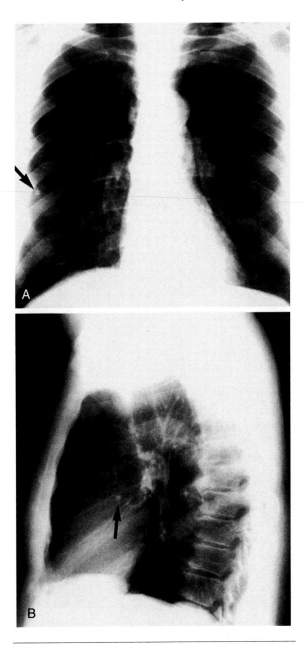

FIGURE 3–55. Solitary calcified granuloma. A very dense pulmonary nodule is seen on both PA *(A)* and lateral *(B)* chest x-rays. This can be confidently called a granuloma; it needs no further work-up, since it is much denser than even the surrounding ribs and therefore is clearly densely calcified.

TABLE 3–4. Common Differential Diagnosis of Pulmonary Nodule(s)

Solitary
  Less than 3 cm
    Granuloma (especially if calcified)
    Lung cancer
    Single nipple shadow
    Wart on the skin
    Benign lung tumors
    Metastasis
    Rounded atelectasis
    Septic embolism
  Large
    Lung cancer
    Round pneumonia
    Large solitary metastases
    Lung abscess
Multiple
  Granulomas
  Metastases
  Septic emboli
Cavitary
  Septic emboli
  Tuberculosis
  Fungal
  Squamous cell cancer
Benign Characteristics
  Small (<3 cm)
  Round
  Well defined edges
  Slow growing (no appreciable change in 2 yr)
  Central calcification
  Solid (not cavitated)
Malignant Characteristics
  Large (>3 cm)
  Irregular shape
  Poorly defined edges
  Obvious growth in <2 yr
  Asymmetric or no calcification
  Cavitated

will grow only to 1.2 cm. A difference this small is hard to appreciate on a chest x-ray.

Further evaluation of a nodule can be obtained by doing a CT scan. In this case, you should ask for thin cuts at the level of the nodule of interest. You should, however, include

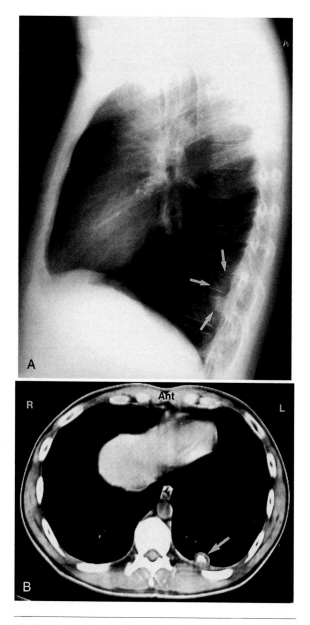

FIGURE 3–56. Granuloma with central calcification. A lateral chest x-ray (A) showed what was thought to be a posterior pleural mass (arrows). No definite calcification is seen on the chest x-ray; however, evaluation with CT scan (B) clearly shows the lesion with dense central calcification. If the calcification were not central in the mass, a neoplasm would need to be excluded.

the entire lungs on the CT scan. Since CT scanning is more sensitive than a chest x-ray for detection of nodules, you may find that what you really have is the presence of multiple nodules; if this is the case, your differential diagnosis changes very quickly.

Lung Cancer. The pathology of lung cancers is a bit confusing. Some confusion arises because a number of tumors exhibit more than one type of pathology; a number are undifferentiated; and the incidence of cell types varies depending upon the type of series (surgical vs. autopsy) quoted. About 40 per cent of lung cancers are adenocarcinomas and 30 per cent or so are squamous. Most of the remainder are small cell carcinomas (which includes oat cell types).

You may erroneously think that a 1 cm lung nodule, which turns out to be a lung cancer, is an early lesion. Nothing could be further from the truth. A 1.0 cm diameter nodule has about 10 billion cells in it. In terms of doubling times it is already two thirds of the way toward filling the entire hemithorax.

Primary lung cancers have a number of appearances. Adenocarcinoma occurs peripherally, whereas squamous cell types are central or peripheral. Squamous cell tumors of any origin tend to cavitate. Small cell carcinomas often present as an indistinct hilar or perihilar mass. A unilateral hilar mass or persistent infiltrate in an adult over the age of 40 should always raise the suspicion of a lung cancer.

A CT scan is the most valuable imaging method for locating and staging lung cancers. Often, intravenous contrast is used with the CT scan, so that the tumor, adenopathy, and pulmonary vessels can be differentiated. However, if you have a good knowledge of anatomy, it is not necessary to use intravenous contrast. Analysis of a CT scan should include not only location and size of the pulmonary lesion but also whether it has a pleural or chest wall involvement and whether hilar or mediastinal lymphadenopathy is present (Fig. 3–57). The accuracy of CT in determining chest wall invasion is only about 50 per cent, but invasion is suggested by pleural thickening, more than 3 cm of contact between pleura and tumor, obtuse angles between tumor and pleura, or an increased density of the extrapleural fat. A pleural effusion usually indicates a poor prognosis; however, only aspiration and cytologic confirmation of malignant cells in the effusion make the tumor unresectable.

There are two classic, although uncommon, appearances of lung carcinoma on the chest radiograph that you should be aware of. The first of these is the "Golden S sign," from a hilar

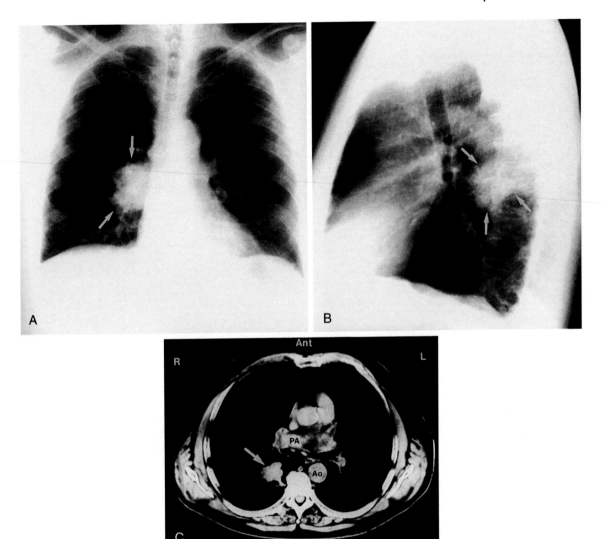

FIGURE 3–57. Lung cancer. An ill-defined mass is noted on the PA chest x-ray *(A)*. While this appears to be located near the right hilum, the lateral chest x-ray *(B)* clearly shows the mass to be posterior to the hilum. Its shaggy appearance is very suggestive of carcinoma. Further evaluation by CT scan *(C)* clearly shows the mass in relationship to the mediastinal structures, such as the pulmonary artery and aorta.

tumor that has caused peripheral atelectasis (most commonly of the right upper lobe). Normally, as the right upper lobe collapses, there is an upward bowing of the minor fissure from the hilum out to the lateral aspect of the chest. With the presence of the hilar mass, there now is inferior and lateral bowing near the hilum, and this creates an S shape to the inferior margin of the collapsing right upper lobe (Fig. 3–58). The second classic appearance is that of the Pancoast tumor. This is an upper lobe carcinoma that has eroded into the pleura and adjacent structures, such as the ribs (Fig. 3–59).

Lung cancers commonly metastasize to the opposite lung, liver, bones, brain, and adrenal glands. The liver is the most common site, and the adrenal glands are involved in about 30 per cent of patients. For this reason, any chest CT scan done for a suspected lung cancer should be extended far enough down to visualize these organs. When there are bony metastases, these are usually purely lytic or destructive. For peripheral lesions (that cannot be reached with a bronchoscope), a percutaneous biopsy can be performed with a thin needle guided by either fluoroscopy or a CT scan. For most lesions, I

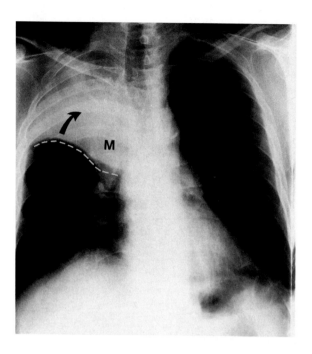

FIGURE 3–58. The "Golden S" sign of lung cancer. Where there is a mass in the region of the hilum that obstructs the upper lobe bronchus, the minor fissure collapses superiorly. With uncomplicated atelectasis, the minor fissure is simply bowed up, but with a mass near the hilum, the inferior margin of the upper lobe takes on an S shape as it goes around the mass.

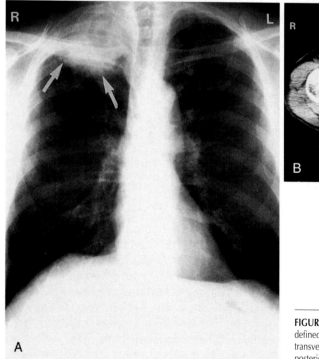

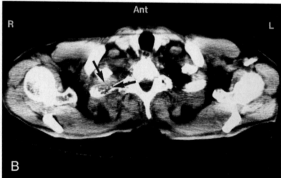

FIGURE 3–59. Pancoast tumor. In this patient with shoulder pain, an ill-defined mass (white arrows) is seen in the right lung apex (A). On a transverse CT scan of the upper thorax (B), permeative destruction of a right posterior rib by the tumor is identified (black arrows).

find fluoroscopy easier, faster, and cheaper. The most common complication of this procedure is a pneumothorax (about 25 per cent of cases); about 5 to 10 per cent of patients will need a chest tube to correct this.

Immunocompromised AIDS patients often have a higher incidence of Kaposi's sarcoma. This usually appears as indistinct focal pulmonary focal infiltrates rather than as well-defined discrete masses (see Fig. 3–47C).

Lymphoma. Lymphomas, and particularly Hodgkin's disease, are most commonly visualized on the chest radiograph either as a large anterior mediastinal mass or as hilar adenopathy. If the lymphomatous mass is large and is up against the aorta, the mass can easily be mistaken for an aortic aneurysm. Hilar adenopathy is often difficult to distinguish from enlarged central pulmonary arteries. Extensive adenopathy can be recognized by multiple lumps or bumps rather than the single one you might expect from a prominent main pulmonary artery. Adenopathy also may fill in the normal concavity between the left main pulmonary artery and the aortic arch. If there is any question, a CT scan can easily sort out the differences (Fig. 3–60). Lymphoma and Hodgkin's disease

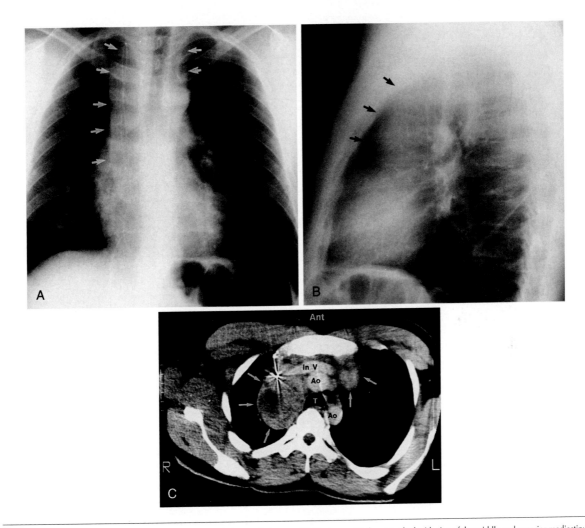

FIGURE 3–60. Hodgkin's disease. In this 20-year-old male with low-grade fevers, a PA chest x-ray (A) shows marked widening of the middle and superior mediastinum (arrows). On the lateral chest x-ray (B), there is filling in of the retrosternal space by an ill-defined anterior mediastinal mass (arrows). The transverse contrast-enhanced CT scan (C) through the upper portion of the chest shows the innominate vein, ascending and descending aorta, and trachea. They are all enveloped by a mass of nodes (arrows).

can cause pulmonary infiltrates or nodules, although this is a relatively uncommon presentation.

Metastatic Lesions. The pulmonary parenchyma is a very common site for metastatic deposits because the lungs act as a filter for large particles or cells. Most metastatic disease has two predominant patterns in the lung. One is the rela-

tively familiar nodular lesions. These are typically referred to as hematogenous metastases. Metastatic lesions in the pulmonary parenchyma vary from being very small nodules to extremely large (cannonball) masses. The pulmonary metastases of thyroid cancer typically create a snowstorm of very small nodular lesions. Other tumors, such as colon and renal cell carcinomas, typically produce metastatic le-

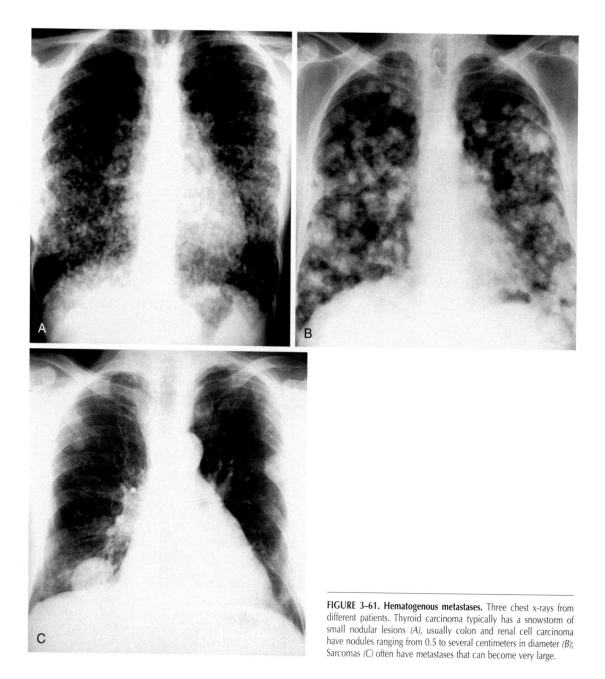

FIGURE 3–61. Hematogenous metastases. Three chest x-rays from different patients. Thyroid carcinoma typically has a snowstorm of small nodular lesions (A), usually colon and renal cell carcinoma have nodules ranging from 0.5 to several centimeters in diameter (B); Sarcomas (C) often have metastases that can become very large.

sions that range from approximately 1 cm to several centimeters in diameter. When there are extremely large multiple masses (about the size of a tennis ball), metastases from a sarcoma should be suspected (Fig. 3–61).

There is a second appearance of metastases in which there are streaky or linear infiltrates throughout the lungs. This is referred to as lymphangitic spread of tumor. In fact, it is not really lymphangitic spread at all, but another appearance of hematogenously spread disease. This particular "lymphangitic" pattern occurs quite commonly with stomach cancer (Fig. 3–62). Breast cancer can produce either the rounded hematogenous metastases or the "lymphangitic" pattern. Of course, remember that if you are looking for metastatic disease, you should carefully examine the mediastinum and hilar regions for evidence of lymphadenopathy, and you should examine the bony structures for evidence of lytic lesions (holes) as well as for sclerotic lesions (areas of ill-defined dense bone).

Clinicians commomly ask how often to get a periodic chest x-ray on a patient with a known cancer in order to exclude pulmonary metastases. It is rarely efficacious to get films monthly, and most oncologists will order chest x-rays only on a 6-month or annual basis and only if the results may affect therapy.

Congestive Heart Failure and Pulmonary Edema. In the upright position, there is substantially more blood flow to the lung bases than to the apices. When you look at an upright chest x-ray, you should assess this normal difference in the pulmonary vascularity. The vessels should be distinct from the peripheral one third of the lung back centrally to the hila, and they should be much more apparent in the lower lung zones than in the upper lung zones.

With congestive failure, a spectrum and progression of findings are normally identified on an upright chest x-ray. In the early stages, there may be minimal cardiomegaly and redistribution of the pulmonary vascularity, with almost equal flow to upper and lower lung zones (with mean capillary wedge pressures of 15 to 25 mm Hg). Also, at this time the diameter of upper lobe vessels will be equal to or greater than that of lower lobe vessels at the same distance from the hilum. Another way to tell is by the presence of pulmonary vessels in the first intercostal space that are greater than 3 mm in diameter. Remember that you cannot use these signs on a supine chest x-ray, since the pulmonary blood flow will change in a normal person as a result of gravity.

As congestive failure increases, fluid may be seen in the interlobular septa at the lateral basal aspects of the lung (25 to 30 mm Hg). These are referred to as Kerley B lines. They are always located just inside the ribs and are horizontal in orientation (Fig. 3–63). Remember, these cannot be blood vessels, because you should not normally see lung markings in the peripheral one fourth of the lungs.

As congestive failure becomes more pronounced, vessels near the hila become indistinct owing to fluid accumulating in the interstitium. Symmetric and bilateral hilar indistinctness should immediately raise the possibility of congestive failure (Fig. 3–64A). Pleural effusions may be present, as evidenced by blunting of the lateral or posterior costophrenic angles. With pronounced congestive failure, fluid accumu-

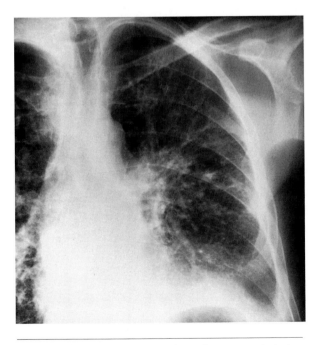

FIGURE 3–62. Lymphangitic metastases. The streaky appearance in the lung parenchyma is due to metastatic disease, in this case stomach carcinoma. The term "lymphangitic" is really a misnomer, since these actually do represent hematogenous metastases in the pulmonary interstitium.

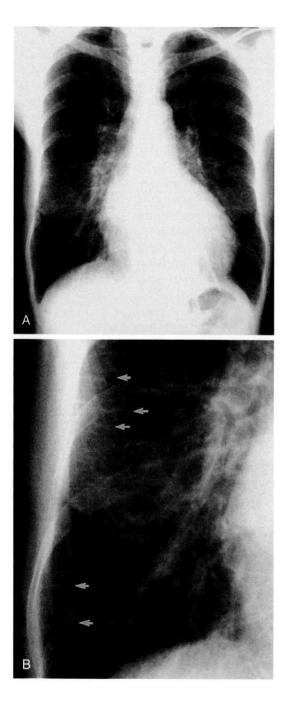

FIGURE 3–63. Early findings of congestive heart failure. The major signs on upright PA chest x-ray *(A)* are cardiomegaly and redistribution of the pulmonary vascularity. Normally, the vessels to the lower lobes are more prominent than those in the upper lobes; however, here they appear at least equally prominent. On a close-up view *(B)*, small horizontal lines can be seen at the very periphery of the lung *(arrows)*. These are known as Kerley B lines and represent fluid in the interlobular septa.

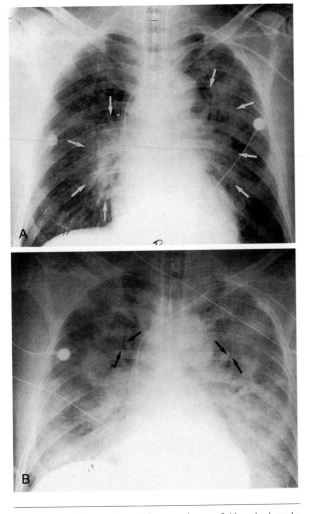

lates in the alveolar spaces, and frank pulmonary edema becomes apparent (Fig. 3–64*B*). This is seen as bilateral, predominantly basilar and perihilar alveolar infiltrates (>30 mm Hg). A note of caution is inserted here, since the changes of minimal cardiomegaly and equalization of the pulmonary vasculature are essentially normal findings on a supine AP chest radiograph. You should not be fooled into making the diagnosis of minimal congestive failure on a supine chest x-ray.

There are some common variations of congestive failure that you should be aware of. In

patients who have been lying down, on either their right or left side, there can be relatively more accumulation of pulmonary edema on the dependent side, since the fluid pressure is greater (Fig. 3–65). Patients who are in renal failure often look as though they are in congestive failure, particularly with a perihilar indistinctness and a sort of butterfly or bat-wing infiltrate centered about the hila. Typically, this is seen pre-dialysis, and after dialysis the infiltrate resolves almost immediately (Fig. 3–66). Remember that pulmonary edema may occur from noncardiogenic causes. In the absence of cardiomegaly you should consider drug overdose, head injury (with central nervous system depression), and acute inhalations of noxious agents as possible etiologies.

PLEURAL PATHOLOGY

Pneumothorax. Pneumothorax refers to air in the pleural space. This is most often caused by trauma (such as stabbings or motor vehicle

FIGURE 3–64. Pulmonary edema. Pulmonary edema, or fluid overload, can be manifested by indistinctness of the pulmonary vessels as they radiate from the hilum *(A)*. This is sometimes termed a "bat wing" infiltrate. As pulmonary edema worsens *(B)*, fluid fills the alveoli, and "air bronchograms" *(arrows)* become apparent.

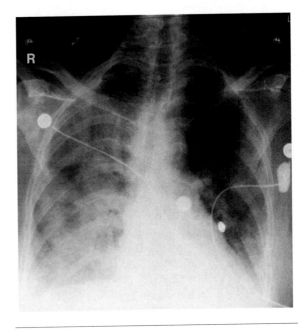

FIGURE 3–65. Dependent pulmonary edema. In debilitated patients who are lying on one side, the increased hydrostatic pressure in the lung that is lower can produce pulmonary edema only in that one lung. In this intensive care unit patient, a right-sided alveolar infiltrate is due to dependent pulmonary edema.

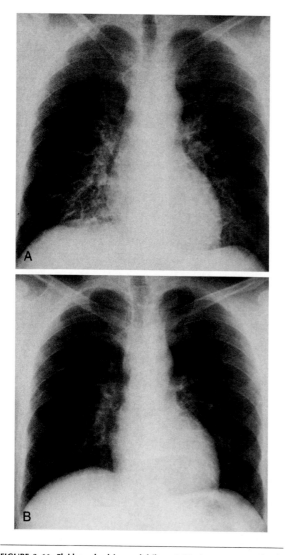

or semi-upright position, air in the pleural space will typically go toward the apex. Thus, the first place to look for a pneumothorax is in the right and left upper hemithorax (Fig. 3–67). The most common appearance is an area adjacent to the ribs where no lung vascularity is seen and where there is a very thin white line, which represents the visceral pleura that has been separated from the parietal pleura by air. You will need to look very carefully for this line, since it is often difficult to distinguish from the bony cortex of nearby ribs. If the pneumothorax is small and the pleural line is behind the rib, it can be almost impossible to see. In such circumstances, it may be useful to obtain an expiration chest radiograph in addition to the usual inspiration chest radiograph. On an expiration view, the lung becomes somewhat denser and smaller as expiration occurs. The amount of air in the pleural space will not change in size or density, and thus the pneumothorax will appear relatively larger during expiration (Fig. 3–68).

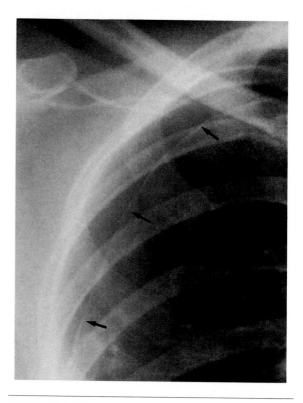

FIGURE 3–67. Apical pneumothorax. A thin line caused by the visceral pleura is seen separated from the lateral chest wall *(arrows)*. Notice that no pulmonary vessels are seen beyond this line and that the line is curved. Notice also that the pleural line is white and that it is almost equally dark on the side of the pneumothorax and the side of the lung.

FIGURE 3–66. Fluid overload in renal failure. A PA chest x-ray immediately prior to dialysis shows what looks like a lot of indistinct pulmonary vessels about the hila. Many of these are not vessels but interstitial fluid. Another chest x-ray obtained 1 hour after dialysis *(B)* shows that all these abnormalities have resolved.

accidents). It also commonly results from attempted introduction of subclavian venous catheters or after liver biopsy (the pleural space extends down quite a way between the liver and the lateral and posterior abdominal wall). A pneumothorax may occur spontaneously (as a result of bleb rupture) or even as a result of some unusual tumors, such as histiocytosis X or metastatic osteogenic sarcoma.

Since the pleural space is continuous around each lung, if the patient is in an upright

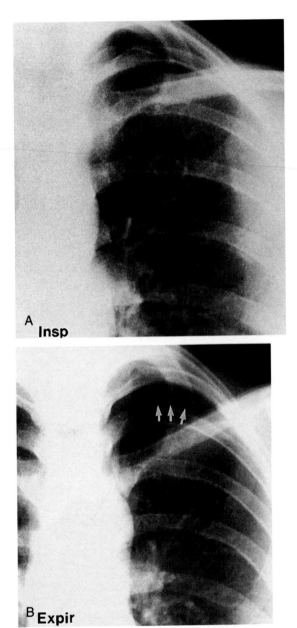

FIGURE 3–68. **Accentuation of the pneumothorax.** In this young male with chest pain, on a typical inspiration chest x-ray *(A)* no pneumothorax is identified. With expiration *(B)*, the lung becomes smaller, but the pneumothorax stays the same size; thus, relatively it appears bigger and can sometimes be easier to see.

How much the lung collapses with a pneumothorax is a function of how much air can get into the pleural space. In patients who have adhesive pleural changes between the visceral and parietal pleura as a result of previous inflammatory disease or scarring, complete col-

lapse of the lung is not possible, even if a large amount of air is available. The same is true of patients who have diffuse lung disease, because their relatively stiff lungs will not allow complete collapse.

Total lung collapse can occur in patients with normal lungs and without adhesions in the pleural space. This may or may not be accompanied by mediastinal shift. If mediastinal shift occurs or if there is depression of the hemidiaphragm with displacement of the heart and trachea away from the side with the pneumothorax, your patient has a potentially lethal condition known as a tension pneumothorax (Fig. 3–69).

Occasionally, a pneumothorax occurs when pleural fluid is present. This gives a rather characteristic, straight horizontal line as a result of the air-fluid level in the pleural space. This is termed a hydropneumothorax. Whenever you see a very straight horizontal line that extends to the chest wall, you should be thinking about

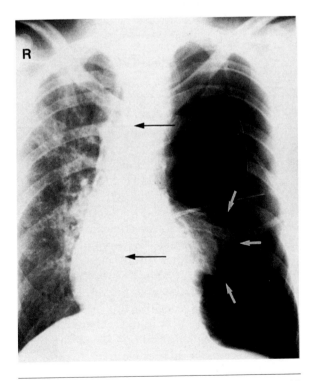

FIGURE 3–69. **Tension pneumothorax.** On this PA chest radiograph, the left hemithorax is very dark or lucent because the left lung has collapsed completely *(white arrows)*. The tension pneumothorax can be identified by the fact that the mediastinal contents, including the heart, are shifted toward the right, and the left hemidiaphragm is flattened and depressed.

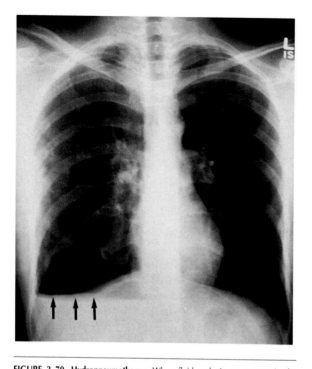

FIGURE 3–70. Hydropneumothorax. When fluid and air are present in the pleural space, on an upright chest x-ray there will be a perfectly straight horizontal line that extends all the way from the spine to the edge of the pleural cavity. In this patient, a loculated right basilar hydropneumothorax is present. The air-fluid interface is easily seen *(arrows)*. If this were a lung abscess, it would be very unlikely that the air-fluid level would extend all the way from the medial to the lateral aspect of the hemithorax.

a hydropneumothorax (Fig. 3–70). Occasionally, you will see an air-fluid level within a lung as a result of an abscess, but this almost always is surrounded by a thick wall and should be easy to distinguish from a hydropneumothorax.

Quite commonly, a skin fold may cause an artifact that looks very much like a pneumothorax. This artifact is caused by the patient's skin being folded over and pressed against the x-ray film cassette. The artifact is seen most often in patients who are either supine or semi-erect. It usually appears as an almost vertical line along the outer third of the upper lung zones. You need to be able to recognize this artifact; otherwise, you will end up putting a chest tube in a patient who does not need one. There are three ways to recognize this artifact: (1) A skin-fold line often extends above the lung apex into the supraclavicular soft tissues. (2) An increasing density or whiteness may become apparent as you look from the hilum toward the periphery of the lung, just before you reach the line that

you think may be a pneumothorax. If there is increasing density (whiteness) as you proceed laterally, followed by sudden decrease in density, this probably represents a skin fold (Fig. 3–71). In the case of a small pneumothorax, both the lung and the pneumothorax are quite dark, and they are separated by a thin white line, which is the visceral pleura. (3) A skin fold line often is relatively straight whereas a pleural line follows the curve of the inner aspect of the chest wall.

Since air tends to go to the highest position that it can find in the pleural space, it can be difficult to appreciate a small or even a moderate-sized pneumothorax on a frontal chest x-ray of a patient who is supine. With a supine AP chest projection, the x-ray beam is vertical and the pneumothorax is layered horizontally along the anterior portion of the chest and probably at least 500 cc of air needs to be in the pleural space. In supine infants and neonates, an anterior pneumothorax is common. Often the only way to see this pneumothorax is to obtain a supine lateral film and look for lucency (or a dark area) in the retrosternal region.

On the supine AP chest radiograph in the adult, one of the most reliable signs of a pneu-

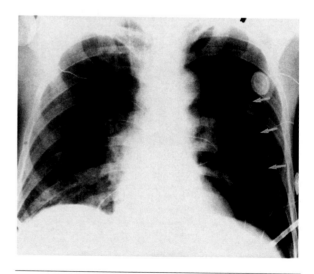

FIGURE 3–71. Skin fold simulating a pneumothorax. A near-vertical line is seen projecting over the left hemithorax *(arrows)*. This is a fold of skin caused by the patient pressing up against the film cassette. A skin fold can be differentiated by noting if it extends outside the normal lung area, by seeing pulmonary vessels beyond this line, or, as in this case, by noting that the lung is increasing in density or getting whiter from the hilum out to this line, then becoming darker. A pneumothorax will be seen as a white line that is dark on both sides.

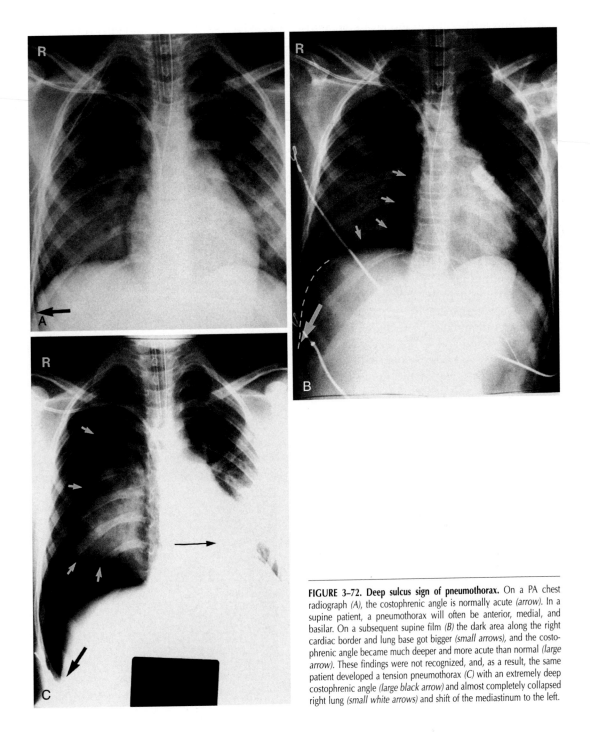

FIGURE 3–72. Deep sulcus sign of pneumothorax. On a PA chest radiograph *(A)*, the costophrenic angle is normally acute *(arrow)*. In a supine patient, a pneumothorax will often be anterior, medial, and basilar. On a subsequent supine film *(B)* the dark area along the right cardiac border and lung base got bigger *(small arrows)*, and the costophrenic angle became much deeper and more acute than normal *(large arrow)*. These findings were not recognized, and, as a result, the same patient developed a tension pneumothorax *(C)* with an extremely deep costophrenic angle *(large black arrow)* and almost completely collapsed right lung *(small white arrows)* and shift of the mediastinum to the left.

mothorax is what is known as the deep sulcus sign. Normally, the lateral costophrenic angles are quite sharp or acute. The pleural space, however, goes much farther down along the edge of the lateral aspect of the liver and spleen than most people think. If air is in the pleural space, it can easily track down, making the costophrenic angle or sulcus much deeper and the angle much more acute than is normally seen. Thus, you should be very careful to look for an extremely sharp or deep costophrenic angle or a costophrenic angle that becomes progressively deeper and sharper on sequential supine chest x-rays. If you see this, a pneumothorax is probably present (Fig. 3–72). If you can sit the patient upright and take another chest radiograph, you will often see an apical pneumothorax, since the air typically will move from the sulcus up to the apex.

Most of the findings that we have discussed describe the situation in which the air in the pleural space can move freely. In patients who have had prior inflammatory processes and adhesions in the pleural space, the air may not be able to move freely, and there may be a loculated pneumothorax. These can be difficult to appreciate, but if you see a dark area of lucency either around the edge of the lung or along the cardiac border, you should consider the possibility of a loculated pneumothorax (Fig. 3–72B).

A number of issues arise with regard to appropriate clinical management of a pneumothorax. Often, clinicians want to know how big the pneumothorax is. A few radiologists will give the volume in terms of percentage, although this is very inaccurate. Personally, I refer to them as small, medium, large, and tension pneumothoraces. Experiments have been done on cadavers indicating that, on an upright film, if 50 cc of air has been placed in the pleural space, the apex of the lung will have dropped approximately to the level between the second and third posterior ribs. One centimeter of space lateral to the lung constitutes about a 10 per cent pneumothorax. One inch of space between the lateral chest wall and the lung margin is about a 30 per cent pneumothorax.

After a chest tube has been placed, you should note not only the size of residual pneumothorax and the position of the tip but also the side port of the chest tube, if it has one. This

is seen as a discontinuity of the opaque line in the catheter; it should be projecting inside the chest cavity and not sitting out in the soft tissues (see Fig. 3–27B). When a chest tube is properly placed, connected to a vacuum, and unobstructed, if there is persistence of the pneumothorax you should consider the possibility of a bronchopleural fistula. This usually is a result of blunt trauma with a tear in the region of a major bronchus. Other possibilities are a loculated pneumothorax or an anterior pneumothorax (with a posteriorly placed chest tube and the patient supine).

After a lung has been fully re-expanded and the chest tube remains in place, there is some slight compressive atelectasis of the lung that abuts the chest tube. As a result, for a day or so

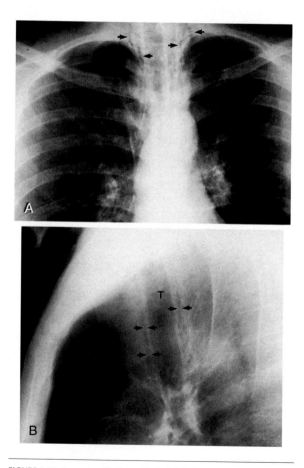

FIGURE 3–73. Pneumomediastinum. Vertical dark (lucent) lines representing air within the mediastinum are usually seen at or above the level of the aortic arch. On the PA view *(A)* these can be seen extending up into the lower cervical soft tissues. On the lateral view *(B)*, dark linear air collections can be seen in front of and behind the trachea (T).

after the chest tube is withdrawn, you can see a linear track where the chest tube had been. This is normal, and it will resolve spontaneously in a day or so.

Pneumomediastinum. Air within the mediastinum often (although not always) is associated with a pneumothorax. With a pneumomediastinum, there are air collections within the upper portion of the mediastinum and lower neck that are typically vertical. On the lateral view, you can sometimes see air in front of or behind the trachea (Fig. 3–73). A pneumomediastinum can be the result of a tracheobronchial tear. This entity carries up to a 50 per cent mortality rate if not treated. You should suspect pneumomediastinum in a post-traumatic patient who has an abnormal air collection in the chest that does not resolve with placement of a chest tube.

Sometimes, people have difficulty distinguishing between a pneumomediastinum and a pneumopericardium. Pneumopericardium in an adult is very rare, typically resulting from a stab wound. You should remember that the pericardium envelops the heart and reaches only as high as the level of the hila. It does not extend around the hila or over the ascending aorta. Thus, in a pneumopericardium, air should be confined to the margins of the major chambers of the heart and not higher.

Subcutaneous Emphysema. Air in the soft tissues of the chest wall is often caused by blunt trauma with a pneumothorax and some broken ribs or by penetration as with a stab wound or placement of a chest tube. Air in the soft tissues is seen as dark linear or ovoid areas. Subcutaneous emphysema can extend into the supraclavicular and lower cervical regions. When this happens, however, you should make very sure that you are seeing subcutaneous emphysema and not a pneumomediastinum that has extended up into the lower cervical area. When subcutaneous emphysema is extensive, it can dissect into the pectoral muscles, producing a bizarre fan-shaped appearance of the air as it outlines the muscle fibers (Fig. 3–74).

Pleural Effusions. The appearance of pleural effusions or other fluid collections depends upon

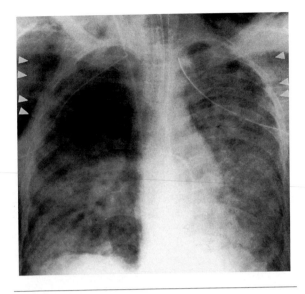

FIGURE 3–74. Subcutaneous emphysema. Air is seen along the lateral soft tissues of the chest outside the rib cage dissecting into the pectoral muscles creating fan-shaped dark lines over the upper chest (*arrowheads*).

their size and location. Pleural effusions usually are at least 100 cc if they are seen on a routine upright chest x-ray. The most typical location of an effusion is in the dependent portions of the pleural space; therefore, they are seen best on upright chest radiographs. There will be blunting of the lateral costophrenic angles identified on the anterior or posterior chest radiograph and blunting of the posterior costophrenic angle seen on the lateral view. Somewhat larger effusions may extend into the inferior aspect of the major fissure (Fig. 3–75) and very large effusions displace and compress lung tissue.

The appearances of larger effusions vary according to the position of the patient when the x-ray was obtained. On the upright chest x-ray, there is increasing basilar density (whiteness) and loss of the normal lung/hemidiaphragm interface (Fig. 3–76A). It can be difficult to figure out whether you are looking at a large or moderate-sized basilar pleural effusion or a basilar alveolar infiltrate. If the patient was supine when the x-ray was obtained, the effusion typically will be layered out horizontally in the posterior pleural space. Since the x-ray beam is vertical for a supine chest x-ray, all you may see is a relatively increased density or whiteness of

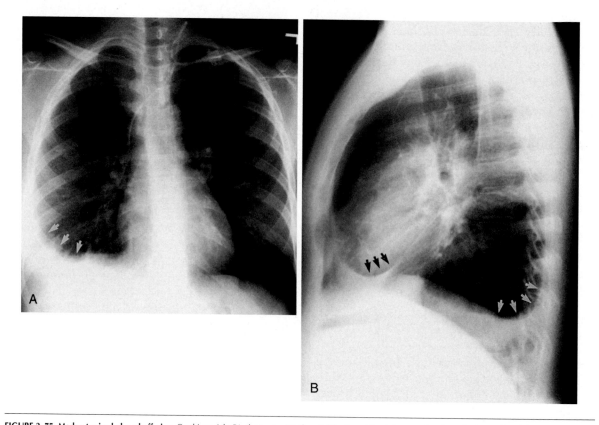

FIGURE 3–75. Moderate-sized pleural effusion. On this upright PA chest x-ray *(A)*, there is blunting of the right costophrenic angle due to pleural fluid. On the lateral view *(B)*, fluid can be seen tracking up into the major fissure *(black arrows)*, and there is blunting of the right posterior costophrenic angle *(white arrows)*.

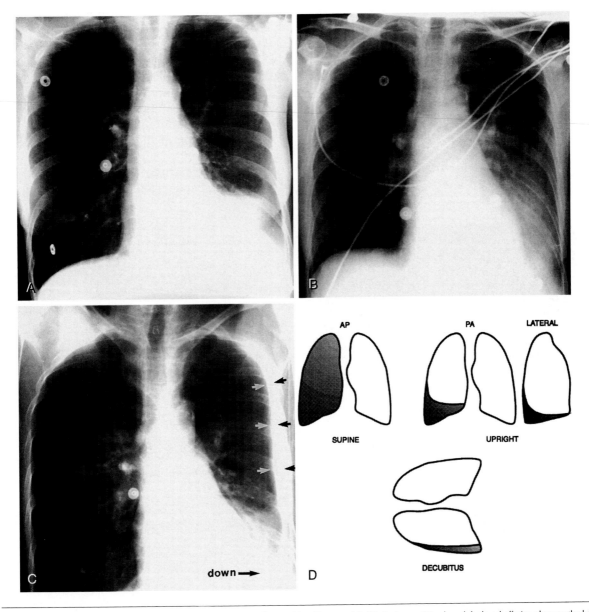

FIGURE 3–76. The appearance of pleural effusions depending upon patient position. On an upright PA chest x-ray *(A)*, a large left pleural effusion obscures the left hemidiaphragm, the left costophrenic angle, and the left cardiac border. On a supine AP view *(B)*, the fluid runs posteriorly, causing a diffuse opacity over the lower two thirds of the left lung; the left hemidiaphragm remains obscured. This can easily mimic left lower lobe infiltrate or left lower lobe atelectasis. With a left lateral decubitus view *(C)*, the left side of the patient is dependent, and the pleural effusion can be seen to be free-moving and layering *(arrows)* along the lateral chest wall. These findings are shown diagrammatically as well for a right pleural effusion *(D)*.

the affected hemithorax as compared with the normal side (Fig. 3–76B). In cases of doubt or to determine if a pleural fluid collection is free-moving, you can obtain a decubitus chest x-ray. If you suspect that there is an effusion on the right, you should order a right lateral decubitus view, that is, with the right side down when the x-ray is taken (Fig. 3–76C).

Pleural effusions have two other appearances sufficiently common that you should be aware of them. The first is a subpulmonic pleural effusion. In my experience, this is more common on the right side. The tip-off to its existence is when you think that the hemidiaphragm on the right is slightly higher than normal, with the highest portion of the dome more lateral than usual. The highest portion of the dome of the right hemidiaphragm is normally in the mid-clavicular line or slightly medial to this. If the highest portion is lateral, you should suspect a subpulmonic effusion (Fig. 3–77).

A loculated pleural effusion located within a fissure may be mistaken for an intrapulmonary lesion (a pseudotumor). On careful examination, loculated effusions in a fissure are typically lenticular or oval (not round) and are located in the expected position of the major or minor fissure (Fig. 3–78).

Chest x-rays cannot be used to differentiate between a transudate and an exudate. The cause

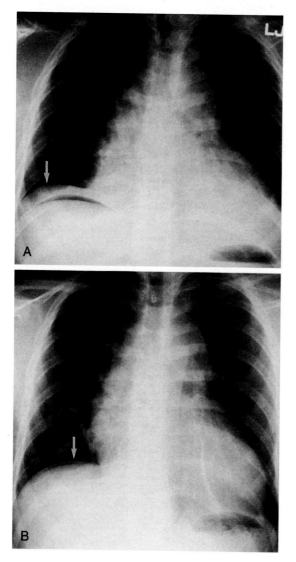

FIGURE 3–77. **Subpulmonic effusion.** The only finding of a subpulmonic effusion on an upright chest film may be that what looks like the superior aspect of the right hemidiaphragm is quite lateral (A). The actual hemidiaphragm can be seen here because this patient has a pneumoperitoneum, or free air, underneath the hemidiaphragm. The normal thickness of the hemidiaphragm and its position can be seen in a patient with a pneumoperitoneum, who does not have a subpulmonic effusion (B).

FIGURE 3–78. **Loculated pleural effusions.** Occasionally, pleural effusions may become loculated in the fissures. These can be seen on the PA view *(A)* as well as on the lateral chest x-ray *(B).* These are lenticular, with a long axis oriented along either the major or the minor fissure.

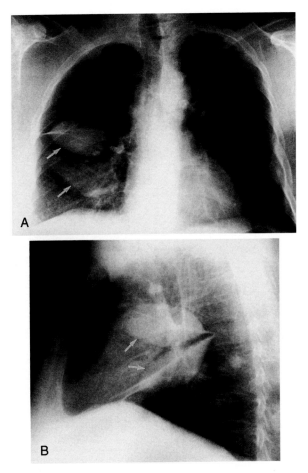

of an effusion, however, can sometimes be inferred. Massive effusions are usually malignant in origin. Pancreatitis is associated with left-sided effusions, whereas cirrhosis is associated with right-sided effusions. Most cardiogenic effusions are bilateral and are associated with cardiomegaly and other signs of congestive failure. About 40 per cent of pneumonias are associated with a small effusion. When there is a moderate or large pleural fluid collection with a pneumonia, an empyema or malignancy should be suspected.

Empyemas. An empyema is pus within the pleural space. It is the result of a postinfectious process 60 per cent of the time, being postsurgical (20 per cent) or post-traumatic (20 per cent) the rest of the time. On a chest radiograph, an empyema may look very much like a pleural effusion or pleural thickening, but it does not move freely and will not layer on a decubitus

chest x-ray. The process is often elliptical, with the long axis along the lateral chest wall, and the lung will be compressed or displaced. Empyemas often are loculated and have septa. A CT scan is the easiest way to visualize empyemas and locate them for potential drainage (Fig. 3–79). Occasionally an empyema may contain gas or air. If this is the case, the air-fluid level is often a different length on the frontal and lateral chest x-rays. The gas is most commonly the result of a bronchopleural fistula and much less frequently due to gas-forming bacteria or a prior thoracentesis.

Pleural Calcification and Pleural Masses. Most pleural calcifications are the result of an old calcified empyema or asbestosis. Calcification from an empyema is almost always unilateral and can be quite dense, whereas after asbestos exposure, calcification is often bilateral and not quite as dense (Fig. 3–80). Asbestosis also can

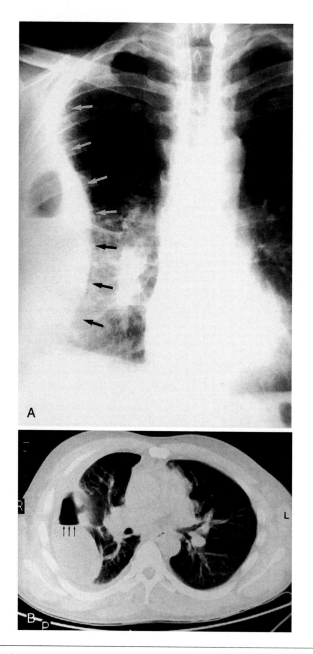

FIGURE 3–79. Empyema. On an upright chest x-ray *(A)*, a lenticular density is seen along the lateral chest wall. An air-fluid level is also seen within this. A transverse CT scan *(B)* also demonstrates the air-fluid level *(arrows)* and shows that the epicenter of the lesion is between the lung and the rib cage, distinguishing this lesion from a lung abscess.

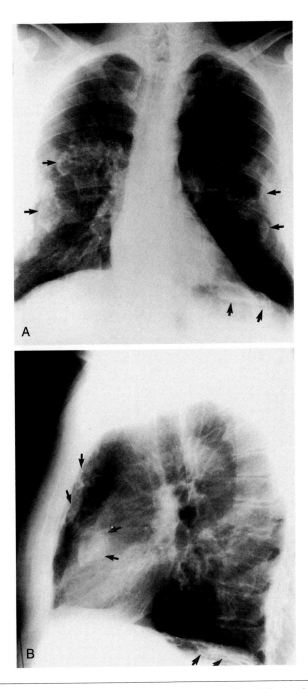

FIGURE 3–80. Asbestosis. Both the PA chest x-ray *(A)* and the lateral view *(B)* show areas of plaquelike calcification along the pleura and the hemidiaphragms *(arrows)*. Pleural lesions often appear to project within the lung parenchyma.

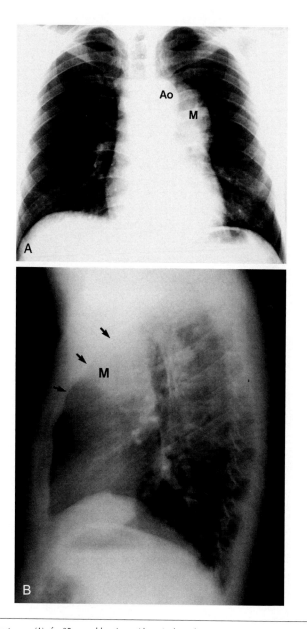

FIGURE 3–81. Seminoma. On the PA chest x-ray *(A)* of a 25-year-old patient with testicular enlargement, a mass can be clearly seen (M). Note that you can still see the outline of the aortic arch (Ao), indicating that this mass must be either in front of or behind the aortic arch but not next to it. A lateral view *(B)* shows an anterior mediastinal mass, in this case metastatic seminoma.

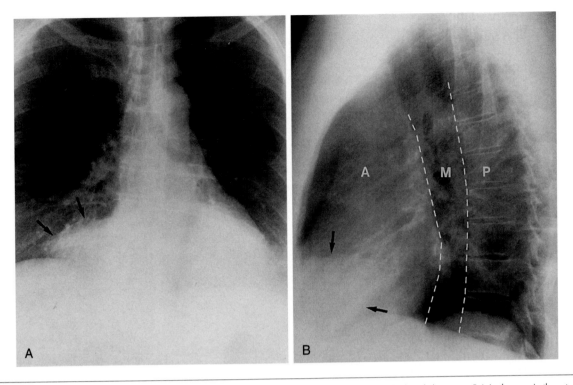

FIGURE 3–82. Pericardial fat pad. *(A),* A soft tissue mass *(arrows)* is seen in the right cardiophrenic angle on the frontal chest x-ray. *B,* It is also seen in the anterior mediastinum on the lateral view. On this view the anterior (A), middle (M), and posterior (P) portions of the mediastinum have been identified.

produce an interstitial or reticulonodular pulmonary parenchymal pattern and occasionally a "shaggy-looking" heart. Mesotheliomas occur after asbestos exposure, and a focal pleural mass or thickening should raise your suspicion of this tumor. You should remember, however, that the most common tumor after asbestos exposure is a lung cancer and not a mesothelioma.

MEDIASTINAL LESIONS

A large number of diseases present in the mediastinum and are seen on the anterior chest radiograph as a widening or bulge in the central soft tissues of the chest. The differential diagnosis will change depending on the location of the lesion in the mediastinum. You need to determine whether the problem is in the anterior, middle, or posterior mediastinum. The "silhouette sign" can be helpful in determining the site of a pathologic process. Normally you can see the border of a soft tissue object (such as the

aorta or heart) in the chest because it is bounded by air. If there is a pathologic soft tissue mass in contiguity with a normal structure, the air interface will be lost. For example, if you are looking at a frontal chest x-ray and a lesion is on the left upper medinstinum and if the descending aorta (in the posterior mediastinum) and the left pulmonary artery (in the middle mediastinum) are seen well, you are probably dealing with an anterior mediastinal lesion.

Probably the next and simplest way to localize the lesion is to look at the lateral chest x-ray. There are several classification schemes of the portions of the mediastinum and its contents. I use anterior, middle, and posterior but some authors include a superior portion. There is also a difference as to whether the heart is in the anterior or middle mediastinum. I put it in the anterior portion. If there is filling-in of the space behind the top of the sternum and the ascending aorta, you are most likely dealing with an anterior mediastinal lesion. There are basically four types of lesions that tend to occur in the anterior mediastinum; these are subster-

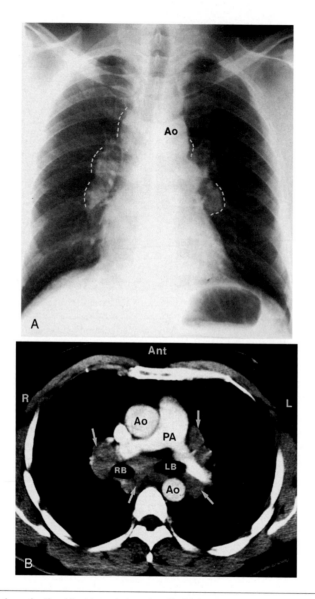

FIGURE 3–83. Sarcoid. Marked lymphadenopathy *(dotted lines)* is seen in the region of both hila in the right paratracheal region *(A)*. The transverse contrast-enhanced CT scan of the upper chest *(B)* clearly shows the ascending and descending aorta (Ao) as well as the pulmonary artery (PA) and superior vena cava. The right and left mainstem bronchus area is also seen. The arrows indicate the extensive lymphadenopathy. (See also Figure 3–54 for the alveolar form of sarcoid.)

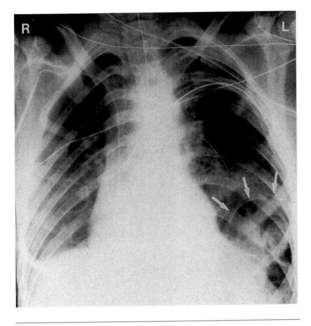

FIGURE 3–84. Diaphragmatic rupture. Six days after an auto accident, bowel loops can be seen in the left lower chest *(arrows)*. Diaphragmatic rupture is more common on the left than on the right.

nal thyroid gland, thymic lesions, germ cell tumors (much more common in males) (Fig. 3–81), and lymphoma. Occasionally, retrosternal and internal mammary lymph nodes can become enlarged from metastases of breast cancer, or from leukemia. Students can remember most of the anterior mediastinal lesions by using the four "T"s. This stands for *t*hymoma, *t*hyroid lesions, *t*eratoma, and *t* cell lymphomas. A benign normal variant that you should be aware of is the pericardial fat pad (Fig. 3–82). This almost always is found at the right cardiophrenic angle.

Lesions in the middle mediastinum include thoracic aortic aneurysms, hematomas, neoplasms, adenopathy (Fig. 3–83), esophageal lesions, diaphragmatic hernias (hiatal or Morgagni type), and duplication cysts. Morgagni hernias tend to be on the right side. Any middle mediastinal lesion associated with the aorta should be considered an aneurysm until proven otherwise.

Posterior mediastinal lesions are seen on the lateral view projecting over the spine and are also paraspinous on the frontal chest x-ray. Most (90 per cent) posterior mediastinal lesions are neurogenic. They may represent neuroblastomas in young children but in adults are more likely to be neurofibromas, schwannomas, or ganglioneuromas. Other posterior mediastinal lesions include hernias (hiatal or Bochdalek type), neoplasms, hematomas, or extramedullary hematopoiesis. Bochdalek hernias are most often on the left side.

DIAPHRAGM

Diaphragmatic Rupture. Rupture of the diaphragm may occur following blunt trauma. The diaphragm most frequently is ruptured on the left side, perhaps because the liver may dissipate some of the force of an abdominal blow, lessening the likelihood of rupture of the right hemidiaphragm. The most common appearance is loops of bowel protruding into the lower chest cavity without the normal dome-shaped structure of the hemidiaphragm (Fig. 3–84). The manifestations of a ruptured diaphragm can be delayed, and sometimes the bowel herniates through the diaphragm only 1 or 2 weeks after the initial accident. The patient may remain asymptomatic for months or years.

Suggested Reading

Fraser RG, Paré J, Paré PD, et al: Diagnosis of Diseases of the Chest, 3rd ed. Philadelphia, WB Saunders, 1989.

Chapter 4
Breast Imaging

Breast imaging generally refers to mammography. There are a number of other methods that have been generally discredited (such as thermography). Ultrasound can be a useful adjunctive method but should not be relied upon as a screening method for breast cancer.

Mammography is complementary to physical examination. Each method can detect a significant number of tumors that are not found by the other. The primary purpose of mammography is to detect small breast cancers and, by so doing, to improve survival. In young women, the breast is extremely dense; the density of the parenchymal tissue is the same as the density of a carcinoma. In young women, not only is the incidence of breast cancer low, but it is also very difficult to tell whether a cancer is present amid the normal dense tissue. As women age, there is fatty infiltration of the breast and atrophy of the parenchyma. Since the fat is lucent (dark) on a mammogram and a cancer is dense (white), tumors are more easily visualized as a woman gets older. The density of the breast is partly due to hormonal stimulation. Following replacement estrogen therapy in older women, the density of the breast tissue increases, making tumors more difficult to see (Fig. 4–1).

There often is great variation in the appearance of the breast tissue between women. Fortunately, most women have very symmetric tissue when one breast is compared with the other. Any asymmetries in density should be examined carefully, since they may represent a cancer (Fig. 4–2). In addition to asymmetric masses, another sign of breast cancer is very tiny grouped calcifications. Often called microcalcifications, these are usually very fine (about 1 mm or less) and sandlike and sometimes can be seen to have a branching structure. Most women, as they age, have calcifications within the breast that are benign. These are usually rounded calcifications greater than 2 mm in diameter (Fig. 4–3). In women over the age of 60 years, serpiginous calcifications can normally be seen within blood vessel walls. There are associated indirect signs of malignancy that you should also look for. These include focal skin thickening or dimpling due to an underlying tumor, unilateral nipple retraction, and vascular asymmetry (increased vascularity due to the tumor).

Mammograms are usually obtained in what are referred to as the craniocaudal (top to bottom) and axillary oblique views. The latter, a somewhat tilted lateral view, allows better visualization of the tail of the breast tissue as it

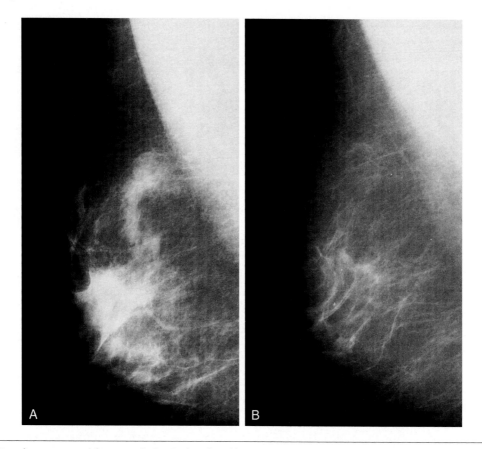

FIGURE 4–1. Normal mammogram and the process of aging. On the axillary oblique view of the right breast *(A)*, the normal breast parenchyma is seen as ill-defined white densities, predominantly located behind the nipple. In young women, the breast tissue can be extremely dense with only a small amount of interspersed fat, making tumors hard to see. Another mammogram *(B)* on the same patient several years later shows fatty replacement of most of the breast tissue. The breast tissue can become dense again if the woman is placed on estrogen therapy.

extends out toward the axilla than is possible on a straight lateral view. On the craniocaudal view, it is often not easy to tell which is the medial and which is the lateral aspect; by convention, the identifying markers or technologist's initials are placed along the lateral edge of the breast.

Once a suspicious lesion is identified on both craniocaudal and axillary oblique views, further investigation usually ensues, in the form of a magnified mammogram, an ultrasound examination, or a biopsy. Ultrasound of the breast should not be considered to be a screening tool, since it cannot differentiate carcinomas from fibroadenomas or other benign solid lesions. It is useful only to differentiate solid lesions from a cyst. If a lesion is solid, asymmetric, or stellate or if there are grouped microcalcifications, an intensive search should be undertaken for prior

mammograms that can be used for comparison. The reason for this is that a surgical biopsy will necessarily result in scar tissue, and scar tissue often leaves an asymmetric radial density that can look like a neoplasm; hence you should obtain biopsies only when necessary. If the solid lesion is new or if old films are not available and the lesion is thought to be suspicious, a biopsy is recommended. If the lesion is palpable, the surgeon may simply proceed.

If the suspicious lesion is not palpable, a procedure called needle localization can be performed by the radiologist. In this procedure the breast is compressed with a holder that has coordinates on the sides, and a mammogram is taken. A thin needle can then be inserted at the coordinates of interest until it is shown that the end of the needle is either at or slightly past the lesion. At this point, a small amount of blue dye

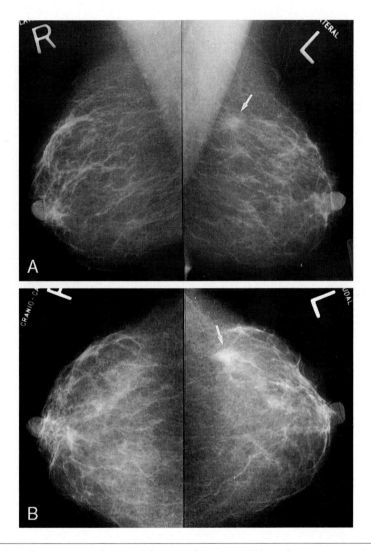

FIGURE 4–2. Breast cancer. Axillary oblique views *(A)* and craniocaudal views *(B)* of the right and left breast show an asymmetric density *(arrows)* in the upper outer aspect of the left breast. Any asymmetric density should raise suspicion of a neoplasm.

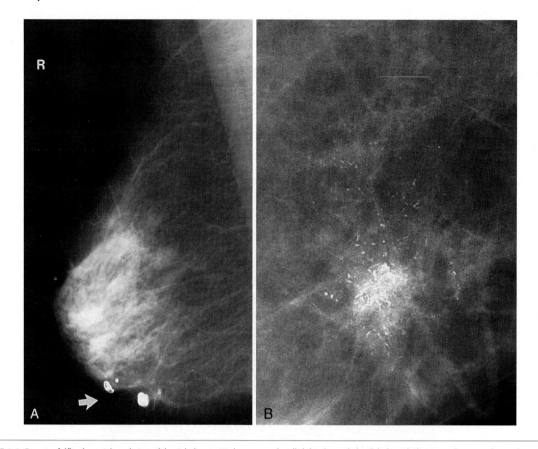

FIGURE 4–3. Breast calcifications. A lateral view of the right breast *(A)* shows several well-defined rounded or lobular calcifications. These are almost always benign. Malignant calcifications *(B)* tend to be very small, sandlike, and clustered as seen in this very enlarged view from a mammogram in a different patient with breast cancer.

is injected and a thin hooked wire is passed through the needle. As the wire exits the point of the needle, it opens and becomes fixed in the tissue. The needle is withdrawn, leaving the wire in place. The surgeon then removes the tissue near the end of the hooked wire (Fig. 4–4). The biopsy specimen is x-rayed to make sure that the lesion of interest has been removed.

There has been great discussion over the last decade as to the indications for screening mammography. Concerns about overutilization revolve about financial issues as well as the

potential of radiation-induced breast carcinoma several decades later. Most screening guidelines currently utilized for non–high risk women call for annual screening over the age of 50 years and a baseline mammogram at age 40. There is controversy about the utility of screening between the ages of 40 and 50 years; at present a number of guidelines produced by different groups suggest biannual screening during this period.

The radiation cancer studies (such as those done for follow-up of atomic bomb survivors at Hiroshima and Nagasaki) show that the risk of

FIGURE 4–4. Localization and biopsy of a breast cancer. A group of suspicious calcifications *(arrows)* is seen on a craniocaudal view of the left breast *(A)*. Needle localization is first performed by repeating the mammogram in the same projection but with an overlying grid that has coordinates *(B)*. A needle is then inserted straight down at the appropriate coordinates. A lateral view of the breast is obtained, and when it is clear that the tip of the needle is in the right location, a hooked wire is inserted through the needle, and the needle is withdrawn *(C)*. The patient is then taken to the operating room, and the specimen of concern at the end of the wire is removed. A magnified specimen radiograph is then obtained *(D)* to ensure that the suspicious calcifications have been removed.

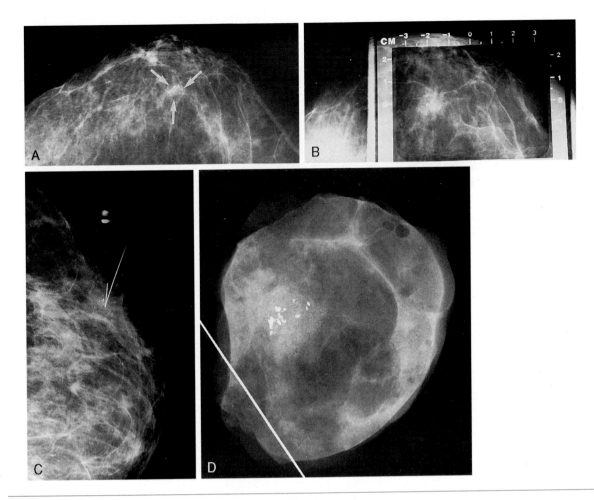

FIGURE 4–4 *See legend on opposite page*

FIGURE 4–5. **Calcification around the breast prosthesis.** On the chest x-ray, a rim of calcification *(arrows)* can occasionally be seen around a breast prosthesis.

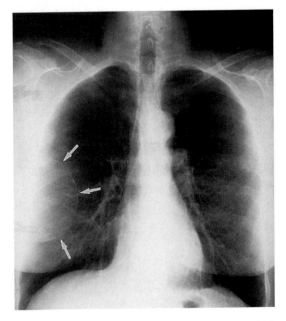

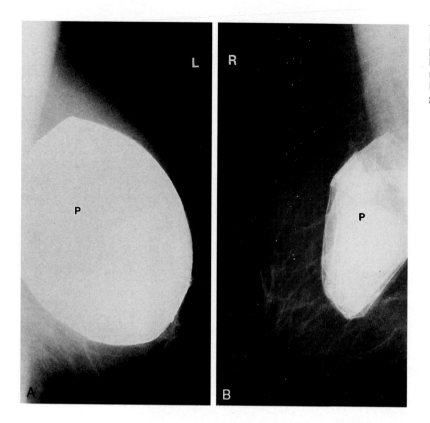

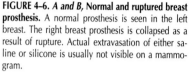

FIGURE 4–6. *A and B,* Normal and ruptured breast prosthesis. A normal prosthesis is seen in the left breast. The right breast prosthesis is collapsed as a result of rupture. Actual extravasation of either saline or silicone is usually not visible on a mammogram.

breast cancer after radiation exposure is greatest when exposure occurs at a young age. There is little, if any, risk from mammograms performed after the age of 45 years. Present guidelines vary as to whether to perform an annual, a semiannual, or only a baseline study in women 40 to 50 years of age. My personal opinion is that biannual examinations may be warranted in this age group and that a baseline study is certainly useful. You should always remember that screening mammography is not a substitute for monthly breast examination by the woman herself. CT scanning is not indicated for examination of the breast, and the role of MRI and nuclear medicine for evaluation or screening for breast cancer remains in the realm or research.

Mammograms can be used in the evaluation of a breast prosthesis. Normally, the prosthesis can be seen as an oval area of increased density in the central portion of the breast. Complications that arise include calcification, which can occur around the prosthesis, and this actually is sometimes visualized on chest radiographs (Fig. 4–5). Leakage of a prosthesis can be identified if the leakage has been enough to cause deflation of the prosthesis (Fig. 4–6). Leaking silicone or saline cannot be visualized directly on a mammogram. Screening mammography for occult breast carcinomas can be quite difficult in patients with prostheses, since the prosthesis can obscure a small cancer.

General Suggested Reading

Kopans D: Breast Imaging. Philadelphia, JB Lippincott, 1989.

Chapter 5

Cardiovascular System

NORMAL ANATOMY AND IMAGING TECHNIQUES

The normal anatomy and configuration of the heart on a chest x-ray and on CT scanning were discussed in Chapter 3. Imaging of the heart can also be done utilizing magnetic resonance imaging (MRI). This modality, although expensive, gives quite good visualization of the cardiac anatomy. The lungs are not well seen on these scans owing to respiratory motion that causes image degradation. The anatomy of the heart at several different levels on an MR scan is shown in Figure 5–1. Both MR and nuclear medicine images can be gated to the cardiac cycle, allowing images to be produced in systole and diastole as well as the phases in between (Fig. 5–2). Transthoracic ultrasound can also be used to image through those portions of the heart that are in contact with the chest wall. This method is generally considered the practice of cardiologists and will be discussed here only when it is the appropriate test to order.

EVALUATION OF THE CARDIAC SILHOUETTE

Generalized Cardiomegaly

Examination of the shape of the heart on a chest x-ray can sometimes provide clues to the type of cardiac disease present. If the heart appears large in most dimensions, it is often difficult to tell whether you are dealing with multichamber enlargement, a myocardiopathy, or a pericardial effusion. If there is acute marked enlargement of the cardiac silhouette (within several days or weeks), the most likely diagnosis is a pericardial effusion. Under these circumstances the heart has a very pendulous appearance and is much wider at the base. This is often referred to as a "water bag" appearance (Fig. 5–3). The causes of a pericardial effusion include autoimmune disease, uremia, congestive failure, postsurgical changes, acute myocardial infarction, viral infections, and metastatic tumor. Pericardial effusions must be greater than 250 ml in order to be detectable radiographically. Effusions are some-

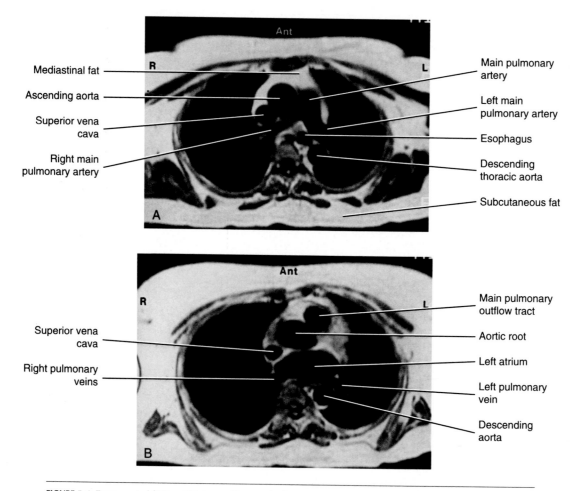

FIGURE 5–1. Transverse (axial) T1 weighted magnetic resonance images *A* to *D* of the thorax in the transverse plane showing normal vascular anatomy.

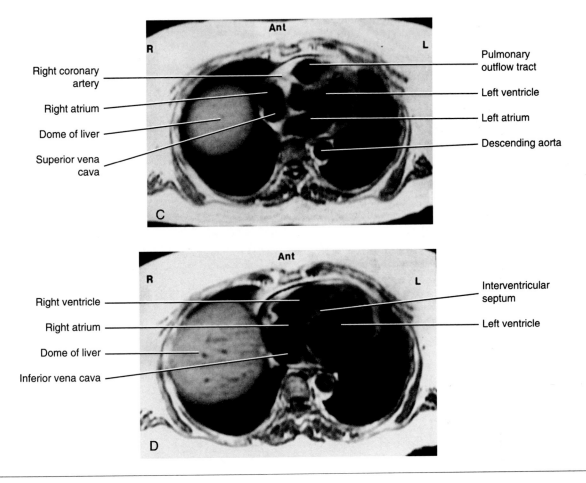

Ant

R   L

Right coronary artery

Right atrium

Dome of liver

Superior vena cava

Pulmonary outflow tract

Left ventricle

Left atrium

Descending aorta

C

Ant

R   L

Right ventricle

Right atrium

Dome of liver

Inferior vena cava

Interventricular septum

Left ventricle

D

FIGURE 5–1 *Continued*

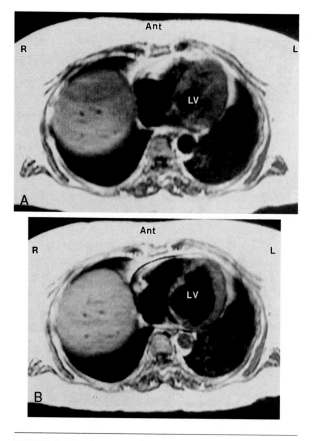

FIGURE 5–2. Magnetic resonance images of the heart in systole and diastole. Transverse images obtained at the level of the right and left ventricle show the left ventricle in systole (A) and in diastole (B).

tive contraction during systole and most commonly result from infections and metabolic disorders. They may also be caused by collagen vascular disease and toxic agents such as alcohol and chemotherapeutic drugs. An example of the latter is doxorubicin, one of the most widely used chemotherapeutic agents (Fig. 5–4).

Since assessment of cardiac function by

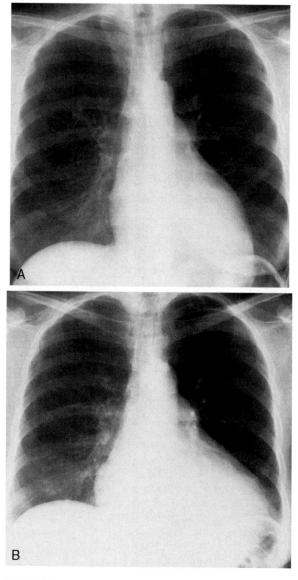

FIGURE 5–3. Pericardial effusion. In a patient with a viral syndrome, a PA chest x-ray (A) shows mild cardiomegaly with prominence of the left cardiac border. One week later (B), there has been a marked and sudden increase in the transverse diameter of the heart due to a pericardial effusion. A definitive diagnosis is best made by utilizing cardiac ultrasound.

times visible on CT scans of the chest, but if you suspect a pericardial effusion, the imaging procedure of choice is echocardiography.

Constrictive pericarditis is most commonly due to tuberculosis and viral and pyogenic infections. It may also occur with radiation therapy. Ninety per cent of patients with constrictive pericarditis will have pericardial calcification (which may be visible only on CT), and 60 per cent will have a pleural effusion. Of those patients with pericardial calcification, 50 per cent will also have constrictive pericarditis.

Cardiomegaly can be due to valvular disease, cardiomyopathy, congenital heart disease, pericardial effusion, and mass lesions. Cardiomyopathies and pericardial effusions both generally lead to symmetric enlargement, whereas valvular disease and congenital heart disease often have specific chamber enlargement. The dilated cardiomyopathies are caused by ineffec-

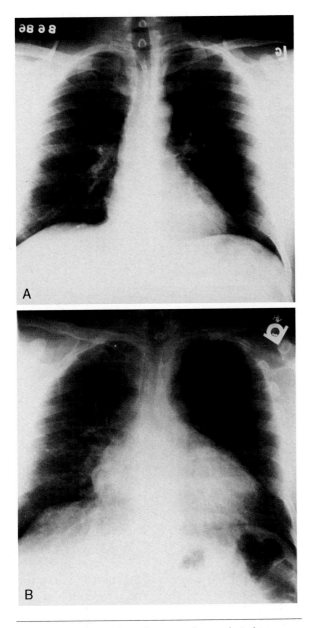

FIGURE 5–4. **Cardiomyopathy.** In this case, cardiomyopathy is due to cancer chemotherapy with doxorubicin. An initial chest x-ray *(A)* demonstrates a normal-sized heart. After several therapeutic courses of doxorubicin *(B)*, there has been marked enlargement in the cardiac silhouette due to multichamber dilatation.

struction of a time-activity curve showing the amount of activity in the left or right ventricle in both diastole and systole, allowing calculation of an ejection fraction. The normal left ventricular ejection fraction (LVEF) is between 55 and 75 per cent. In older persons, the lower limit of LVEF is probably about 50 per cent. Evaluation of the gated blood pool studies also allows computer analysis of the outline of the left ventricle in order to look for regional wall motion abnormalities (Fig. 5–5). If all that you are interested in is a regional wall motion abnormality, this can also sometimes be imaged by echocardiography.

Use of the cardiothoracic ratio to assess heart size and the effect of cardiac failure on the appearance of the pulmonary vessels and lungs was discussed in Chapter 3. The width of the heart should not exceed half the width of the chest at its widest point. This measurement is reliable only on an upright PA chest film; on an AP chest x-ray the heart will often exceed this measurement owing to magnification. On a supine film there is even more magnification and high position of the hemidiaphragms. This high position will push the heart upward and outward, making it appear wide. A note of caution should be inserted here about patients who have chronic obstructive pulmonary disease (COPD). The shape of the heart is determined by external forces and by internal factors. One factor relates to the level of the hemidiaphragms. The measurement of cardiothoracic ratio assumes that the hemidiaphragms are in normal position. With COPD the hemidiaphragms are driven inferiorly (often to the level of the posterior twelfth rib). The heart then sags and elongates. This can make an enlarged heart appear normal in size, especially if you are considering the cardiothoracic ratio. It follows, then, that if the heart appears too wide in a patient who has COPD, it is really very large.

Left Atrial Enlargement

Isolated left atrial enlargement occurs most commonly in mitral stenosis. The earliest sign is displacement of the esophagus posteriorly (Fig. 5–6*A*). Enlargement of the left atrial appendage on the PA view is the next sign to appear (Fig.

chest film is rather crude and insensitive, quantitative evaluations of cardiac ejection fraction are usually made by nuclear medicine gated blood pool (MUGA) studies. In this procedure the red cells are labeled with radioactive material, and images of the heart are obtained in a gated fashion. Computer analysis enables con-

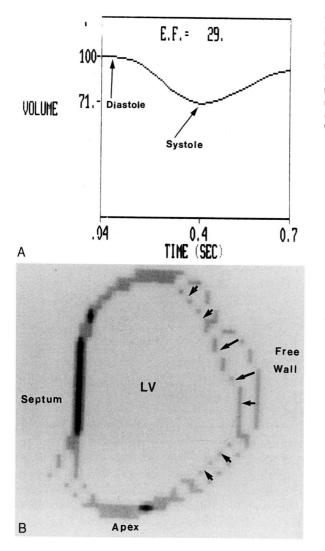

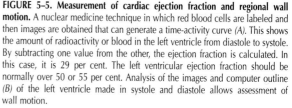

FIGURE 5–5. Measurement of cardiac ejection fraction and regional wall motion. A nuclear medicine technique in which red blood cells are labeled and then images are obtained that can generate a time-activity curve (A). This shows the amount of radioactivity or blood in the left ventricle from diastole to systole. By subtracting one value from the other, the ejection fraction is calculated. In this case, it is 29 per cent. The left ventricular ejection fraction should be normally over 50 or 55 per cent. Analysis of the images and computer outline (B) of the left ventricle made in systole and diastole allows assessment of wall motion.

5–6B). As the left atrium enlarges further the esophagus becomes more posteriorly displaced; there is splaying or widening of the inferior carinal angle; and the enlarged left atrium can be seen on the PA radiograph as a double density behind the heart and below the carina (Fig. 5–6C). The normal inferior carinal angle should not exceed 75 degrees.

Rheumatic heart disease most often affects the mitral valve and to a lesser extent the aortic valve. The classic appearance of a mitral heart on a PA chest radiograph is easily recognized by four bumps along the left cardiac border. This also is sometimes called the "ski mogul" heart. Going from superior to inferior, the bumps represent the aortic arch, pulmonary artery, left

atrium, and left ventricle (Fig. 5–6B). Left atrial enlargement also is seen with congenital cardiac lesions that have intracardiac shunts as well as in patients who have left ventricular failure.

As rheumatic heart disease progresses there is not only mitral stenosis but also development of mitral insufficiency. The heart becomes very large owing to dilatation and hypertrophy of the left ventricle. In the combined form of mitral disease, the left atrium becomes even larger than is seen in mitral stenosis alone. Typical findings are a straightening of the left cardiac border due to left atrial enlargement; left ventricular enlargement as evidenced by leftward and downward displacement of the cardiac apex; and, if left ventricular dilatation becomes mas-

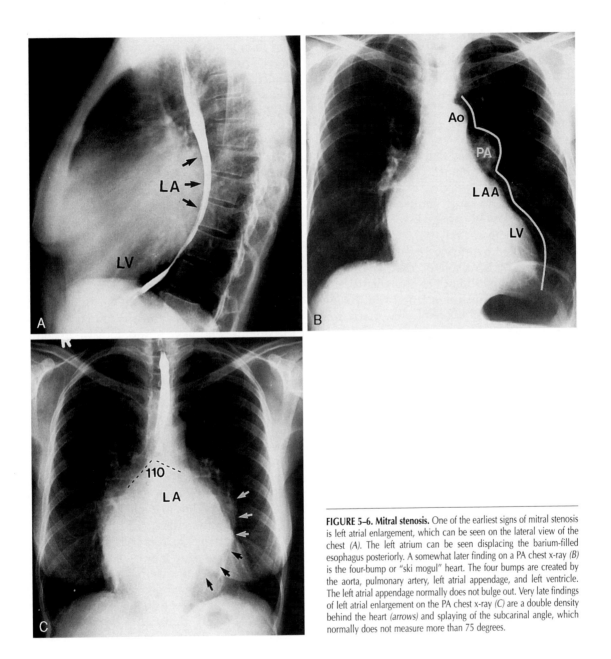

FIGURE 5–6. Mitral stenosis. One of the earliest signs of mitral stenosis is left atrial enlargement, which can be seen on the lateral view of the chest *(A)*. The left atrium can be seen displacing the barium-filled esophagus posteriorly. A somewhat later finding on a PA chest x-ray *(B)* is the four-bump or "ski mogul" heart. The four bumps are created by the aorta, pulmonary artery, left atrial appendage, and left ventricle. The left atrial appendage normally does not bulge out. Very late findings of left atrial enlargement on the PA chest x-ray *(C)* are a double density behind the heart *(arrows)* and splaying of the subcarinal angle, which normally does not measure more than 75 degrees.

sive, rightward displacement of the right ventricle. On the lateral view, in addition to the obvious left atrial enlargement, the posterior displacement of the heart continues down inferiorly, indicating left ventricular enlargement as well. In severe mitral disease, not only is the mitral valve affected but also the aortic and tricuspid valves. In general, the manifestations of the more proximal valve lesion are the most prominent. With mitral and tricuspid disease, there will be enlargement of the left atrium and left ventricle and also of the right atrium and right ventricle.

Many radiologists say that you cannot differentiate right atrial from right ventricular enlargement on a chest x-ray, and this is probably true. Fortunately, in most adults, when one of the right chambers is enlarged, so is the other. On the frontal chest x-ray, right atrial enlargement is suggested by an increased convexity of the right heart border. Isolated right ventricular enlargement is very difficult to appreciate, since it overlaps the right atrium and left ventricle on the frontal view. On the lateral view, both right ventricular and right atrial enlargement will cause a filling in of the anterior clear space behind the sternum (Fig. 5–7). Normally on the lateral view, the anterior portion of the heart fills in only approximately one third or less of the anterior clear space, unless there is enlargement of the right atrium or right ventricle.

Prosthetic tricuspid and mitral valves are often utilized in treatment of rheumatic heart disease. You should be able to recognize these valves by their size, location, and orientation (see Fig. 5–8). The valve with the largest area is the tricuspid valve; the mitral valve is intermediate sized; and the smallest is the aortic valve. You should also be able to recognize prosthetic mitral and tricuspid valves. As expected, the mitral valve is located posteriorly and to the left in the heart and the tricuspid valve is anterior and toward the right side.

Left Ventricular Enlargement

On a frontal chest radiograph, left ventricular enlargement, as already mentioned, produces a round left cardiac border as well as downward displacement of the apex. On the lateral view,

the posterior aspect of the heart, where it intersects the hemidiaphragm, is usually posteriorly displaced behind the inferior vena cava. The Hoffman-Rigler sign also can be used. To use this, find the intersection of the inferior vena cava with the hemidiaphragm on the lateral film and then measure 2 cm up and 2 cm back. If the heart projects posteriorly, there is probably left ventricular enlargement. A note of caution should be inserted here because an enlarged right heart can sometimes push the left ventricle back. To exclude this, look at the space behind the sternum—only the lower one third should be filled by soft tissue.

Left ventricular dilatation can be due to a number of causes, including coronary artery disease, aortic stenosis, and aortic regurgitation. You should take care to consider the possibility of a left ventricular aneurysm before you suggest left ventricular enlargement and quit. Ventricular aneurysms most commonly occur near the apex and anteriorly and have a high rate of mortality. Left ventricular hypertrophy is difficult to detect radiographically. It may be present in patients who have a normal cardiac configuration on chest x-ray. If this is suspected, a cardiac echo (ultrasound) is the test of choice.

Aortic Stenosis and Insufficiency

Aortic stenosis is most commonly valvular, although in a smaller number of patients it may be either subvalvular or supravalvular. Valvular stenosis can be due to rheumatic heart disease, a bicuspid (rather than tricuspid) aortic valve, or degenerative changes (usually in patients over 70 years of age). It may be difficult to detect this condition from findings on a plain film of the chest, and sometimes the only finding is a calcified aortic valve. Initially, with aortic stenosis, there is left ventricular hypertrophy. The heart will be normal in size and may show slight rounding of the cardiac apex. When left ventricular dilatation occurs, the left cardiac border elongates, and the apex of the heart moves downward toward the left hemidiaphragm. The aortic knob will be normal in size, although the ascending aortic arch is enlarged, causing a convexity of the right upper cardiac margin. The

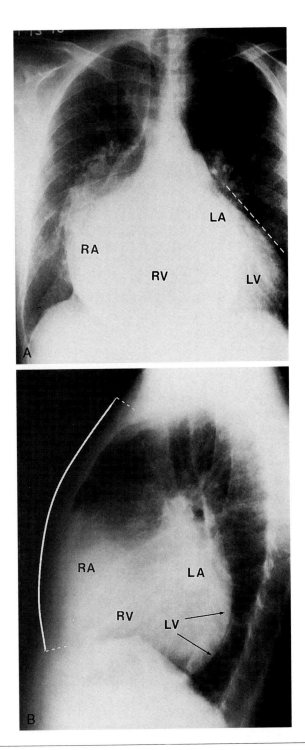

FIGURE 5–7. Mitral and tricuspid insufficiency. As a late finding in rheumatic heart disease, mitral and sometimes tricuspid insufficiency develops. On the PA chest x-ray *(A)*, there is marked enlargement of not only the left atrium but also the left ventricle (seen as straightening of the left cardiac border) as well as right-sided enlargement, particularly of the right atrium (seen by marked prominence of the right cardiac border). On the lateral view of the chest *(B)*, the left ventricle can be seen overlapping the spine, and the right atrium and right ventricle have filled in the retrosternal space to more than the usual lower one third.

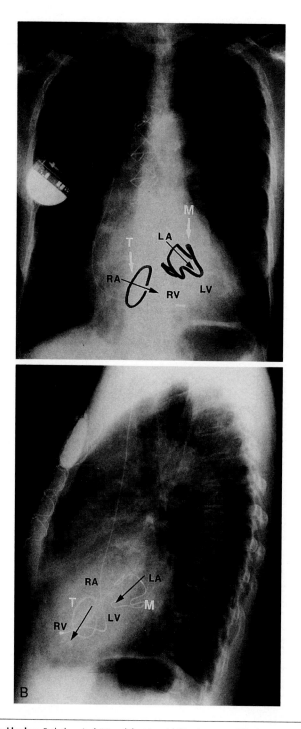

FIGURE 5–8. Prosthetic mitral and tricuspid valves. Both the mitral (M) and the tricuspid (T) valves were difficult to appreciate on the PA view of the chest *(A)* and were, therefore, drawn in. They are easily seen on the lateral view *(B)* in the expected regions between the left atrium and left ventricle and the right atrium and right ventricle. Also note that there is a cardiac pacer that comes down the superior vena cava through the right atrium and into the right ventricle. These two valves are normally relatively large owing to relatively low pressure gradients across these valves.

enlargement of the ascending aorta is due to poststenotic dilatation.

With aortic insufficiency, the left ventricle becomes much larger, and on a PA chest x-ray the apex of the heart may project below the most superior portion of the left hemidiaphragm. The ascending aorta still shows some enlargement (Fig. 5–9). Prosthetic aortic valves are relatively easy to recognize by their relatively small size and the fact that they are located at the root of the ascending aorta (Fig. 5–10).

Pulmonary Artery Enlargement

Enlargement of the pulmonary artery is fairly easy to recognize on the PA chest radiograph by a bulging along the left cardiac border just below the aortic arch (Fig. 5–11). Pulmonary artery enlargement can be due to a number of causes, but probably the three most common are pulmonic stenosis (with poststenotic dilatation), pulmonary artery hypertension, and abnormalities in which there is increased flow through the pulmonary artery, such as a patent ductus arteriosus or an atrial septal defect.

If enlargement of both the left and the right main pulmonary arteries is present, you should consider the diagnosis of pulmonary arterial hypertension. In this entity, in addition to the very large central pulmonary arteries, there is rapid "pruning" of the vessels as they proceed peripherally in the lung. Even though the central vessels are very large, it is unusual to be able to see vessels at the very edge of the lung. Pulmonary hypertension may be due to a number of causes, including atrial and ventricular septal defect, patent ductus arteriosus, arteriovenous shunt, left ventricular failure, mitral valve disease, pulmonary emboli, parenchymal lung disease, chronic obstructive lung disease, and other less common entities.

Congenital Cardiac Disease

Rather than including every entity, a few examples are presented here in order to give you an approach to interpretation. There are several very important factors to assess in the evaluation of congenital cardiac disease. These include the age of the individual; the clinical findings, such as murmurs; whether the patient is cyanotic or acyanotic; specific chamber enlargement; and pulmonary vascularity (increased, decreased, or normal).

Probably the easiest place to begin is in the determination of whether the individual is cyanotic or not. A cyanotic infant who has normal or decreased pulmonary vascularity and a normal heart size probably has a tetralogy of Fallot. Tetralogy of Fallot includes pulmonic stenosis, ventricular septal defect, an overriding aorta, and right ventricular hypertrophy. On x-ray, there is usually decreased pulmonary vascularity and a boot-shaped heart with an uplifted apex and a concavity along the left cardiac border (Fig. 5–12). If there is cardiomegaly with the right atrium enlarged, the differential diagnosis includes Ebstein's malformation, tricuspid atresia, and pulmonic atresia. In Ebstein's anomaly, there is a giant right atrium, with a shoulder along the right side of the heart, and a very small pulmonary artery. In this entity, there is downward displacement of the tricuspid valve, with the right ventricle being partially atrialized (Fig. 5–13).

Cyanotic heart disease with increased pulmonary vascularity includes transposition of the great vessels (which is most common), truncus arteriosus, total anomalous pulmonary venous return (TAPVR), tricuspid atresia, and a single ventricle. Radiographic features of transposition of the great vessels include a heart that is said to have an "egg-on-side" shape and a narrow superior mediastinum secondary to a hypoplastic thymus (Fig. 5–14).

Acyanotic congenital heart disease similarly should initially be evaluated by determination of pulmonary vascularity. In those with normal vascularity, aortic stenosis, pulmonic stenosis, coarctation, and interruption of the aortic arch should be considered. Acyanotic heart disease with increased pulmonary vascularity should next be investigated by looking for left atrial enlargement. This is not present in atrial septal defect, and an endocardial cushion defect may be considered.

An atrial septal defect (ASD) is the most common congenital cardiac anomaly in adults and rarely is symptomatic in infancy or childhood. The common radiologic findings in an

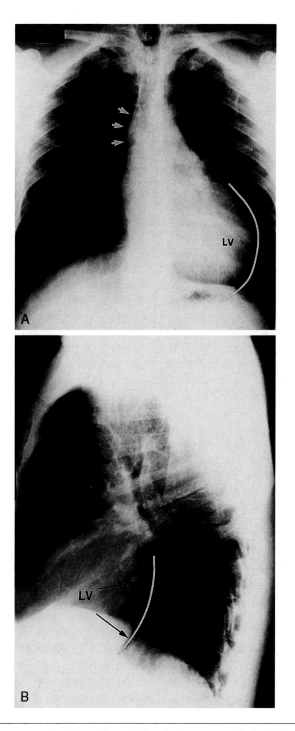

FIGURE 5–9. Aortic insufficiency. There is a very prominent left ventricle seen both on the PA view *(A)* and the lateral view *(B)*. In addition, there is convexity in the region of the ascending aorta *(arrows)* due to poststenotic dilatation.

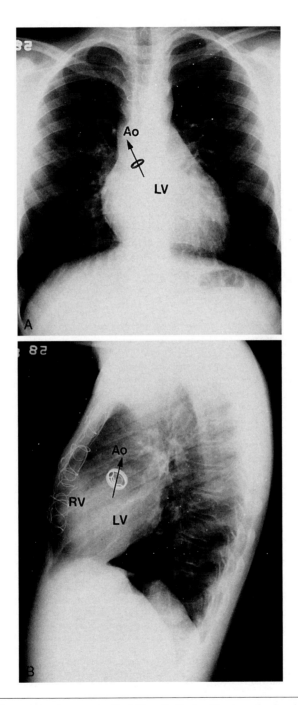

FIGURE 5–10. Prosthetic aortic valve. The prosthetic valve was not easily visible on the PA view *(A)* and was, therefore, drawn in. On the lateral view *(B),* the valve is easily seen in the expected region between the left ventricle and the ascending aorta. Also note its relatively small size. The arrows indicate the direction of blood flow.

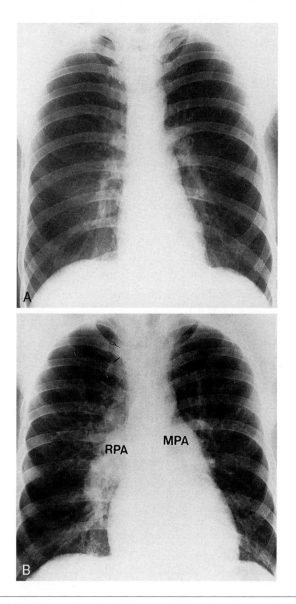

FIGURE 5–11. Progressive pulmonary arterial hypertension. This patient initially presented with a relatively normal chest x-ray *(A)*. However, several years later *(B)*, there is increasing heart size as well as marked dilatation of the main pulmonary artery (MPA) and right pulmonary artery. Rapid tapering of the arteries as they proceed peripherally is suggestive of pulmonary hypertension and is sometimes referred to as "pruning."

ASD, in addition to enlargement of the pulmonary artery, are an increase in the size of the right atrium and right ventricle. This is often best seen as filling in of the retrosternal clear space on the lateral view (Fig. 5–15). The imaging modality of choice, if an ASD is suspected, is echocardiography.

If there is acyanotic heart disease with increased pulmonary vascularity and left atrial enlargement, you should next look at the aorta. If the aorta is enlarged, a patent ductus arteriosus should be suspected, because there is excess blood flow through the aortic arch that is shunted to the pulmonary arteries. If the aorta is not enlarged, consider a ventricular septal defect.

Pulmonary Embolism

Pulmonary embolism (PE) is a potentially fatal entity. Typical symptoms include dyspnea (80 per cent), tachypnea (>16 resp/min, 80 per cent) pleuritic chest pain (70 per cent), rales (60 per cent), fever (45 per cent), tachycardia (40 per cent), and hemoptysis (20 per cent). Patients who present without dyspnea, pleuritic chest pain, or tachypnea are unlikely to have PE. A

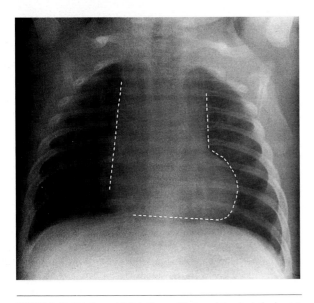

FIGURE 5–12. Tetralogy of Fallot. On an AP view of the chest, the heart is shaped like a boot seen from the side. This is due to the uplifted apex of the heart. Also note that there is a concavity on the left cardiac border and decreased pulmonary vascularity.

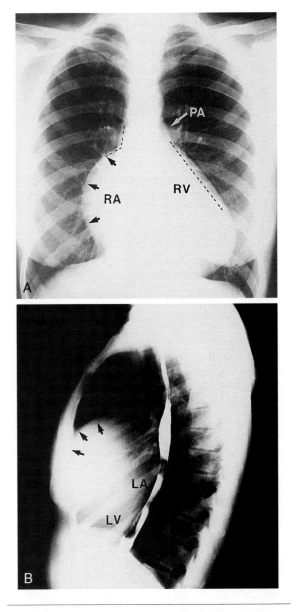

FIGURE 5–13. Ebstein's anomaly. On the PA view of the heart *(A)*, there is a giant right atrium causing a shoulder along the right cardiac silhouette. There is a giant right ventricular outflow tract that causes the left cardiac border to be straight, and the pulmonary artery is very small. On the lateral view *(B)*, the left atrium and left ventricle are essentially normal, but the right atrium and right ventricle are filling in the retrosternal space *(arrows)*.

low-grade fever may occur with PE, but a high-grade fever and leukocytosis suggest a pneumonia. About 35 per cent of patients with PE will also have clinically evident phlebitis. The converse is more important, however; that is, about two thirds of patients with PE will not show evidence of phlebitis.

The chest x-ray findings in a patient with pulmonary emboli are relatively nonspecific, and the major reason for ordering a chest x-ray is to exclude other causes of the patient's symptoms. Occasionally, a small pleural effusion, atelectasis, or an elevated hemidiaphragm may be present. If there has been infarction of a portion of the lung as a result of the embolism, there may be a wedge-shaped infiltrate present (Fig. 5–16).

After a chest x-ray, the next essential study to be performed is a nuclear medicine ventilation/perfusion (V/Q) lung scan. Ventilation is assessed by having the patient inhale and then exhale a radioactive gas or an aerosol containing radioactive particles (Fig. 5–17). Perfusion is assessed by intravenously injecting a number of biodegradable radioactive particles that are unable to pass through the pulmonary capillary bed. These are trapped in the capillary bed, and since they give off radiation, images of the lungs can be obtained in various projections (Fig. 5–18). The V/Q lung scans are then compared. You are looking for a defect on the perfusion scan that is not seen on the ventilation scan (a mismatch). The reason is that a pulmonary embolism generally does not interfere much with ventilation. Abnormalities such as tumors and bullae

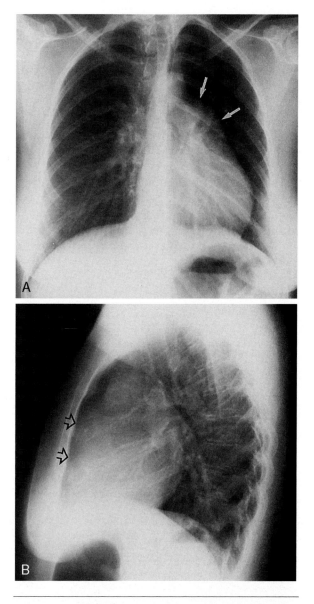

FIGURE 5–15. **Atrial septal defect.** Extra blood flow from the left side of the heart back to the right side increases the size of the main pulmonary artery (seen best on the PA chest x-ray) *(A)*. There is also an increase in the size of the right ventricle (seen best on the lateral view *(B)* as soft tissue filling in the lower and middle retrosternal space).

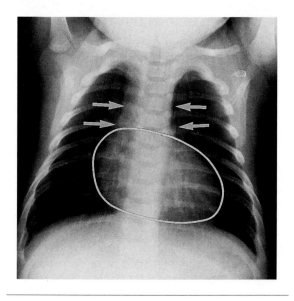

FIGURE 5–14. **Transposition of the great vessels.** With this entity, the heart is classically described as looking like an "egg lying on its side." There is a very narrow vascular pedicle or upper mediastinum *(arrows)*, and pulmonary vascularity is usually increased.

would cause both a ventilation abnormality and a perfusion abnormality (a matched defect).

If a number of segmental defects are seen on the perfusion scan and are not identified on the ventilation scan, the images will be interpreted as high probability for pulmonary embolism (Fig. 5–19). Under these circumstances there is a greater than 80 per cent chance that the patient has pulmonary emboli. There is rarely any need to perform pulmonary angiography on a patient with a high probability scan unless there is a significant contraindication to anticoagulation.

If the perfusion scan is normal or shows only very tiny subsegmental defects, the examination is interpreted as either low probability or normal. Under these circumstances there is less than a 15 per cent chance that the individual has pulmonary emboli, and it is unlikely that these defects are the cause of your patient's symptoms.

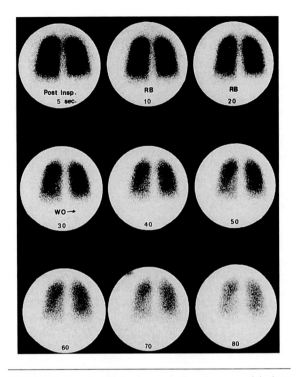

FIGURE 5–17. Normal ventilation lung scan. These are images of the lungs made from the patient's back. The patient inhales radioactive gas and rebreathes it for several seconds (RB); then additional images are made as the radioactive gas is allowed to wash (WO) out of the lungs, during 30 to 80 seconds.

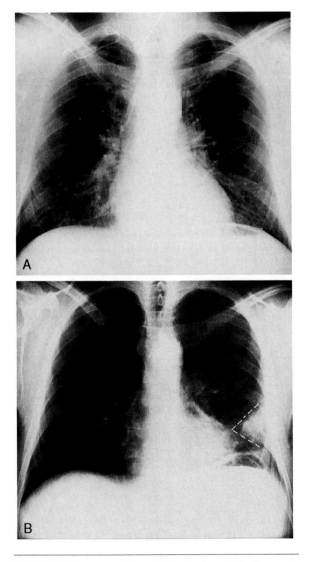

FIGURE 5–16. Pulmonary embolism and infarction. Immediately after an acute episode of shortness of breath due to a pulmonary embolism, the PA chest x-ray is essentially normal (A). If the pulmonary embolism actually leads to infarction, there is development of a peripheral wedge-shaped infiltrate (B).

Occasionally, mismatched (large but not completely segmental) defects are seen, or the patient has a large amount of chronic obstructive lung disease, making the scan difficult to interpret. These scans are interpreted as intermediate probability for pulmonary embolus. If a patient has positive tests for deep venous thrombosis, and clinical suspicion is high, the individual usually is treated. If tests for deep venous thrombosis are negative, yet clinical suspicion remains high, then pulmonary angiography is usually performed.

Some clinicians believe that in a patient with severe COPD, a ventilation scan should not be performed. Their reasoning is that the ventilation/perfusion scan will most likely be interpreted as intermediate. In fact, if the ventilation/perfusion scan is done and multiple segmental defects are seen, there can be an interpretation of high probability, obviating the need for pulmonary angiography. In addition, there is a high complication rate of pulmonary arteriography in patients with COPD and elevated pul-

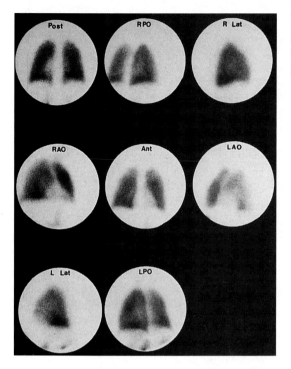

FIGURE 5–18. Normal perfusion lung scan. This nuclear medicine study is performed by intravenously injecting numerous, very tiny particles that lodge in the pulmonary capillary bed. This allows perfusion images of the lungs to be obtained in a number of projections. The defect, or lack of activity between the lungs, is due to the spine and the heart.

FIGURE 5–19. Multiple pulmonary emboli. This young lady with shortness of breath had a normal chest x-ray and a normal ventilation lung scan. The images here are from the perfusion portion of the nuclear medicine lung scan. Note that there are multiple segmental and subsegmental areas without perfusion *(arrows)* throughout both lungs. This is indicative of a high probability of pulmonary emboli.

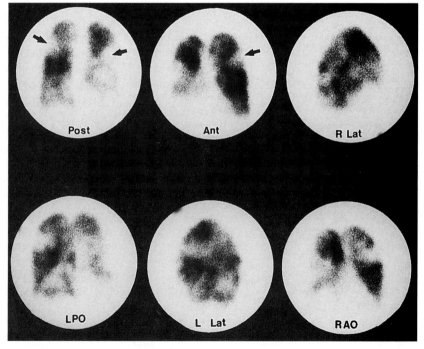

monary artery pressures. The ventilation/perfusion lung scan may identify a particular lung segment of interest, enabling the radiologist to perform a selective arteriogram on that segment. Performance of the V/Q scan will also allow the radiologist to choose the optimal projection, since a single view of a pulmonary arteriogram shows a lot of overlying vessels that can obscure each other. Signs of a pulmonary embolism on an arteriogram include an abrupt termination of a vessel or an intraluminal filling defect (Fig. 5–20). An area where no perfusion was identified does not necessarily mean that there is a pulmonary embolus, since there can be a bulla in this area.

A correlation can be made between the likelihood of pulmonary embolism based on the size of an infiltrate seen on the chest radiograph and the size of a defect seen on a nuclear medicine lung perfusion study. An embolus typically has a larger area of nonperfusion than the size of the resultant infiltrate. If there is an infiltrate on the chest x-ray, it represents infarcted lung. With a pneumonia, there usually is a large area of infiltrate on chest x-ray, but on the perfusion lung scan the area of decreased perfusion is relatively smaller. If the perfusion defect and the infiltrate are almost the same size, the probability of pulmonary embolus is intermediate.

Septic pulmonary emboli are common in drug addicts. They are usually seen as ill-defined pulmonary nodules, but they can cavitate (Fig. 5–21). Differentiation from metastatic disease is made mostly on the basis of patient history, and, in the case of septic emboli, positive blood cultures and presence of fever.

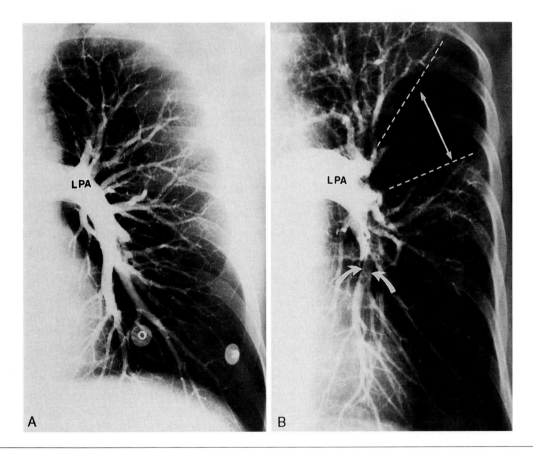

FIGURE 5–20. Pulmonary emboli. The gold standard for evaluation of pulmonary emboli is pulmonary angiography. In this, contrast is injected directly into the left main pulmonary artery. A normal angiogram *(A)* shows the typical branching structures of the pulmonary artery. The pulmonary arteriogram in a patient with pulmonary emboli *(B)* shows a large area of nonperfusion. This is suggestive of, but not specific for, pulmonary emboli. What is much more specific is the filling defect seen within the lumen of the left lower lobe pulmonary artery *(curved arrows).*

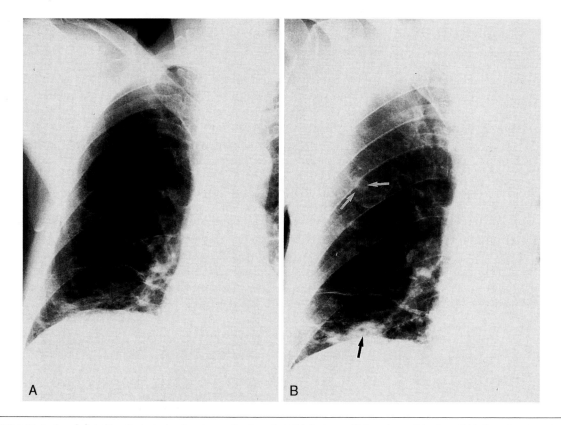

FIGURE 5–21. Septic emboli. In this patient, who is a drug abuser with a fever, the initial chest x-ray *(A)* showed some linear interstitial infiltrates just above the right hemidiaphragm. Several days later, a repeat chest x-ray *(B)* showed that a nodule had developed *(white arrows)* as well as an ill-defined lesion at the right lung base with a central area of cavitation *(black arrow).*

Coronary Artery Disease

Most patients with coronary artery disease have relatively normal chest x-rays. As coronary artery disease progresses, however, there may be cardiac decompensation with enlargement of the cardiac silhouette and signs within the pulmonary parenchyma of congestive failure. Although it is quite rare, occasionally you can see tram-track or parallel calcifications in the coronary arteries on a plain film (Fig. 5–22). Coronary artery calcification is associated with intimal atheroma. Although calcification is a reliable marker for atherosclerosis, it does not indicate a significant coronary artery stenosis. Calcification is seen best on CT scans, seen less well on fluoroscopy, and not seen on a chest x-ray unless it is very extensive. With conventional CT about 90 per cent of patients who had coronary artery calcification had some stenosis, although not necessarily of significant size (more than 50 per cent reduction in diameter). The major lesson is that if a chest CT does not show any coronary calcification, the risk of coronary artery disease is low but that presence of calcification does not imply a significant stenosis.

Evaluation of coronary artery disease usually involves a determination of whether the patient simply has angina, a significant stenosis and ischemia, or a myocardial infarction. The normal initial work-up includes tests of cardiac enzymes and an electrocardiogram (EKG). A stress EKG is also frequently performed. The least invasive imaging methods for evaluation of coronary artery disease are echocardiography and nuclear medicine myocardial perfusion studies. Echocardiography is based upon stressing the patient and then looking for a regional wall motion abnormality, caused either by induced ischemia or by a previous infarction. Al-

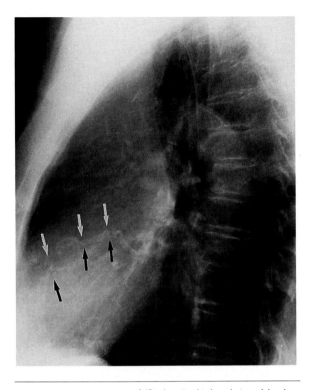

FIGURE 5–22. Coronary artery calcification. On this lateral view of the chest, calcification of the coronary arteries can be easily seen *(arrows)*. CT scanning is much more sensitive for detection of calcification in the coronary artery. Unfortunately, calcification is not well related to the presence of a significant stenosis.

though this method is used in many institutions, it is very operator dependent, and therefore, nuclear medicine studies are much more commonly performed.

A nuclear medicine study can utilize a number of radioactive myocardial agents (such as thallium and sestamibi) to image the musculature of the left ventricle. Images are typically obtained in "slice" or tomographic cuts. With computer analysis, these images may be displayed in the short axis, that is, looking down the barrel of the left ventricle; in the horizontal long axis, essentially slicing the left ventricle horizontally lengthwise; or in the vertical long axis (e.g., slicing the left ventricle from top to bottom in the long axis). Patients are typically imaged with and without the heart having been stressed either by exercise or by chemical agents. If a defect is seen on both exercise and rest images, there is a high probability of myo-

cardial infarction; if a defect is seen only on stress images, this implies ischemia (Fig. 5–23).

Coronary artery stenosis occurs most commonly in the left anterior descending artery, next most commonly in the right coronary artery, and least commonly in the left circumflex artery. The degree of stenosis is directly related to the amount of blood flow reduction. A decrease of less than 50 per cent in the diameter of a vessel or less than 75 per cent in the cross-sectional area is not considered significant. A greater than 75 per cent decrease in the diameter of a vessel is equivalent to a greater than 95 per cent decrease in cross-sectional area, and this is regarded as a severe stenosis. As a rule of thumb, a decrease of 50 per cent or more in diameter of a vessel is equivalent to a 75 per cent or greater decrease in cross-sectional area and flow, and this level or more is regarded as significant.

Visualization of the individual coronary arteries is best done by coronary angiography. Since this is an invasive, expensive procedure and the radiation dose is high, it is not utilized as a screening test. It often is done only following positive results of nuclear medicine study or echocardiogram. Obviously, it also must be done if bypass surgery is contemplated. Coronary angiograms are almost always performed and interpreted by cardiologists. At the present time, cardiologists can utilize coronary angiography to place a catheter either to dilate a particular area of coronary stenosis (angioplasty) or to infuse a clot-lysing agent in an area of recent occlusion.

AORTA

Anatomy and Imaging Techniques

There are a number of anomalies of the aortic arch, the most common of which is a right-sided aortic arch (Fig. 5–24). There are several different types. Some have the arch on the right, with simple mirror-image branching of the innominate, common carotid, and right subclavian arteries. This type also descends along the right side of the spine and can be associated with

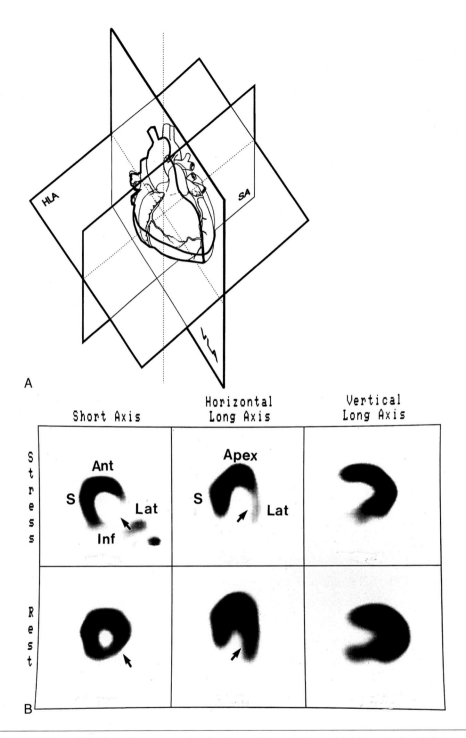

FIGURE 5–23. Assessment of myocardial perfusion. There are a number of nuclear medicine agents that can label the myocardium. Utilizing computer techniques, images of the left ventricular wall can be obtained in the short axis, horizontal long axis, and vertical long axis *(A)*. By imaging during stress and rest, it is possible to tell whether there is an area of reversibility (ischemia), or whether there is a fixed defect (scar or infarction). In this case *(B)*, the arrows demonstrate the defect during stress that reverses or "fills in" during rest images, indicating ischemia of the inferolateral wall of the left ventricle.

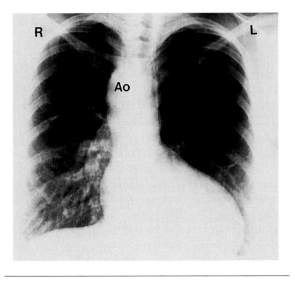

FIGURE 5–24. Right-sided aortic arch. While the heart is in its normal left-sided configuration, the ascending, transverse, and descending thoracic aorta are on the right side.

tion can be seen in the aortic arch and also often in the great vessels (Fig. 5–25).

Injection of contrast directly into the aorta (contrast angiography) yields the most definitive evaluation of normal and anomalous anatomy (Fig. 5–26). The left anterior oblique view is the most useful, since this lays out the anatomy better without much overlap of the great vessels or of the ascending and descending aorta. Imaging can also be done with CT or MR scanning.

Coarctation of the Aorta

Coarctation is a congenital narrowing of the proximal descending thoracic aorta, which usually occurs in the vicinity of the ductus arteriosus. Symptoms are rarely, if ever, present during

tetralogy of Fallot or truncus arteriosus. Right aortic arches are associated with congenital heart disease in 5 per cent of cases. Other variants of right-sided aortic arch include anomalous origins of the pulmonary artery off the ascending or descending aorta; however, these are impossible to differentiate on plain chest x-ray.

Calcification of the aortic arch is very common in persons over the age of 60 years. It is fairly unusual between the ages of 40 and 50 and calcification suggests a higher than average incidence of atherosclerotic disease. Calcifica-

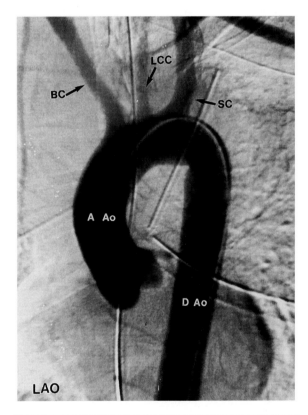

FIGURE 5–26. Normal thoracic aortogram. This angiogram was done with a catheter in the aortic arch and contrast injection. Digital subtraction computer techniques were used to eliminate the bony structures. You can clearly see the ascending and descending thoracic aorta as well as the brachiocephalic, left common carotid, and left subclavian arteries. The projection utilized here is a left anterior oblique because the great vessels do not project over each other in this view.

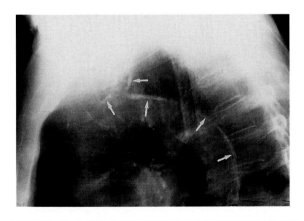

FIGURE 5–25. Calcification of the aortic arch and great vessels. The lateral view of the upper chest clearly shows areas of increased density in the walls of the aortic arch (white arrows) and in the great vessels.

childhood. The diagnosis is usually arrived at by accident during a physical examination by noting diminished or absent femoral pulses or by finding that the patient has hypertension of the upper extremities.

On the chest x-ray, the heart may be normal or may have slight left ventricular enlargement. There is prominence of the ascending aorta. Occasionally the actual site of the coarctation can be visualized as narrowing in the proximal portion of the descending aorta. In addition, there often is prominence along the left paratracheal region in continuity with the outline of the aortic knob caused by dilatation of the left subclavian artery. A rather characteristic finding is notching of the inferior aspect of the ribs due to erosion by tortuous and dilated intercostal arteries (Fig. 5–27). The actual site of stenosis is best visualized by either contrast angiography (Fig. 5–28) or MR scanning. Treatment is surgical, consisting of resection of the coarcted segment.

Aortic Tears

Traumatic disruption of the aorta usually occurs as a result of an automobile accident with the driver's chest striking the steering wheel. In fact, rupture of the aorta causes 15 to 40 per cent of the fatalities due to motor vehicle accidents. Rapid deceleration can cause the aorta to tear, usually in the proximal portion of the descending aorta at the level of the attachment of the ligamentum arteriosum. Ninety five per cent occur at this level, and approximately 5 per cent occur at the level of the aortic root. Signs of a tear on a frontal chest x-ray include a mediastinal width of more than 8 to 10 cm at or above the level of the aortic arch, apical pleural density (capping) due to blood above the apical portion of the lung, and deviation of the trachea or nasogastric tube to the right. Usually there is also poor definition of the aortic arch and opacification of the aortopulmonary window (Fig. 5–29).

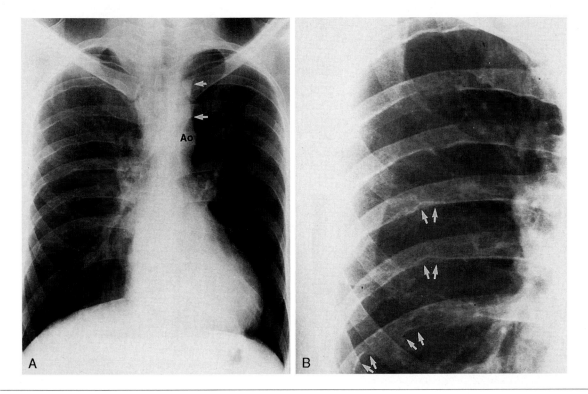

FIGURE 5–27. Coarctation of the aorta. A chest x-ray was obtained in this patient who had very high blood pressure in both upper extremities. *(A)*. It demonstrates prominence of the left cardiac border (due to left ventricular hypertrophy). There is also a dilated left subclavian artery *(arrows)* due to increased flow, since blood has difficulty getting down the descending aorta. A close-up view *(B)* of the chest shows notching along the inferior aspects of the ribs *(arrows)* due to dilated intercostal arteries.

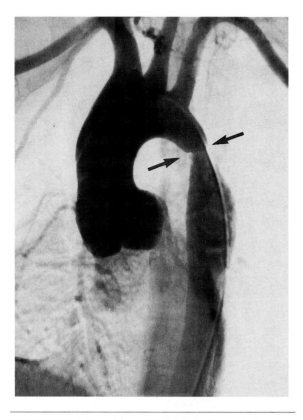

FIGURE 5–28. **Coarctation of the aorta.** A digital subtraction contrast aortogram clearly shows the area of coarctation, or narrowing, distal to the left subclavian artery.

Thoracic Aortic Aneurysms

Aneurysms may be the result of atherosclerosis; inflammatory, mechanical, traumatic, or congenital causes; fibromuscular dysplasia; and cystic medial necrosis. An aneurysm of the ascending aorta historically was most likely due to syphilis. This is very rare at the present time, and Marfan's syndrome is a more likely cause.

With aneurysms of either the thoracic or the abdominal aorta, surgery is usually performed, since there is a marked increase in risk of aortic rupture. Aneurysms may be discovered incidentally, or the patient may present with pain, rupture, or thromboembolic complications. Aneurysms of the thoracic aorta are fairly easy to identify on chest x-rays as widening of the ascending aorta or aortic arch (Fig. 5–30). Sudden onset of chest pain in a patient with an aneurysm should suggest rupture or ongoing dissection.

Detailed evaluation of an aneurysm can be easily performed utilizing CT scanning with a bolus of intravenous contrast. This will allow the lumen to be visualized as well as clot along the inner wall of the aneurysm. Many patients have portions of the clot that come loose and lead to distal thromboembolic events (Fig. 5–30*C*). An arteriogram is not the best initial method for evaluation of aneurysms, since usually all that is visualized is the patent lumen and not the outer wall or the thickness of intraluminal clot. In addition, a catheter in the aorta raises the possibility of knocking portions of clot loose. MRI can be used, but imaging times are longer than on CT scanning. Further, if the patient is unstable, it is difficult to manage life support owing to the high magnetic field strength and the inability to bring ferromagnetic materials into the room.

Aortic Dissection

Aortic dissection is the result of an intimal tear causing separation of the layers of the wall of the aorta. It is more common in men than in women and usually occurs between the ages of 45 and 70 years. The incidence is higher in patients with Marfan's syndrome, coarctation of the aorta, and bicuspid aortic valve disease. Aortic dissection also commonly occurs in patients with aortic atherosclerosis, particularly those who are hypertensive. Dissection carries a very high mortality if undiagnosed and untreated. Dissection of the thoracic aorta proximal to the left subclavian artery is a surgical emergency, whereas dissections of the descending thoracic aorta are usually managed by medical treatment of the patient's hypertension.

The dissection can allow blood to flow in between the layers of the aortic wall, causing a false lumen. Sometimes, this false lumen will re-enter the true lumen farther down the aorta. Generally, aortic dissection begins either in the ascending aorta or in the descending aorta just distal to the left subclavian in the upper back and chest. About one third of patients will have extremity pain, and another one third will have a CNS abnormality if the dissection involves the ascending aorta and great vessels.

Aortic dissection should be suspected on a

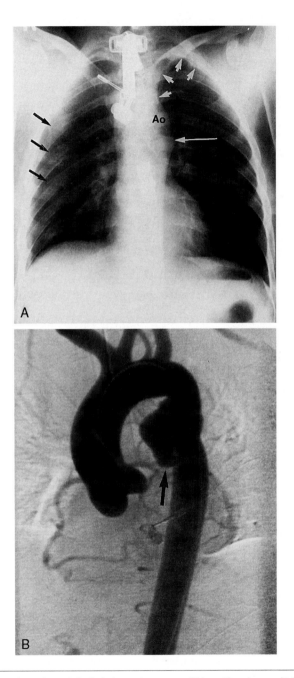

FIGURE 5–29. Aortic tear. A chest x-ray *(A)* obtained in an individual who was in a motor vehicle accident shows multiple rib fractures *(black arrows)*, filling in of the normal concavity of the AP window *(long white arrow)*, and fluid over the apex of the left lung. These latter two findings are suspicious for mediastinal hemorrhage. A digital subtraction contrast aortogram *(B)* shows a bulge of contrast *(arrow)* due to a tear in a very typical location.

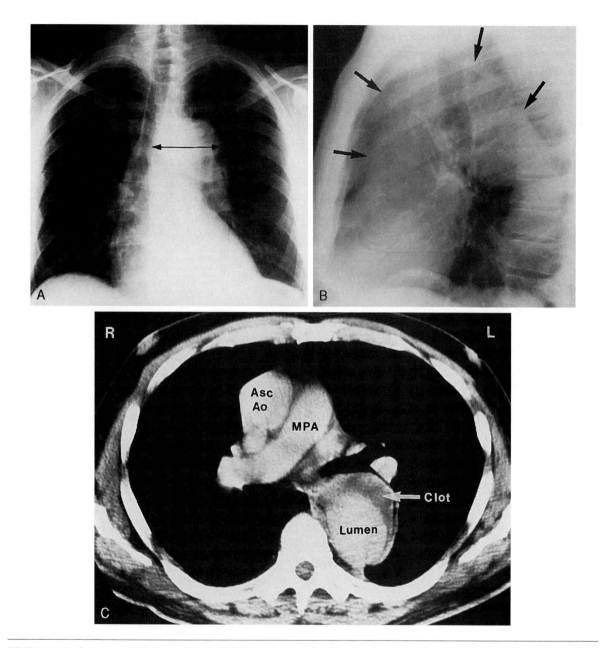

FIGURE 5–30. Aortic aneurysm. A PA chest radiograph *(A)* demonstrates a markedly widened aortic arch *(double-ended arrow).* The lateral view *(B)* also shows marked dilatation of the entire aortic arch. A contrast-enhanced transverse CT scan *(C)* shows the ascending aorta, the main pulmonary artery, and marked dilatation of the proximal portion of the descending thoracic aorta. The contrast-enhanced lumen is seen as well as mural clot.

chest x-ray if there is a double contour of the aortic arch, if there is progressive serial enlargement, or if there is displacement of intimal calcification more than 6 mm from the outer aortic margin. This last sign has to be interpreted with caution, since a minor degree of rotation of the chest may cause anterior arch calcification to project eccentrically over the posterior arch. On chest x-ray, most patients with a dissection will have a dilated aorta with a widened mediastinum and cardiomegaly.

Enlargement of the aortic arch on a single film is not specific for a dissection, inasmuch as the aortic arch can frequently be enlarged in patients with hypertension or atherosclerosis. Lack of enlargement of the aortic arch should not be taken as evidence that a dissection is not present, since the arch is of normal size in 25 per cent of dissection cases.

An angiogram can sometimes show the true and false lumens (Fig. 5–31). Care must be taken not to do a power injection of contrast if the end of the catheter is in the false lumen. A slow hand injection is made prior to the actual arteriogram in order to visually assess the flow rates. The diagnosis of dissection can also be made by a contrasted CT or an MR study. CT scanning is somewhat quicker, and it is easier to manage a patient who may suddenly decompensate. Demonstration of an intimal flap on CT is conclusive evidence of a dissection. An intimal flap and the false lumen can be seen in 70 per cent of patients. Transesophageal ultrasound can be utilized to evaluate dissections or aneurysms of the descending thoracic aorta, since the esophagus is in such close proximity. Generally, however, surgeons want a more complete evaluation, such as that provided by CT, before they will operate on a patient.

PERIPHERAL VESSELS

Head and Neck

Evaluation of vessels of the head and neck classically is done by utilizing contrast angiography. This involves percutaneous access to the femoral artery and placement of the catheter up the aorta with selective catheterization of the indi-

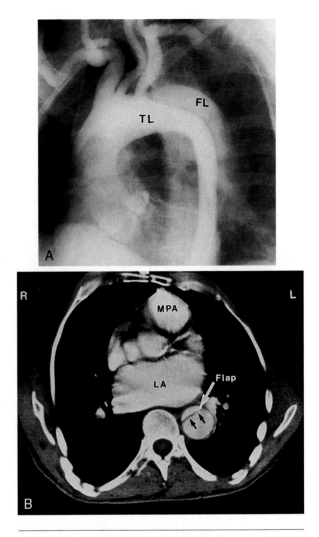

FIGURE 5–31. Aortic dissection. A standard contrast aortogram in the left anterior oblique projection *(A)* shows contrast in the true lumen (tl) as well as the great vessels. Contrast is also seen in the false lumen (fl), which is a channel within the wall of the aorta. A contrast-enhanced transverse CT scan *(B)* easily shows the intimal flap between the true lumen and the false lumen.

vidual great vessels, including the carotid and vertebral arteries. The typical contrast angiogram shows exquisite detail of the vessels of the neck, face, and brain and can easily demonstrate areas of stenosis or aneurysm. One of the difficulties of standard contrast angiography is that vessels can be obscured by nearby dense bone, but it is now possible to utilize computer subtraction techniques to produce what is referred to as a digital angiogram. This can be performed utilizing intravenous contrast but the images are better with an arterial injection. What happens is that an initial picture is taken prior to the injection of contrast; then this "mask" of the bony structures can be subtracted from later images, leaving only the vessels (Fig. 5–32).

All contrast angiography of the vessels of the head and neck carries a small risk of stroke, due to injection of air bubbles, or of vascular spasm or clotting, due to the catheter. Recently, advances in MR scanning have allowed magnetic resonance angiography to be performed. A different signal is obtained from moving blood as opposed to stationary structures, and the computer is able to reconstruct an angiogram. This method is most satisfactory for imaging the head, since there is little or no movement of nonvascular structures during the time it takes to acquire the necessary information. Because of motion artifacts, MR angiography is much less satisfactory for imaging vessels of the abdomen, pelvis, and proximal extremities.

Abdominal and Pelvic Vessels

In patients with extensive atherosclerosis, there can be striking calcification of the abdominal aorta and iliac arteries (Fig. 5–33*A*). You should remember that atherosclerosis is a common cause of aneurysm formation, and you should therefore be assessing the diameter of the vessels. Since on the AP view of the abdomen the aorta overlies the spine, it can be difficult to assess calcification in the aortic wall. The lateral view of the abdomen or of the lumbar spine often gives you a better appreciation of the calcified abdominal aorta (Fig. 5–33*B*). The abdominal aorta should not exceed 2.5 cm in diameter; as with the thoracic aorta, once the diameter exceeds 5 cm there is an increased likelihood of rupture. The diameter of the aorta should be measured from the anterior wall back

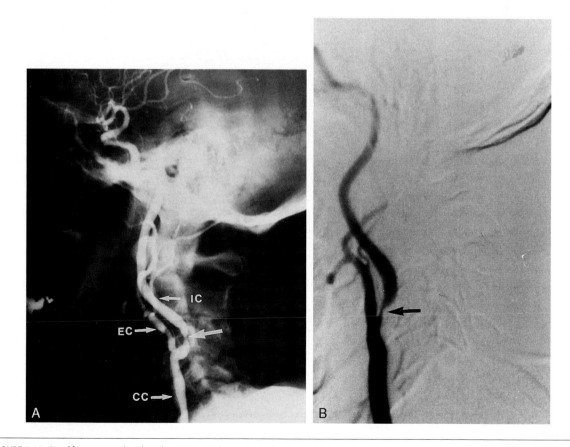

FIGURE 5–32. Carotid artery stenosis. A lateral projection *(A)* from a standard contrast arteriogram shows the common carotid (CC), the external carotid (EC), and the internal carotid (IC) arteries. An area of stenosis can be identified at the base of the internal carotid artery *(large arrow)*. A digital subtraction angiogram *(B)* makes areas of stenosis much easier to see, since the bones have been subtracted off the image.

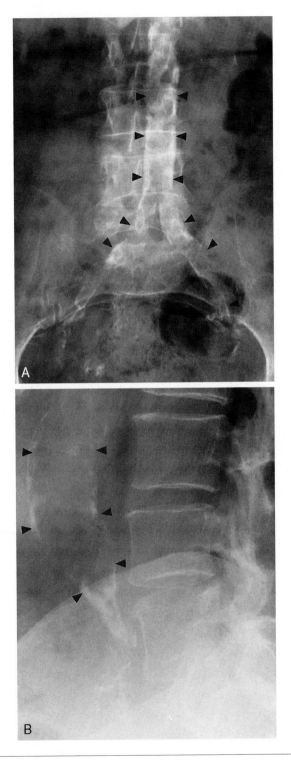

FIGURE 5–33. Calcification of the abdominal aorta. A plain x-ray of the abdomen *(A)* shows extensive calcification of the abdominal aorta and iliac vessels. Calcification of the abdominal aorta is usually much easier to see on the lateral view *(B)*. If the distance from the anterior calcified wall back to a vertebral body exceeds 5 cm, an abdominal aortic aneurysm is present.

to the vertebral bodies and not just to the posterior calcified wall. Sometimes the calcification in an abdominal aneurysm can be somewhat subtle and, on the AP view, may be seen as curvilinear streaks along the lateral aspects of the vertebral bodies (Fig. 5–34).

A very easy noninvasive examination of the abdominal aorta can be done utilizing abdominal ultrasound. Not only can the aorta be visualized, but also other vessels, such as superior mesenteric artery and vein, can be seen (Fig. 5–35). Abdominal ultrasound is the imaging test of choice if (1) you suspect that there is an abdominal aortic aneurysm or (2) you need to follow a patient who has a dilated aorta that has not yet reached 5 cm in diameter. In a symptomatic patient whose condition raises fear of clot within the aorta, dissection, or rupture, a CT scan with an intravenous bolus of contrast material is the test of choice (Fig. 5–36).

Evaluation of abdominal and pelvic vessels other than the aorta is best done by contrast angiography. Not only can the major vessels, such as hepatic artery and renal arteries, be identified, but also all their branches can be seen in great detail. Even small lumbar arteries can be visualized (Fig. 5–37). Atherosclerotic changes and areas of stenosis also are easily identified.

After identification of areas of stenosis, it is possible to insert a catheter that has a balloon on the end and to dilate the areas of stenosis. This is called percutaneous transluminal angioplasty. The method involves fracturing the vascular intima and media and stretching the adventitia, thus expanding the outer diameter of the vessel. Atherosclerotic plaques themselves are very hard and are rarely fractured by dilatation. The success rate actually depends upon the vessel, and the success of angioplasty is greatest in the larger vessels, such as the iliac arteries (Fig. 5–38). Five-year patency rates are usually quoted as 70 to 90 per cent. Occasionally, it is also possible to insert a metallic stent. This is an expandable wire mesh tube that is placed inside the vessel to keep it from restenosing.

Another relatively new procedure is the creation of an intrahepatic portal shunt. This method is used on patients with end-stage cirrhosis and portal hypertension who are not candidates for surgery. The approach involves puncturing the right jugular vein and passing a catheter down the superior vena cava into the inferior vena cava and then into the hepatic vein. A needle is pushed through the liver into the portal system; the needle tract is dilated with a balloon; and a stent is placed in the dilated tract. This is called a transjugular intrahepatic portal shunt (TIPS) procedure.

Peripheral Veins

Evaluation of the veins of the lower extremities is particularly important, since this is a very common site for development of thrombi that can lead to potentially fatal pulmonary emboli. The standard approach for imaging veins over the years has been contrast venography. With this approach, contrast material is injected into the veins on the dorsum of the foot and the contrast visualized as it proceeds up the veins of the leg and into the pelvis. Contrast venography allows visualization of the deep venous system but not of the superficial venous system. Clots can be seen as intraluminal defects with contrast material surrounding them. Total obstruction with visualization of collateral veins also can be seen with thrombosis (Figs. 5–39 and 5–40). One of the problems with contrast venography is that it involves the use of iodinated and intravenously administered contrast material. Sometimes venous access is difficult in patients who have a grossly swollen leg. It is possible that the contrast itself may cause some inflammation of the vein and may carry a low but real complication rate of thrombophlebitis.

Deep venous thrombosis fails to produce clinical signs in half the patients who have it. Thrombosis in calf veins is usually insignificant; however, in the femoral veins and pelvic veins, thrombi are significant. Risk factors include prolonged bed rest, immobilization of an extremity, pregnancy, oral contraceptives, malignancy, and postoperative and traumatic circumstances.

The initial imaging test of choice for a patient with suspected deep venous thrombosis is ultrasonography. Ultrasound has a sensitivity and specificity of approximately 95 per cent.
Text continued on page 161

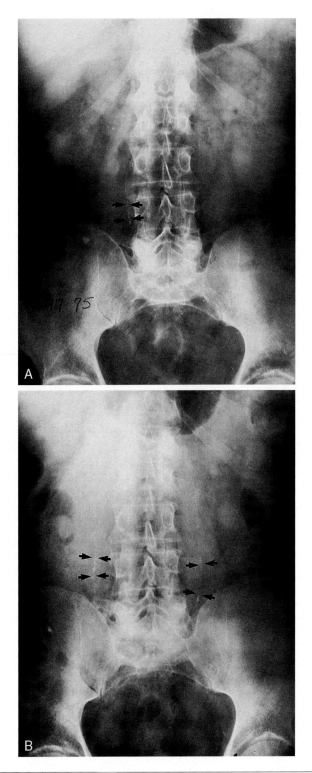

FIGURE 5–34. Progressive development of an abdominal aortic aneurysm. A plain x-ray of the abdomen of a patient done in 1975 *(A)* showed a small area of linear calcification overlying the right side of L5 *(arrows)*. This represents calcification within the wall of the aorta. A repeat x-ray 10 years later *(B)* showed bilateral linear areas of calcification *(arrows)*. The distance between these two linear calcifications represents the width of the aneurysm.

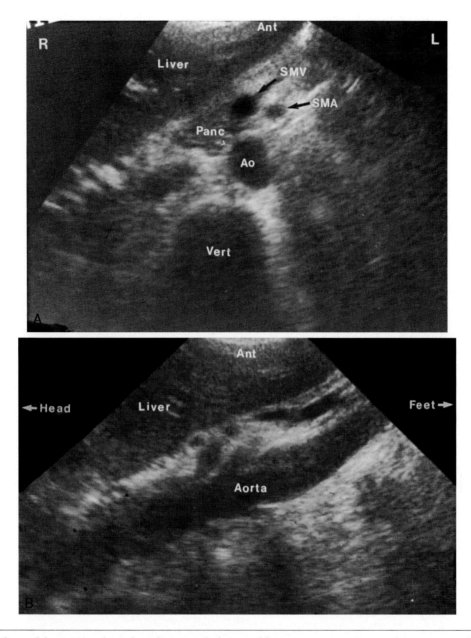

FIGURE 5-35. Ultrasound demonstration of normal vascular anatomy in the upper abdomen. A transverse sonogram *(A)* shows structures, such as the liver and pancreas and vertebral body, but also the superior mesenteric artery, vein, and abdominal aorta. A longitudinal view just to the left of midline *(B)* shows the liver and abdominal aorta as well as the origin of the celiac axis and superior mesenteric artery.

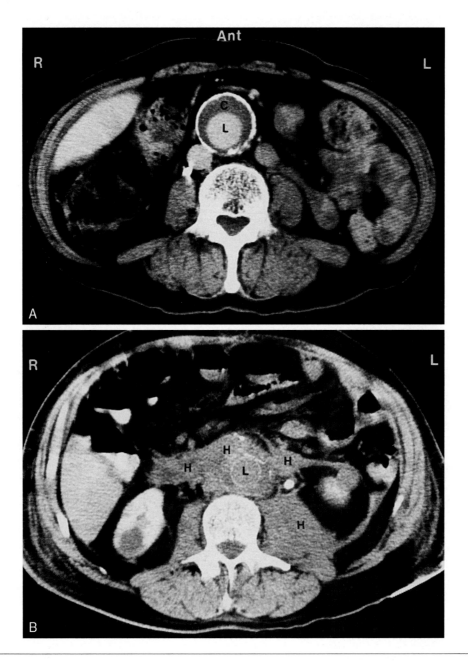

FIGURE 5–36. Abdominal aortic aneurysm and rupture. A transverse contrast-enhanced CT scan *(A)* of the lower portion of the abdomen shows the aorta with a calcified rim and the lumen filled with contrast and mural clot. In a different patient who presented with abdominal pain, a noncontrasted CT scan *(B)* shows the true lumen of the aorta (L), which is visible because of the calcified aortic wall. What looks like soft tissue surrounding the aorta and extending into the left psoas region is hemorrhage due to a leak.

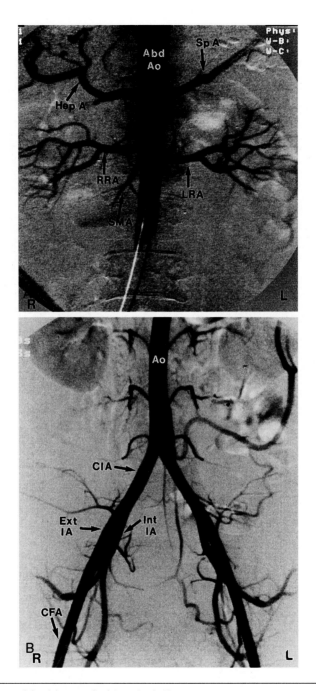

FIGURE 5–37. Normal vascular anatomy of the abdomen and pelvis. A digital subtraction angiogram in an AP projection of the upper abdomen *(A)* shows the abdominal aorta, the hepatic and splenic arteries, the right and left renal arteries, and the superior mesenteric artery. A subsequent image over the lower abdomen and pelvis *(B)* a few seconds later shows the distal abdominal aorta with small lumbar branches, the common iliac artery, the internal and external iliac arteries, and the common femoral artery.

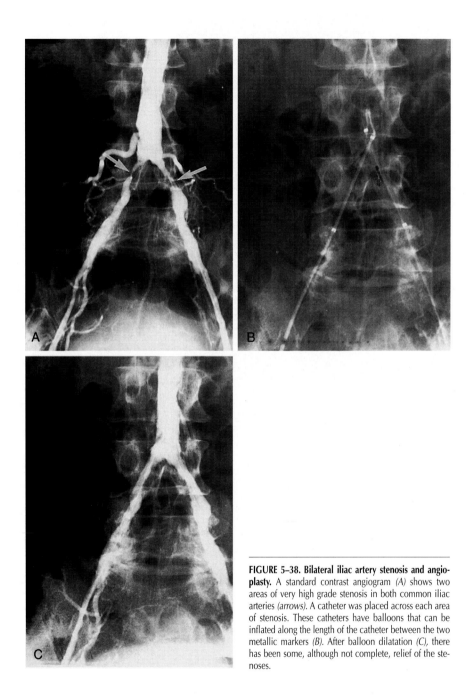

FIGURE 5–38. Bilateral iliac artery stenosis and angio-plasty. A standard contrast angiogram *(A)* shows two areas of very high grade stenosis in both common iliac arteries *(arrows)*. A catheter was placed across each area of stenosis. These catheters have balloons that can be inflated along the length of the catheter between the two metallic markers *(B)*. After balloon dilatation *(C)*, there has been some, although not complete, relief of the stenoses.

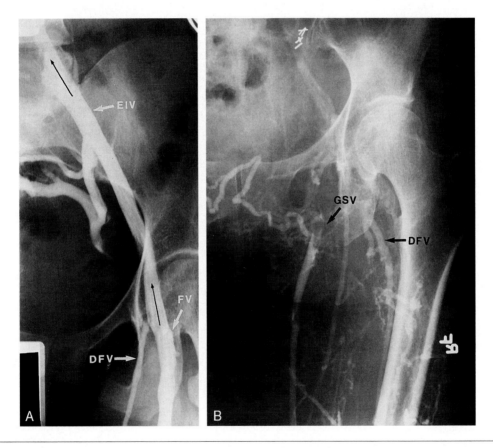

FIGURE 5–39. Thrombosis of the femoral vein. A normal contrast venogram *(A)* shows the contrast coming up the femoral vein and into the external iliac vein. There is some normal reflux into the pelvic vessels. In a postsurgical patient with leg swelling, a contrast venogram *(B)* demonstrates only the deep femoral vein and collateral veins. The greater saphenous vein is obstructed. The femoral vein is not visualized at all owing to complete thrombosis.

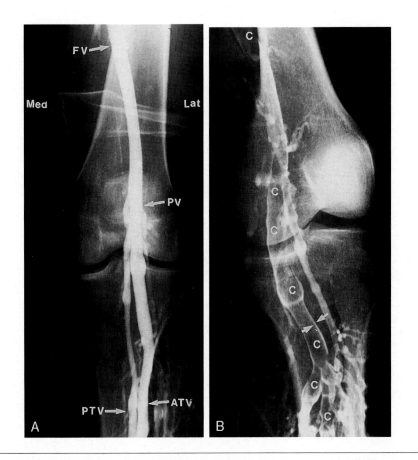

FIGURE 5–40. Venous thrombosis about the knee. A normal contrast venogram *(A)* near the knee shows the contrast coming up the anterior and posterior tibial veins into the popliteal vein and then into the femoral vein. A venogram *(B)* in a different patient with leg swelling shows that the veins are filled with clot (C). A small amount of contrast is able to pass by and outline the clot in some veins *(arrows).*

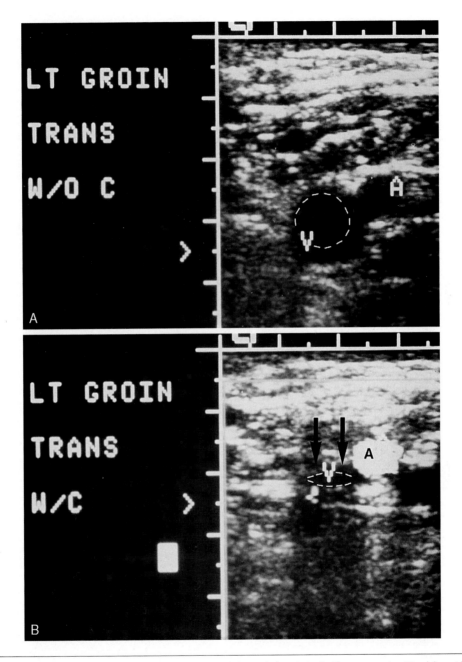

FIGURE 5–41. Normal ultrasound of the femoral vein. A transverse view of the left inner thigh is obtained without compression *(A)* and then with compression *(B)*. Without compression, the vein is seen to be round, but with compression the vein is easily flattened. The artery is seen just lateral to the vein.

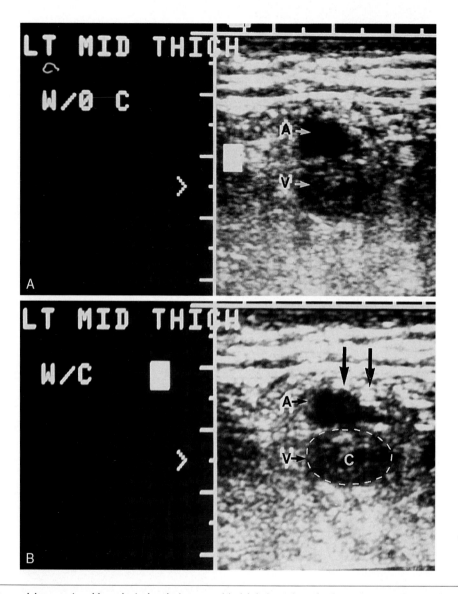

FIGURE 5–42. Ultrasound demonstration of femoral vein thrombosis. Images of the left thigh are obtained without compression *(A)* and with compression *(B)*. The vein could be seen in both instances, and it is not compressible because it contains clot. Additionally, there are echoes within the vein as a result of clot.

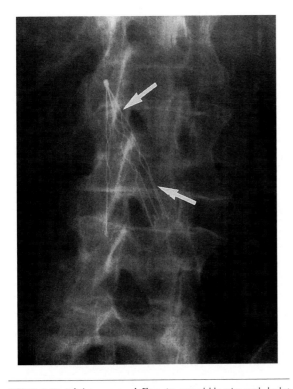

FIGURE 5–43. Inferior vena caval filter. An expandable wire mesh basket *(arrows)* has been placed in the inferior vena cava. This can be done by pushing the device out of a catheter and allowing it to expand in place. This will keep the large clots from traveling from the lower extremities and pelvis up the inferior vena cava and into the lung.

The femoral artery and vein can both easily be visualized utilizing ultrasound. With pressure, the femoral vein will normally be compressed (Fig. 5–41). If there is a clot within the vein,

echoes will be seen within the lumen, and no compression will be identified (Fig. 5–42). Color Doppler ultrasound can be utilized to classify flow in the vein into none or partial flow.

Recurrent deep venous thrombosis or deep venous thrombosis that is not successfully treated with heparin can result in multiple episodes of pulmonary emboli. Owing to the life-threatening nature of this problem, methods have been developed to keep the thrombi from migrating into the lung. Probably the most frequently employed method is placement of a filter in the inferior vena cava. Access is gained through the femoral vein, and contrast is injected to make sure that no clot is in the iliac vein or inferior vena cava itself. After this, a catheter is advanced to the level just below the renal veins, and an expandable wire net or basket is pushed out the end of the catheter. At this time the most commonly used device is a Greenfield filter, and if it is present, it is easily seen on an AP radiograph of the abdomen projecting over the right side of the upper lumbar vertebra (Fig. 5–43).

General Suggested Readings

Kadir S: Current Practice of Interventional Radiology. Philadelphia, BC Decker, 1991.

Amplatz K, Moller J: Radiology of Congenital Heart Disease. St. Louis, Mosby Year Book, 1993.

Higgins C: Essentials of Cardiac Radiology and Imaging. Philadelphia, JB Lippincott, 1991.

Chapter 6

Gastrointestinal System

ANATOMY AND IMAGING TECHNIQUES

The most common imaging study of the abdomen is referred to as a KUB, or plain film of the abdomen. The term "KUB" is historical nonsense. It stands for *k*idneys, *u*reter, and *b*ladder, none of which are usually seen on a regular x-ray of the abdomen; nevertheless, the term remains widely used. A KUB is usually done with the patient supine (Fig. 6–1). When examining this film, you should look at the bony structures, the lung bases, and then at the soft tissue and gas patterns (Table 6–1). The soft tissue pattern should include evaluation of the lateral psoas margins. Whether or not you see them bilaterally, only faintly, or throughout their length depends upon the shape of the psoas and the amount of retroperitoneal fat in that particular individual (it is all right if you do not see the psoas margin on either side). If you see the psoas margin on one side but not on the other, this is most commonly due to normal anatomic variation. In about 25 per cent of cases, however, there will be pathology on the side of the obscured psoas margin.

Even though it is difficult to see, you should look for the outline of the kidneys. Again, if you cannot see the outlines, you should not be terribly concerned, because they are often obscured by overlying bowel gas. The liver is seen as a homogeneous soft tissue density in the right upper quadrant. The spleen can sometimes be seen as a smaller homogeneous density in the left upper quadrant. Although you will be able to appreciate massive enlargement of either one of these organs, minimal to moderate enlargement is very difficult to ascertain, and you should think twice before you suggest it. Clinical palpation and percussion are at least as accurate.

Evaluation of the gas pattern is also important (Table 6–2). Since people routinely swallow air and drink lots of carbonated beverages, the stomach almost always has some gas within it. When a person is lying on his or her back, the air will go to the most anterior portion

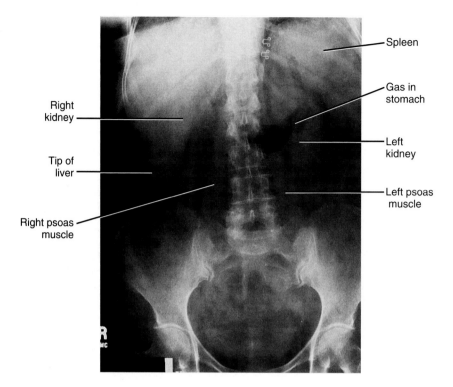

FIGURE 6–1. Normal anatomy seen on a supine x-ray (KUB) of the abdomen.

Right kidney

Tip of liver

Right psoas muscle

Spleen

Gas in stomach

Left kidney

Left psoas muscle

of the stomach, which is the body and antrum; this will be seen as a curvilinear air collection, just along the left side of the upper lumbar spine (Fig. 6–2). If the person has swallowed a lot of air, you may see gas bubbles within the entire gastrointestinal tract extending from the stomach to the rectum. The origin of almost all these bubbles is swallowed air and not gas produced by intestinal bacteria. You should be able to identify the air patterns in the stomach, small

bowel, colon, sigmoid, and rectum. Gas in the small bowel usually can be identified, because small bowel mucosa has very fine lines that cross all the way across the lumen. Most small bowel gas is located in the left midabdomen and the lower central abdomen. The colon often can be traced from the cecum in the right lower quadrant to both the hepatic and the splenic flexures and down to the sigmoid. The cecum and the colon often have a bubbly appearance representing a mixture of gas and fecal material. Colonic air often has a somewhat cloverleaf-shaped appearance caused by the haustra of the

---

TABLE 6–1. Items to Look For on a Plain Abdominal Film (KUB)

Gas Patterns
Stomach, small bowel, and rectosigmoid
Abnormal or ectopic collections

Organ Shapes and Sizes
Liver
Spleen
Kidneys
Soft tissue pelvic masses

Calcifications

Asymmetric Psoas Margins

Skeleton

Basilar Lung Abnormalities

TABLE 6–2. Evaluation of Gas Patterns on a Plain Film of the Abdomen

Collections Normally Present
Look for dilatation of structure and assessment of wall or mucosal thickness in stomach, small bowel, colon, and rectosigmoid

Collections Not Normally Present
Free air under the diaphragm (upright film)
Free air on supine films (double bowel wall sign)
Right upper quadrant: Portal vein (peripheral in liver), biliary system (central in liver)
Small bubbles in an abscess
Emphysematous cholecystitis, pyelonephritis, or cystitis

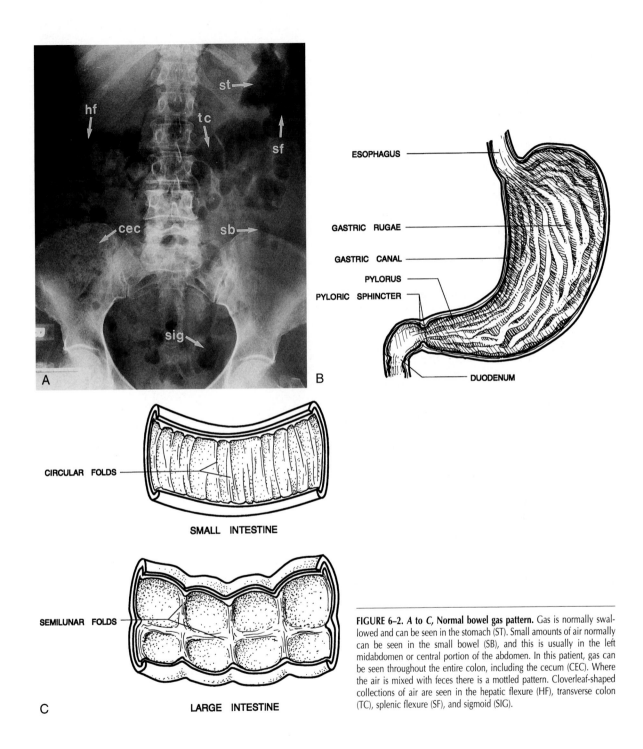

FIGURE 6–2. *A to C,* **Normal bowel gas pattern.** Gas is normally swallowed and can be seen in the stomach (ST). Small amounts of air normally can be seen in the small bowel (SB), and this is usually in the left midabdomen or central portion of the abdomen. In this patient, gas can be seen throughout the entire colon, including the cecum (CEC). Where the air is mixed with feces there is a mottled pattern. Cloverleaf-shaped collections of air are seen in the hepatic flexure (HF), transverse colon (TC), splenic flexure (SF), and sigmoid (SIG).

colon. Normal small bowel should not exceed 3 cm in diameter, and the colon should not exceed 6 cm. The cecum can normally be somewhat larger than the rest of the colon and may be up to 8 cm in diameter.

In addition to a supine abdominal film, a "three-way" view of the abdomen is often obtained. The additional two views are an upright PA chest x-ray and a view of the abdomen taken with the patient standing upright. The reason for taking the PA view of the chest is to look for chest pathology that may be mimicking or causing abdominal symptoms as well as to look for free air underneath the hemidiaphragms. The reason for the standing view of the abdomen is to look at the air-fluid levels within the bowel in order to differentiate between an obstruction and ileus.

There is a common variant that you should be aware of, which is called colonic interposition (also called Chilaiditi's syndrome). In this normal variant, the hepatic flexure of the colon can slip up between the superior aspect of the liver and the dome of the right hemidiaphragm (Fig. 6–3). This should not be mistaken for free air. When colonic interposition occurs, you can almost always see the haustral markings of the colon.

It is very important that you understand the cross-sectional anatomy of both the abdomen and the pelvis. Computed tomographic (CT) scanning is commonly used to image nonintestinal abdominal pathology. CT anatomy is presented in Figure 6–4.

Pneumoperitoneum

It is easiest to identify small amounts of free air in the peritoneal cavity by doing an upright chest x-ray. In this manner, as little as 3 or 4 cc of air may be visualized (Fig. 6–5A). An upright abdominal film is usually not very useful to look for free air, since the domes of the diaphragms are often off the upper edge of the film. It is very difficult to appreciate even relatively large amounts of free air within the peritoneal cavity by looking at a supine (KUB) view of the abdomen. If there is a lot of free air you may be able to see the bowel wall outlined by air (Fig. 6–5B). If the patient is too sick to stand up, and you suspect a small pneumoperitoneum, you should

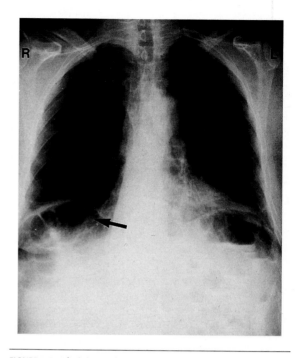

FIGURE 6–3. Colonic interposition. This is a normal variant in which the hepatic flexure can get up above the liver. This is seen as a gas collection under the right hemidiaphragm (arrow), but it is clearly identified as colon, owing to the transverse haustral markings.

order a left lateral decubitus view of the abdomen. In this manner, with the patient lying on the left side (for 10 to 15 minutes), small amounts of air can be seen tracking up over the lateral aspect of the right lobe of the liver.

Abscesses

Air can be seen within some, but by no means all, abscesses. While a very large abscess may be appreciated on a plain film, it is often difficult to tell whether you are looking at air within the bowel or in some other structure. For this reason, the imaging test of choice when an abdominal or pelvic abscess is suspected is a CT scan (Fig. 6–6). It is very important that under these circumstances you order a CT scan with gastrointestinal contrast so that the entire bowel can be filled with contrast. If this is not done, it may be difficult, even on a CT scan, to differentiate a collection of bowel that has air and fluid within it from an abscess. If you suspect an infection but do not know where it is, a nuclear medicine abscess scan can be done with radio-
Text continued on page 170

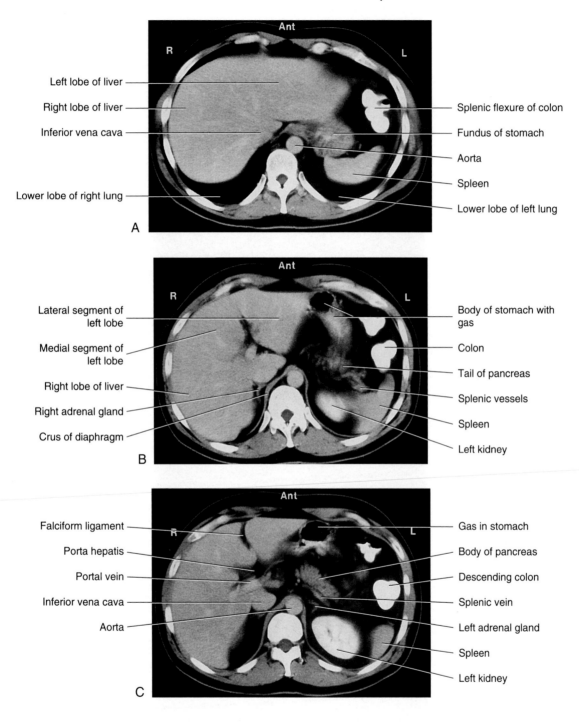

FIGURE 6–4. *A* to *L*, Normal transverse CT anatomy of the abdomen and pelvis. The patient has been given oral, rectal, and intravenous contrast media.

Illustration continued on following page

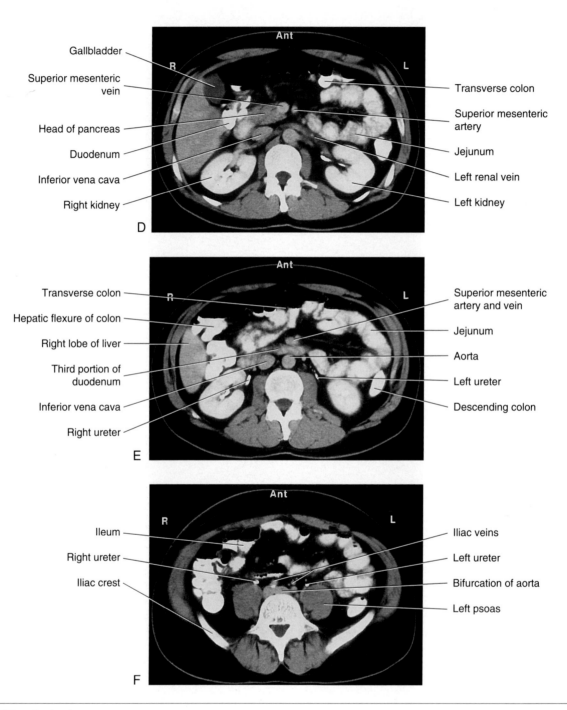

FIGURE 6–4 *Continued*

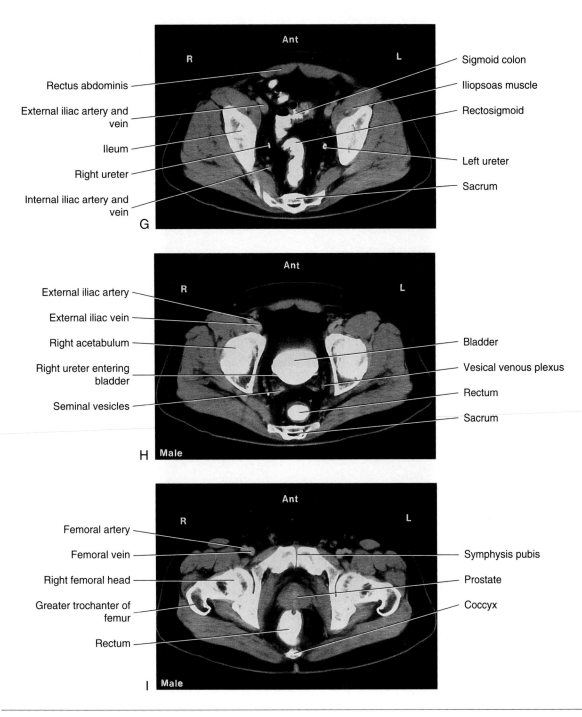

FIGURE 6–4 *Continued*

Illustration continued on following page

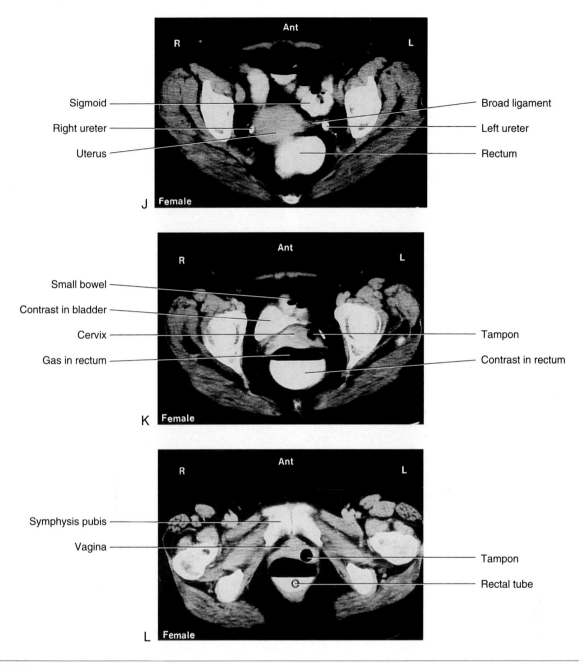

FIGURE 6–4 *Continued*

actively labeled white cells. This allows a look at the entire body.

Feeding Tubes

As mentioned in Chapter 3, feeding tubes or nasogastric tubes are particularly recalcitrant medical devices. Not only can they inadvertently be passed into the trachea and major bronchus, but also they love to coil within the stomach. On the plain film, a well-placed enteric (Dobbhoff) feeding tube can be seen coming down the esophagus, passing in an arc through the stomach toward the right of midline, and then progressing downward in a reverse arc through the duodenum, back to the left, across the vertebral column. It is best to have the tip of these feeding tubes near the junction of the

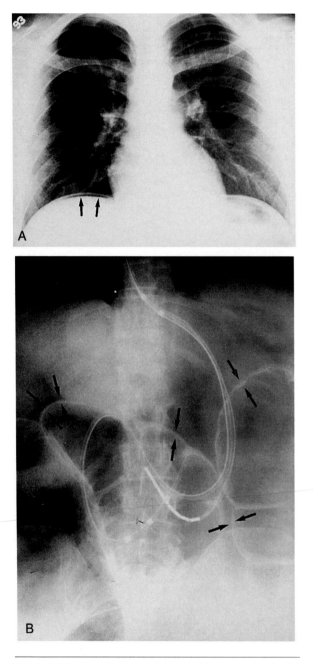

FIGURE 6–5 **Pneumoperitoneum.** *A,* A few mL of free air can be identified under the right hemidiaphragm on this upright PA chest x-ray. *B,* A supine abdominal film obtained on a different patient with massive pneumoperitoneum shows the bowel wall *(arrows)* outlined by air.

duodenum and jejunum (ligament of Treitz) (Fig. 6–7). An unacceptable position of a feeding tube tip is in the esophagus or at the gastro-esophageal junction (Fig. 6–8). If you feed patients with a tube in these positions, there can be esophageal reflux and the potential for aspiration.

Abdominal Calcifications

Abdominal calcifications are quite common, and you should be familiar with them so that you know which ones are important and which ones to discount (Table 6–3). Fortunately, most of them have some characteristics that make this task relatively easy. Calcifications in the right upper quadrant are usually gallstones or kidney

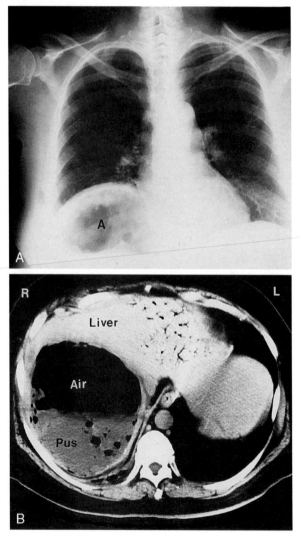

FIGURE 6–6. **Hepatic abscess.** This drug abuser presented with right upper quadrant pain and fever. On the upright chest film *(A),* a collection of air is seen in the right upper quadrant. Notice that there is a thick and irregular margin between the air and the hemidiaphragm, indicating that this is not free air. A transverse CT scan *(B)* shows an air and pus collection due to a large abscess in the right lobe of the liver.

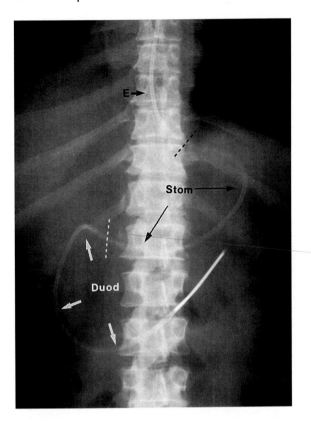

FIGURE 6–7. Optimal positioning for an enteric feeding tube. On an AP film of the upper abdomen, the feeding tube should be seen extending down the esophagus slightly to the left of midline, taking a gentle curve to the right through the stomach, and then reversing its curve through the duodenum and going back to the left across the spine to the junction of the fourth portion of the duodenum and the jejunum (ligament of Treitz).

FIGURE 6–8. Unacceptable position of feeding tube. In this case, the tip of the feeding tube is in the distal esophagus with the remainder coiled within the body of the stomach. Feeding with the tube in this position is likely to cause aspiration.

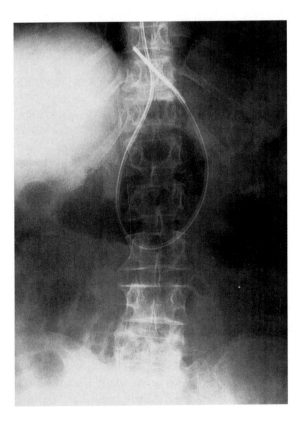

TABLE 6–3. Differential Diagnosis of Abdominal Calcifications

Right Upper Quadrant
Gallstones
Renal calculus, cyst, or tumor
Adrenal calcification

Right Midabdomen or Right Lower Quadrant
Ureteral calculi
Mesenteric lymph node
Appendicolith

Left Upper Quadrant
Splenic artery
Splenic cyst
Splenic histoplasmosis (multiple and small)
Renal calculus, cyst, or tumor
Adrenal calcification
Tail of pancreas

Central Abdomen
Aorta or aortic aneurysm
Pancreas (chronic pancreatitis)
Calcified metastatic nodes

Pelvis
Phleboliths (low in pelvis)
Uterine fibroids (popcorn appearance)
Dermoid
Bladder stone
Calcification in buttocks from injections
Prostatic (behind symphysis)
Vas deferens (diabetic)
Iliac or femoral vessels

related to splenic artery calcification or to a splenic artery aneurysm, respectively (Fig. 6–12).

With chronic pancreatitis, there is often calcification of the pancreas. This can be seen as spotted or mottled calcification, usually lying in a somewhat horizontal distribution over the vertebral bodies of L1 and L2 and extending to the left. Remember, however, that on a plain abdominal x-ray most people with chronic pancreatitis do not have visible calcifications. CT scanning can identify calcifications much more easily than a standard x-ray (Fig. 6–13A), but you should rely on clinical and laboratory history, not a CT scan (Fig. 6–13B), for the diagnosis of chronic pancreatitis.

Calcification of mesenteric lymph nodes can occur as a result of previous infections. These are usually seen as somewhat rounded or popcorn-shaped calcifications in the right midabdomen. A tip-off is the significant downward movement of these calcifications on the upright views, since the mesentery is very mobile (Fig. 6–14).

In a patient who has right lower quadrant

stones. If the calcifications are multiple, are very close together, and lie outside the normal expected area of the kidney, you can be reasonably assured that they are gallstones (Fig. 6–9). A single calcification in the right upper quadrant may be due either to a kidney stone or to a gallstone. A simple way to tell the difference is to take a right posterior oblique view. A gallstone will rotate anteriorly and will not move with the outline of the kidney. Another way to tell the difference is to order a right upper quadrant ultrasound study, on which gallstones are very easily identified (Fig. 6–10). In addition, if the patient has right upper quadrant pain or jaundice, the ultrasound image will allow you to assess whether the common bile duct is dilated and look at the internal architecture of the liver and pancreas.

Left upper quadrant calcifications are essentially always related to the spleen. Multiple small punctate calcifications are the result of histoplasmosis (Fig. 6–11). Serpiginous or rounded calcifications in the left upper quadrant usually are

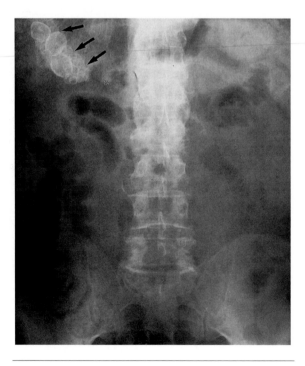

FIGURE 6–9. Multiple gallstones. Any collection of grouped calcifications in the right upper quadrant *(arrows)* is most likely due to gallstones but does not indicate acute cholecystitis.

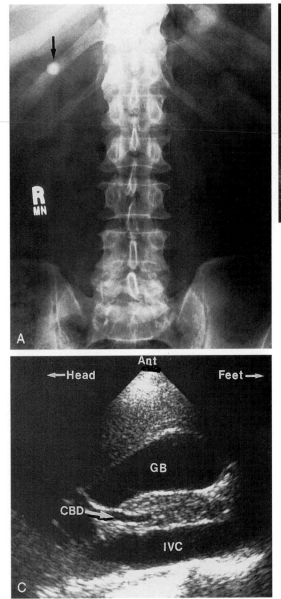

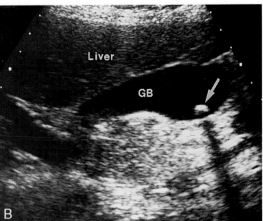

FIGURE 6–10. Single gallstone. *A,* On the KUB (plain film of the abdomen), a single calcification is seen in the right upper quadrant. It is not possible to tell from this one picture whether this is a gallstone, kidney stone, or calcification in some other structure. *B,* A longitudinal ultrasound image in this patient clearly shows the liver, gallbladder, and an echogenic focus *(arrow)* within the gallbladder lumen, representing the single gallstone. Also note that there is a dark shadow behind the gallstone. *C,* Another longitudinal ultrasound image slightly more medial also shows the inferior vena cava and the common bile duct, which can be measured. Here it is of normal diameter.

FIGURE 6–11. Splenic histoplasmosis. Multiple small rounded calcifications in the left upper quadrant (some of which are shown with small arrows) are very specific, representing previous infection with histoplasmosis. These are of little, if any, clinical significance.

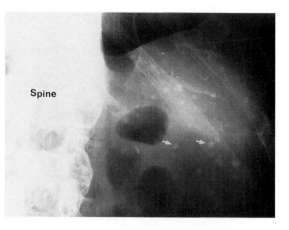

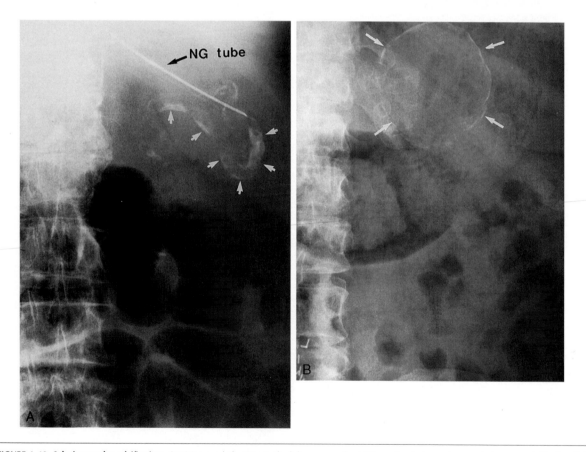

FIGURE 6–12. Splenic vascular calcifications. Serpiginous calcifications in the left upper quadrant *(A)* are almost always due to splenic artery calcification. This finding is of no clinical significance. Occasionally, there can be splenic artery aneurysms, which may cause a shell-like, rounded left upper quadrant calcification *(B)*.

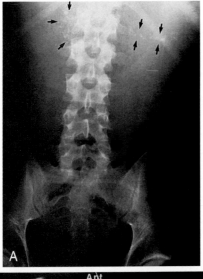

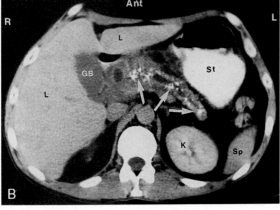

FIGURE 6–13. Calcification in chronic pancreatitis. Rarely, on a plain film of the abdomen (A), a horizontal band of calcifications can be seen extending across the upper midabdomen (arrows). Calcification within the pancreas is much easier to see on a transverse CT scan of the upper abdomen (B). Calcification is seen as white speckled areas within the pancreas (arrows). The darker areas within the pancreas represent dilated common and pancreatic ducts.

pain, you should look very carefully in this area for calcifications. A stone within the appendix (appendicolith) often projects over the right side of the sacrum (Fig. 6–15) and can be difficult to see unless you look carefully. An appendicolith is present in approximately 10 per cent of patients with appendicitis, and if you see an appendicolith, there is a very high probability of appendicitis. Other signs of appendicitis are a bubbly gas collection (appendiceal abscess) in the left lower quadrant or a focal ileus (dilatation) of the nearby small bowel caused by the inflammatory reaction.

In adults, it is very common to see rounded calcifications in the lower half of the pelvis. These almost always are 1 cm or less in diameter, and they are phleboliths (calcifications within pelvic venous structures). They are easy

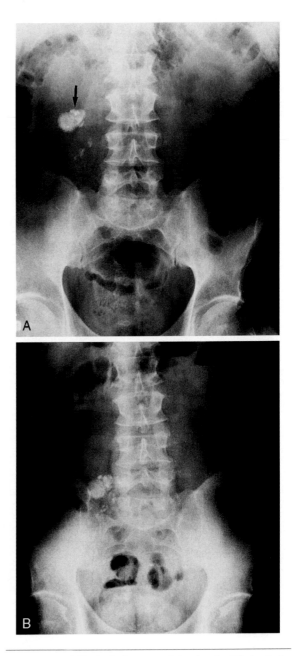

FIGURE 6–14. Calcification in the mesenteric lymph nodes. This is a benign finding. The calcifications are typically located in the midabdomen to the right of midline, are somewhat popcorn shaped (arrow), and are relatively easy to see on a supine KUB (A). On an upright view of the abdomen (B), these calcifications drop substantially owing to the mobility of the mesentery.

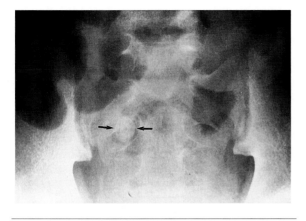

FIGURE 6–15. Appendicolith. This calcification within the appendix can be seen almost anywhere in the right lower quadrant but is especially difficult to see when it overlies the sacrum *(arrows)*. A right lower quadrant calcification in a patient with pain in this area should carry an extremely high clinical suspicion of acute appendicitis.

to identify, since they often have a lucent or dark center (Fig. 6–16). They can occasionally be confused with stones in the distal ureter, and if a patient has symptoms of renal colic or obstruction, it is often necessary to perform an intravenous pyelogram to determine which of the calcifications in the lower pelvis may be a phlebolith or a calculus.

Uterine fibroids can often be calcified. The type of calcification is very similar to the popcorn type seen in the mesenteric lymph nodes.

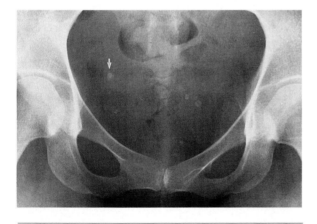

FIGURE 6–16. Phleboliths. These rounded vascular calcifications within the pelvis are very common and are of no clinical significance. They are usually round and less than 1 cm in diameter. They often have a lucent or dark center. They are typically seen in the lower half of the pelvic brim and can occasionally be difficult to differentiate from a ureteral calculus without an intravenous pyelogram.

The difference is that fibroids are located in a suprapubic position and centrally in the pelvis. On occasion, these can be quite large and spectacular (Fig. 6–17).

Two special types of calcification can be seen in the male pelvis. The first, found immediately behind the symphysis pubis, is quite common and is the result of benign inflammatory disease (Fig. 6–18). The second, and more rare, type of calcification looks like a little set of antlers in the middle of the pelvis, projecting slightly above the symphysis pubis. This represents calcification of the vas deferens and almost always indicates that the patient is a diabetic (Fig. 6–19).

ESOPHAGUS

Anatomy and Imaging Techniques

The appropriate initial imaging study for a number of suspected clinical problems is shown in Table 6–4. Imaging of the esophagus for many problems is best done by direct visualization (endoscopy). Since this is a major procedure requiring sedation, many physicians begin by ordering an upper gastrointestinal (GI) examination or a contrast esophagogram. In addition to barium, other contrast materials that are water soluble can be used. If a tear or perforation of the esophagus is suspected, it is best to initially use water-soluble contrast material rather than

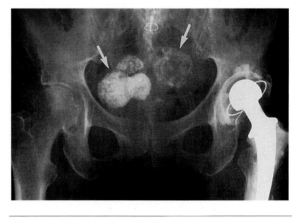

FIGURE 6–17. Calcified fibroids. Central pelvic calcifications, which are somewhat amorphous, most commonly represent fibroids *(arrows)*.

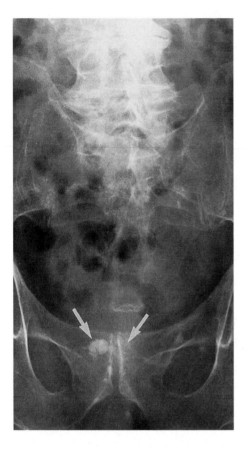

FIGURE 6–18. Prostatic calcification. Calcification situated immediately behind the pubis *(arrows)* in a male usually represents the sequelae of previous prostatitis.

FIGURE 6–19. Calcification of the vas deferens. These bilateral asymmetric calcifications occur in the lower to middle portion of the male pelvis. When they are seen, they almost always indicate that the patient is diabetic.

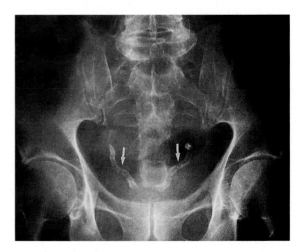

TABLE 6–4. Initial Study to Order for Various Clinical Problems

Suspected Clinical Problem	Imaging Study
Esophageal obstruction	Barium swallow
Esophageal tear	Gastrografin swallow
Bowel perforation or free air	Upright chest and supine abdominal plain film
	Supine and left lateral decubitus if patient is unable to stand
Hematemesis	Endoscopy
	Upper GI series
Gastric or duodenal ulcer	Upper GI series
Trauma	CT
Aortic aneurysm	KUB and lateral
	US or CT
Pancreatic pathology	CT (intravenous and GI contrast)
Abscess	CT (intravenous and GI contrast)
Right upper quadrant pain	
Rule out cholelithiasis	Right upper quadrant ultrasound
Rule out common duct obstruction	Right upper quadrant ultrasound or ERCP
Rule out acute cholecystitis	Nuclear medicine hepatobiliary study
Suspected bile leak	Nuclear medicine hepatobiliary study
Intestinal obstruction	KUB and upright plain film of abdomen
Rule out proximal obstruction	Upper GI and small bowel series
Rule out colon obstruction	Barium enema
Right lower quadrant pain	KUB
Rule out appendicitis	Ultrasound
Rule out abscess	CT
Rule out ureteral stone	IVP
Pelvic pain	
Ureteral stone	IVP
Bladder pathology	Cystogram
Uterine or ovarian pathology	US
Tumor	CT
Trauma	CT
Diverticulitis	Barium enema
Rectal bleeding	
Dark red	Upper GI series
Bright red	Colonoscopy
Unknown source	Barium enema
	Nuclear medicine bleeding study

barium. If aspiration is suspected, barium is used, since water-soluble contrast can irritate the lung.

The normal esophagus has a rather smooth lining. Two indentations, due to impression by the aortic arch and the left mainstem bronchus, can be seen along the left side (Fig. 6–20). Normally, there is a peristaltic wave, initiated by swallowing, which propels food down the esophagus. You should not diagnose a stricture on the basis of one image alone, since you may be looking at a normal area of peristaltic contraction. Sometimes in the distal portion of the esophagus, a **Z** line can be seen going across the

esophagus. This represents the junction between the mucosa of the esophagus and the stomach (Fig. 6–21).

Esophageal Diverticula

In the lower cervical region, there sometimes is a pharyngeal diverticulum (known as Zenker's diverticulum) that projects posteriorly. Food can be caught in this, and it can cause dysphagia (Fig. 6–22). In the middle of the esophagus (near the carina) there may be a traction diverticulum caused by scarring from mediastinal granulomatous disease. Just above the stomach, a pulsion diverticulum can sometimes be found. The two latter types are rarely symptomatic.

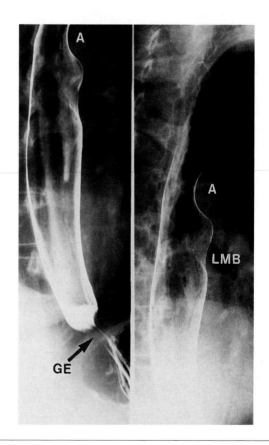

FIGURE 6–20. Normal anatomy of the esophagus. The upper portion of the esophagus is seen on the image on the right and the lower half in the image on the left. An indentation along the left side of the esophagus occurs from the aorta (A) and another less significant one from the left mainstem bronchus (LMB). As the distal aspect of the esophagus goes through the diaphragm, the gastroesophageal junction (GE) can also be identified.

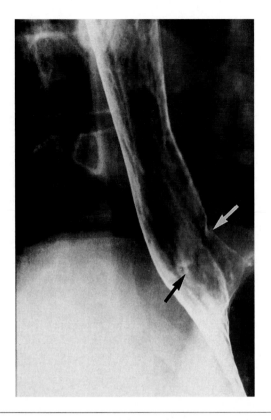

FIGURE 6–21. Junction of the esophageal and gastric mucosa. In the distal esophagus, it is sometimes possible to see a dark horizontal zigzag line (between the two arrows). This is called the **Z** line and represents the normal junction between the two different types of mucosa.

Presbyesophagus

As a function of aging, there may be development of tertiary deep contractions within the esophagus. These are usually disordered and can interfere with the normal peristaltic process and swallowing. These tertiary contractions are easily visualized as multiple transverse or ring-like contractions of the esophagus (Fig. 6–23). No specific therapy is indicated for this condition, and it is very common in persons over the age of 60 years.

Hiatal Hernia

A large number of people suffer from "heartburn" or dysphagia as a result of reflux of gastric contents into the esophagus. This most often occurs because of a hiatal hernia. The most common

type of hiatal hernia is the sliding type, in which the gastroesophageal junction and a portion of the fundus of the stomach slide upward into the thorax. Small hiatal hernias can be identified by noting an indentation at the distal esophagus known as Schatzki's ring as well as longitudinal gastric mucosa folds distal to the ring (Fig. 6–24). Large hiatal hernias can be identified by seeing the fundus of the stomach projecting up into the retrocardiac space (Fig. 6–25). Another type of hiatal hernia occurs more rarely. This is the paraesophageal type, in which the fundus of the stomach slips up past the gastroesophageal junction, which remains in the normal location. Large hiatal hernias can be seen on the chest x-ray, even without the use of barium. The typical finding is an air-fluid level or soft tissue mass located behind the heart but in front of the spine (Fig. 6–26).

Esophageal reflux can sometimes be seen on an upper GI examination, but if it is not seen, the patient may still be refluxing at other times and under other conditions. There is a more

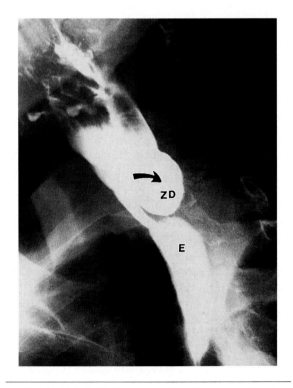

FIGURE 6–22. Zenker's diverticulum. This is basically an outpouching of mucosa (ZD) in the pharynx. Food can be caught in this and cause symptoms. The esophagus (E) can be seen distally.

FIGURE 6–23. Presbyesophagus. These tertiary or ringlike contractions are commonly seen in older persons, and they can disrupt the normal peristaltic motility of the esophagus.

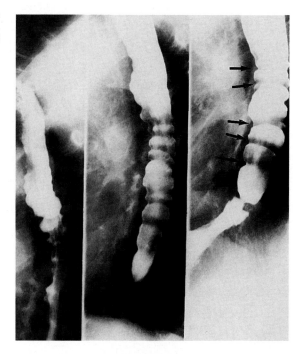

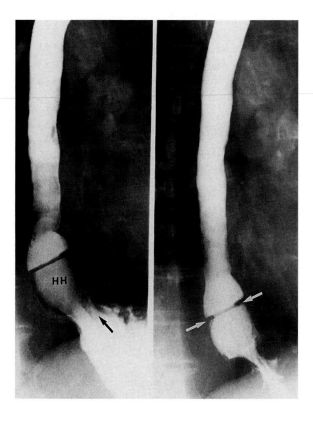

FIGURE 6–24. Small sliding type hiatal hernia. When a small portion of the fundus of the stomach slips up through the hemidiaphragm, a small hiatal hernia (HH) can be identified. The two keys to identification are (1) a very sharp ringlike construction (called Schatzki's ring, which is seen between the two white arrows); and (2) the normal longitudinal lines of gastric mucosa *(black arrow)*, which can be seen projecting up above the hemidiaphragm.

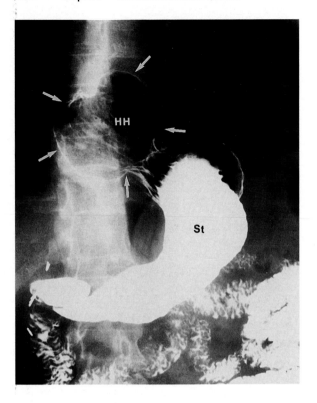

FIGURE 6–25. **Large sliding type hiatal hernia.** A large portion of the fundus of the stomach has slipped up through the hemidiaphragm into the retrocardiac region *(arrows)* and can easily be identified on an upper gastrointestinal examination.

sensitive imaging method using nuclear medicine. A small amount of radioactive material is mixed with orange juice, which the patient drinks. A computer region of interest is set up over the chest, abdominal compression is applied and the patient is followed for about 1 hour. If the study is positive there is reflux, but if it is negative the same caveat applies. A more invasive but more accurate method used by gastroenterologists is to put a pH probe on the end of a tube and station this for some time above the gastroesophageal junction.

Foreign Bodies of the Esophagus

The foreign bodies lodged in the esophagus of children are most commonly coins. They often stick just above the level of the aortic arch (Fig. 6–27). A number of other foreign bodies lodge at the gastroesophageal junction (Fig. 6–28). In adults the most common object is a piece of unchewed meat. Meat will not be visualized on a plain x-ray but can easily be seen during a contrast esophagogram.

Strictures and Dilatation

Strictures in the esophagus are a common cause of food lodging at a specific level. High esophageal strictures can occur as a result of scarring after suicide attempts in which the individual swallowed lye or corrosive alkaline material (Fig. 6–29). Mid- and distal esophageal strictures may develop from scarring due to gastroesophageal reflux or may result from a tumor. Most benign strictures have a smooth appearance. The diameter of a stricture can be assessed during a barium swallow by giving the patient a radiopaque pill of known diameter. These pills will quickly dissolve (Fig. 6–30). Strictures due to carcinomas most commonly are irregular and have overhanging edges (Fig. 6–31). Even benign appearing strictures are usually biopsied to exclude malignancy.

There are two entities that can cause marked dilatation of the esophagus. These are achalasia and scleroderma. The esophagus may be so dilated that it can be visualized on chest x-ray as a tortuous structure in the post-tracheal and retrocardiac regions, and often a horizontal air-

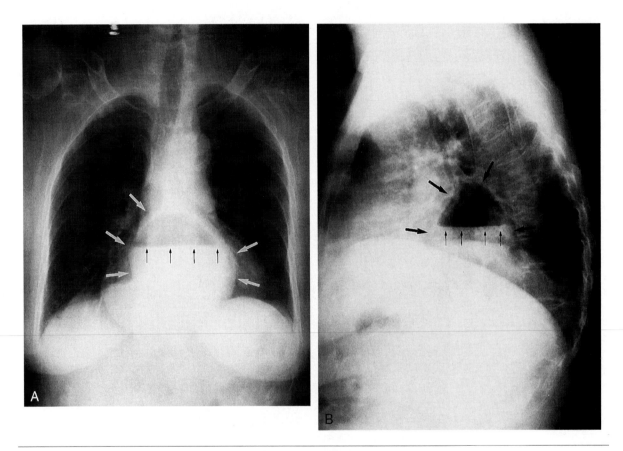

FIGURE 6–26. Large hiatal hernia. Hiatal hernias can sometimes be seen on a plain chest x-ray. On an upright PA chest x-ray *(A)*, a mass with an air-fluid level within it can be seen behind the heart *(large arrows)*. This can also be easily seen on the lateral chest x-ray *(B)*.

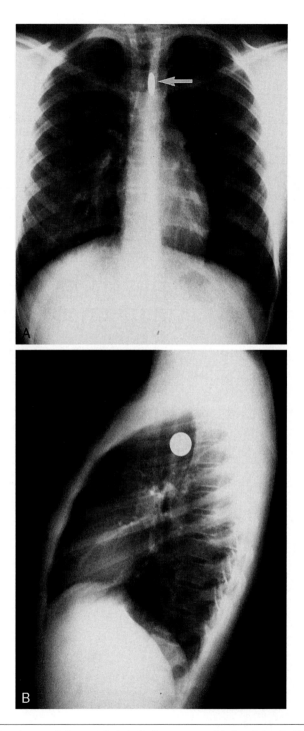

FIGURE 6–27. Coin in the esophagus. The coin can easily be seen in both the PA chest x-ray *(A)* and the lateral view *(B)*. Objects often stick at this level because the esophagus is somewhat narrowed here by the impression of the aortic arch.

FIGURE 6–28. Steak knife lodged at the esophagogastric junction. This mentally ill patient claimed to have swallowed his steak knife at dinnertime. The chest x-ray shows the metallic blade *(arrow)* at the gastroesophageal junction. The wooden handle of the knife, which is down in the stomach, is not seen because wood typically is not visible on an x-ray. Metallic surgical clips are seen to the left of the stomach gas bubble. These are from a previous surgery to remove other swallowed objects.

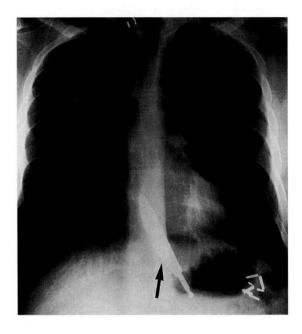

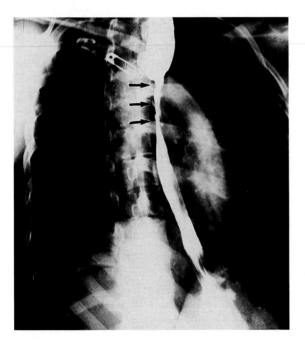

FIGURE 6–29. Benign esophageal stricture. This upper esophageal stricture *(arrows)* was due to attempted suicide by lye ingestion. Notice that the stricture does not have any overhanging edges and is relatively smooth and tapered. Essentially all patients with esophageal strictures should have esophagoscopy and biopsy to rule out malignancy.

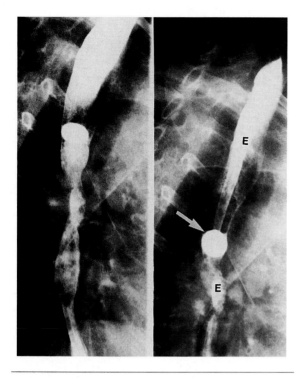

FIGURE 6–30. Measurement of an esophageal stricture. During a barium swallow, a radiopaque pill of known diameter *(arrow)* can be given. This will lodge above a stricture, but it will quickly dissolve. Knowing the size of the pill allows measurement of a stricture.

fluid level can be seen in the upper esophagus. Air-fluid levels within the esophagus are definitely abnormal.

In achalasia (Fig. 6–32), the gastroesophageal sphincter fails to relax. The esophagus becomes massively dilated and tapers distally to a beaklike shape. There usually is no evidence of gastroesophageal reflux. A massively dilated esophagus that looks like achalasia can also be seen in Chagas' disease, which is caused by an infection with *Trypanosoma cruzi*. This parasite releases a neurotoxin that destroys ganglion cells in the myenteric plexus. Scleroderma is a collagen vascular disease involving the smooth muscle. The esophagus is usually only mildly dilated and has no primary contractions. Gastroesophageal reflux can occur with this condition, causing stricture and ultimately proximal dilatation.

Esophagitis and Tears

Ulceration and irregularity of the esophageal mucosa can be the result of reflux esophagitis,

and in these circumstances the irregularities are very fine. In patients who are immunocompromised, there may be *Candida albicans (Monilia)* infection of the esophagus that creates a very coarse irregular pattern (Fig. 6–33).

Tears of the esophagus occur in Boerhaave's syndrome as well as in Mallory-Weiss syndrome. In Boerhaave's syndrome, there is spontaneous perforation of the esophagus due to a sudden increase in intraluminal esophageal pressure, and the patient clinically has severe epigastric pain. Overall mortality in this syndrome is approximately 25 per cent, but it approaches 100 per cent if diagnosis is delayed 24 hours. Severe epigastric pain and dyspnea are common. An erect chest film is useful, since it may demonstrate a left pleural fluid collection, left pneumothorax, or mediastinal air.

A Mallory-Weiss tear is usually a longitudi-

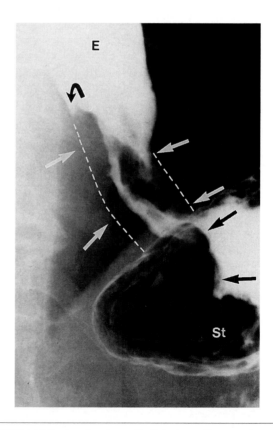

FIGURE 6–31. Esophageal carcinoma. On this barium swallow, a spot image at the gastroesophageal junction clearly shows a dilated distal esophagus (E) as well as the fundus of the stomach (ST). A thin, irregular column of barium is seen joining the two, and there are overhanging beaklike edges *(dark curved arrow)*, which suggest a malignancy. The normal contour of the esophagus is outlined, and the dark straight arrows indicate a mass protruding into the fundus of the stomach.

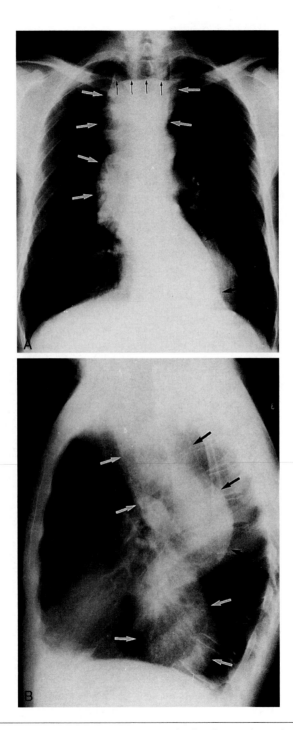

FIGURE 6–32. Achalasia. On the frontal chest x-ray *(A)*, a tortuous structure is seen extending from the cervical region down into the retrocardiac region *(arrows)*. An air-fluid level is also seen near the top *(small arrows)*. This represents a massively dilated esophagus due to achalasia. The dilated esophagus is also seen on the lateral chest x-ray *(B)*, since it is dilated and filled with fluid.

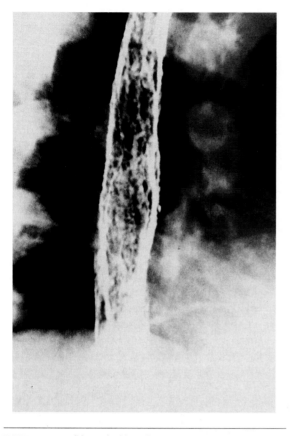

FIGURE 6–33. Candida esophagitis. In this immunocompromised AIDS patient, the normal smooth esophageal mucosa has been replaced by a rough and irregular ulcerated mucosa extending the length of the esophagus. Very tiny ulcerations can be seen in tangent along the edge of the esophagus.

nal nontransmural tear in the lesser curvature of the stomach, often extending across the gastroesophageal junction. These tears are produced by prolonged vomiting in alcoholics, are usually self-limited, and are not painful. There should be no evidence of a pneumomediastinum, although there is hematemesis.

Varices

Long, tortuous, longitudinal or vertical wormlike filling defects in the distal esophagus can be the result of varices. The large vascular channels in the esophageal wall are large enough to displace barium (Fig. 6–34). The best way to appreciate varices is by endoscopy, since only when the varices are large and extensive are they seen on a barium swallow.

Tumors

Malignant tumors of the esophagus are squamous cell carcinoma 95 per cent of the time and adenocarcinoma about 5 per cent of the time. Adenocarcinomas usually arise in the region of the gastroesophageal junction or have grown out of the stomach to involve the lower esophagus (see Figure 6–31). Adenocarcinomas also occur somewhat higher up in the esophagus in patients with chronic gastroesophageal reflux who develop islands of columnar mucosa (Barrett's esophagus).

STOMACH AND DUODENUM

Anatomy and Imaging Techniques

Lesions of the stomach and duodenum are most appropriately visualized utilizing an upper GI

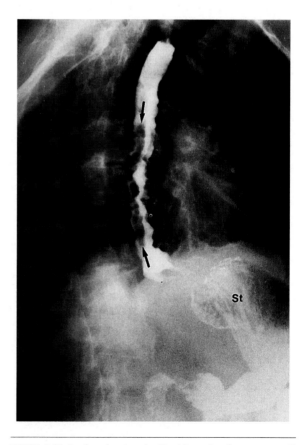

FIGURE 6–34. Esophageal varices. In this oblique view from an upper GI examination performed on an alcoholic patient, a large, dark, wormlike filling density (arrows) is seen in the distal esophagus. It is caused by varices protruding into the lumen of the esophagus. The stomach (St) is also seen.

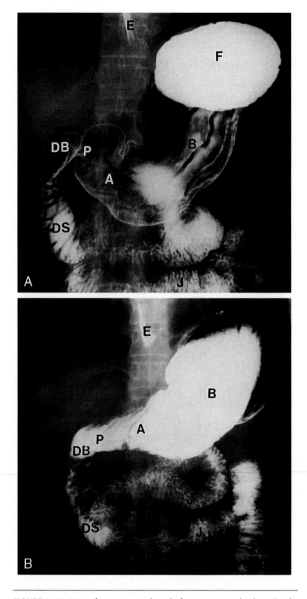

FIGURE 6–35. Normal upper gastrointestinal contrast examination. On the supine view (A), the barium layers in the most dependent portions. The esophagus (e), fundus (f), body (b), antrum (a), and pylorus (p) of the stomach are all easily identified. The normal longitudinal gastric mucosa is also seen. The duodenal bulb, duodenal sweep, and jejunum are also identified with their predominantly transverse mucosal pattern. On a prone view (B), the barium collects in the body and antrum of the stomach, since these are more dependent in that particular projection.

examination or endoscopy. If a perforated viscus is suspected, Gastrografin (meglumine diatrizoate) or another water-soluble material should be used as a contrast agent rather than barium. CT scanning is usually not an appropriate initial imaging modality for most stomach or intestinal pathology.

The appearance of the stomach on an upper GI study can be variable depending on whether the patient is prone or supine. With the patient supine, barium collects in the most dependent position, which is the fundus of the stomach, and the normal mucosal patterns of the body and antrum are easily visualized (Fig. 6–35). In the prone position, the body and antrum of the stomach are the most dependent, and barium will collect there. The duodenal bulb projects upward to the right and posteriorly relative to the gastric antrum. It is important to obtain images with the bulb distended. Radiologists will almost always take several pictures of the bulb in different stages of peristalsis (Fig. 6–36).

The duodenum has a C loop configuration and extends to the ligament of Treitz near the body of the stomach. The jejunum is usually located in the left midabdomen and the ileum in the lower central and right abdomen. There are two normal variants that you should be aware of. The first is malrotation of the small bowel, with a number of variations. The stom-

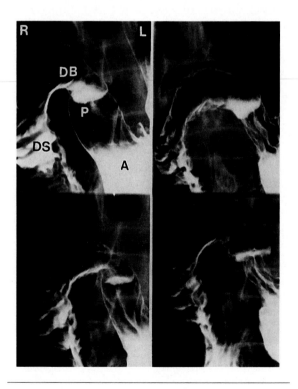

FIGURE 6–36. Spot views of the duodenal bulb. Several views of the duodenal bulb are typically obtained, since it is undergoing active peristalsis during examination. Here, four similar spot views taken several seconds apart are shown indicating the antrum, pylorus, duodenal bulb, and duodenal sweep.

ach and duodenal bulb may be in a normal position, but the third and fourth portions of the duodenum may be on the right side of the spine rather than swinging across the spine and behind the stomach in the region of the ligament of Treitz (Fig. 6–37). Sometimes the duodenum is positioned normally, but all the small bowel is on the right side and the cecum and colon are on the left side. Another, much less common, variant is situs inversus, in which the liver, stomach, and all abdominal organs are reversed between right and left, and the heart is on the right (Fig. 6–38).

Gastritis and Gastric Ulcer Disease

Large gastric folds may be the result of simple gastritis, although they are also seen with lymphoma, Menetrier's disease (giant hypertrophic gastritis), and Zollinger-Ellison syndrome. Simple gastritis may be present without ulceration, and the only finding on an upper GI examination may be enlarged gastric folds (Fig. 6–39).

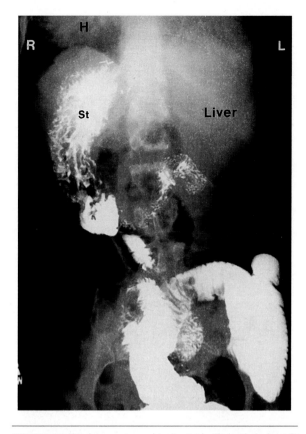

FIGURE 6–38. Situs inversus. A complete situs is identified with the heart (h) and stomach (st) on the right and the liver on the left.

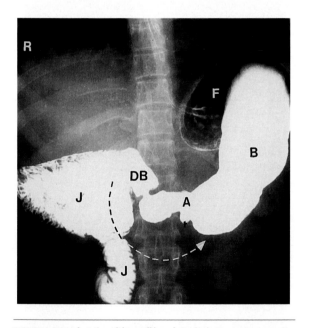

FIGURE 6–37. Malrotation of the small bowel. On this barium contrast examination, the fundus (f), body (b), and antrum (a) of the stomach as well as the duodenal bulb (db) are in normal position. However, the duodenal sweep and jejunum (j) should normally sweep across in the direction of the dotted arrow to the left behind the gastric antrum. In this case, owing to a congenital malrotation, the jejunum is on the right side of the spine.

Ulcers are unusual in Menetrier's disease but are quite common in Zollinger-Ellison syndrome.

The detection rate of gastric ulcers by upper GI examination is only approximately 70 per cent. The nondetectable ulcers are often too superficial or too small to see. Occasionally the ulcers are so large that the crater is overlooked.

Ulcers that are identified on upper GI examination should be characterized as benign, indeterminate, or malignant. In general, benign ulcers decrease to half their original size with several weeks of therapy and should show almost complete healing within 6 weeks. Unless an ulcer has all benign features, endoscopy with biopsy is usually recommended. There are four radiographic signs of a benign ulcer. If the mucosal folds are thin and regular and extend up to the margin of the ulcer crater, the lesion is probably benign. Benign ulcers typically extend beyond the projected margin of the stomach (Fig. 6–40A). There may be a 1 to 2 mm lucent

FIGURE 6–39. Gastritis. In the body of the stomach, thickened mucosal folds *(arrows)*, the result of inflammation, can be seen.

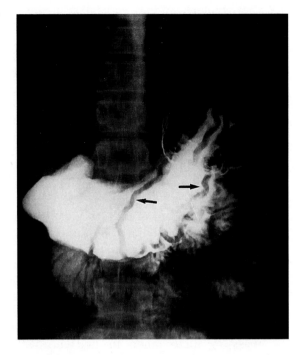

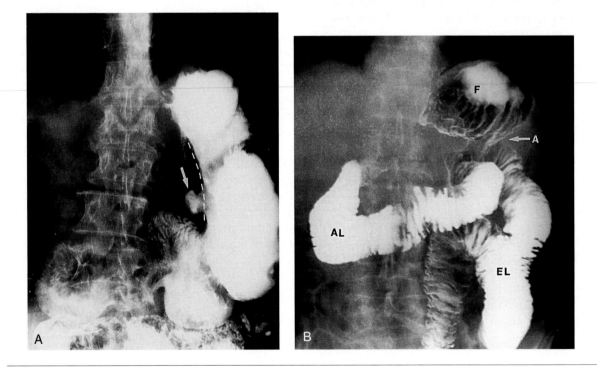

FIGURE 6–40. Benign gastric ulcer. *A,* A large ulcer *(arrow)* is seen along the lesser curvature of the stomach. Notice that the ulcer projects out beyond the normal expected lesser curvature *(dotted lines);* this is one sign that the lesion is benign. *B,* A Billroth II operation was performed for recurrent ulcers and shows the residual fundus (F) of the stomach as well as the anastomosis (A) and the afferent (AL) and efferent (EL) loops of small bowel.

line around the mouth of the ulcer on a tangential view. Finally, normal peristalsis in the region and invagination of the wall opposite the ulcer are helpful signs to indicate benignity. Historically, a treatment for recurrent ulcer disease was a Billroth II operation. In this, there is resection of the distal aspect of the stomach, with an anastomosis made between the fundus of the stomach and the small bowel at the level of the ligament of Treitz. This leaves a blind-ending afferent loop composed of second, third, and fourth portions of the duodenum (see Fig. 6–40B). At the present time most benign ulcers are treated with H_2 blocking agents.

In fact, 95 per cent of all ulcers are benign, and 5 per cent are malignant. Of the malignant ulcers, 90 per cent are due to carcinoma and a lesser extent to lymphoma and other rare malignancies or metastases. With a cancer, there is usually a thickened and markedly irregular wall. Peristalsis is limited or decreased. The stomach may have decreased distensibility, and the mass or ulcer tends to lie within the projected outline of the stomach, rather than projecting beyond it (Fig. 6–41). If the tumor becomes large enough to involve most of the stomach, the stomach becomes rigid and nondistensible, and this is termed "linitis plastica" (leather bottle stomach).

Duodenal Ulcers

Ulcers that arise within the first portion of the duodenum are benign at least 90 per cent of the time. These may have an infectious origin, and the spiral organism *Helicobacter pylori* has been implicated. Ulcers that occur distal to the duodenal bulb should be considered malignant until proved otherwise. Duodenal ulcers are two to three times more common than gastric ulcers. Their location is bulbar in 95 per cent of cases and postbulbar in 5 per cent. In the duodenal bulb, the anterior wall is the most common site of ulceration, and these anterior ulcers can lead to perforation, peritonitis, and pneumoperitoneum. Ulcers in the posterior wall of the duodenal bulb may penetrate into the pancreas. Duodenal ulcers can be difficult to appreciate if you have not seen a lot of upper GI examinations. The key to identification is a duodenal defect

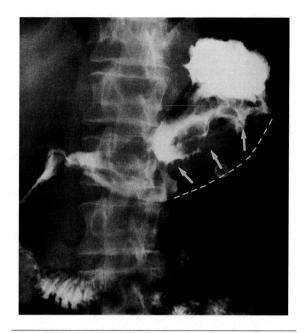

FIGURE 6–41. Malignant gastric ulceration. A large series of ulcers is seen along the greater curvature of the stomach. Notice that, in addition, there is a mass projecting into the lumen from the expected normal greater curvature *(dotted lines)*. This is a sign of malignancy.

that contains barium and remains essentially unchanged on the multiple spot films that are obtained. There is generally edema or thickening of the mucosal folds in the proximal duodenum. Duodenal ulcers often heal with a scar that is accompanied by deformity and shrinking of the duodenal bulb. This is sometimes referred to as an "hourglass" or "cloverleaf" deformity (Fig. 6–42).

A duodenal diverticulum should not be confused with a duodenal ulcer. Duodenal diverticula are reasonably common and are seen as an outpouching of barium along the inner curvature of the duodenal sweep. The most common location is near the ampulla of Vater. There is no associated mucosal thickening or spasm, and these diverticula are asymptomatic.

Gastric Emptying

Patients with abnormal gastric motility may have either accelerated emptying of gastric contents (dumping) or delayed gastric emptying. The latter is quite common in diabetics. Since barium is not physiologic, nuclear medicine

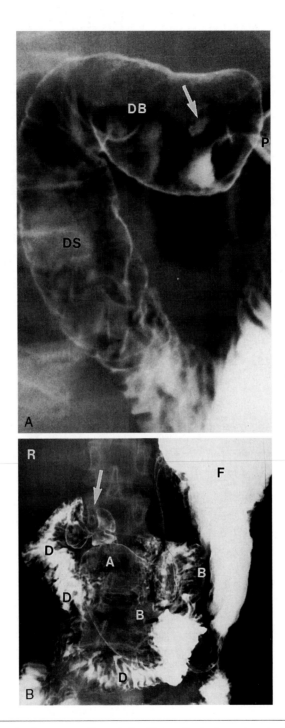

FIGURE 6–42. Duodenal ulceration. A spot view from an upper GI examination *(A)* shows the duodenum. An acute ulcer is seen as a persistent barium collection *(arrow)* just distal to the pylorus. This was seen on multiple views. A different patient with a healed ulcer and scarring had an upper GI examination *(B)*. The fundus, body, and antrum of the stomach are normal as is most of the duodenal sweep. The duodenal bulb, however, has a cloverleaf deformity *(arrow)* due to scarring.

studies that tag food or liquid with a small amount of radioactive material are used to quantitate gastric emptying. Computer regions of interest are drawn over the stomach, and the emptying rate is calculated. For solid foods, half the material should leave the stomach in less than 90 minutes (Fig. 6–43).

LIVER

Today the most common method of imaging the liver and spleen is with a CT scan. In many institutions CT scans are done with and without the use of intravenous contrast. For most situations, however, a single CT scan utilizing intravenous contrast is often adequate and cheaper. The liver or spleen can also be imaged using ultrasound or nuclear medicine, but there is less anatomic resolution and less complete imaging of other nearby structures.

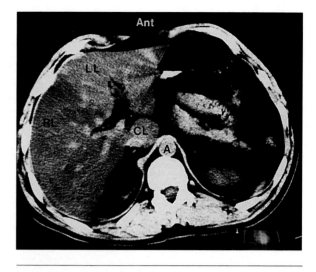

FIGURE 6–44. Focal fatty infiltration of the liver. On this transverse CT scan (done without intravenous contrast), the right lobe of the liver (RL) is darker than the left lobe (LL). This is due to fatty infiltration of the right lobe. Notice also that there has been sparing of the caudate lobe (CL). Normal vascular structures are seen in the right lobe, even without contrast enhancement, because they are surrounded by fat.

Alcoholic Liver Disease

Probably the most common imaging manifestation of alcoholic liver disease is fatty infiltration. On a noncontrasted CT scan, the liver and spleen should be of the same density. If the liver is darker than the spleen or muscle, you can suspect fatty infiltration. Often the fatty infiltration is focal and not uniform, especially since portal venous flow delivers more alcohol to the right lobe of the liver than to the left lobe (Fig. 6–44).

Obesity is the most common cause of a fatty liver. The low density in the area can usually be differentiated from low density due to malignancy or other abnormality because fatty infiltration is usually geographic or has straight borders in its distribution. There is also lack of a mass effect, with normal vessels and architecture being preserved in the areas of the fat, and, finally, the periportal region or medial segment of the left lobe is often spared. Even without the use of intravenous contrast, the hepatic and portal veins in the area of fatty infiltration will appear prominent (whiter) because of the surrounding low density.

Ascites is another common manifestation of alcoholic liver disease. If ascites is massive, gas

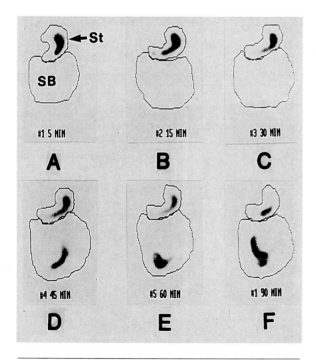

FIGURE 6–43. Quantitative gastric emptying. Evaluation of gastric emptying can be done by giving the patient a small amount of radioactively labeled scrambled eggs or oatmeal. Computer regions of interest are drawn about the stomach (St) and over the small bowel (SB). Quantitation by computer of the two regions allows determination of the amount of time it takes for half the food to leave the stomach. This is used to determine if various therapies or interventions have been effective.

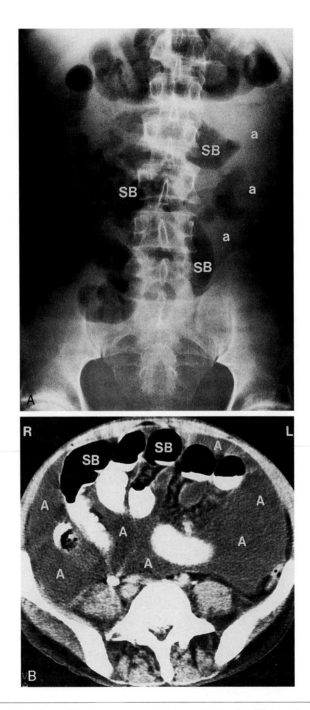

FIGURE 6–45. Ascites. On a plain film of the abdomen *(A)*, only gross amounts of ascites can be identified. This is usually seen because the ascites (a) has caused a rather gray appearance of the abdomen and pushed the gas-containing loops of small bowel toward the most nondependent and central portion of the abdomen. A transverse CT scan *(B)* shows a cross-sectional view of the same appearance with the air- and contrast-filled small bowel floating in the ascitic fluid.

in the small bowel will be seen floating centrally or concentrated in the mid- and anterior abdomen on a supine plain film of the abdomen. You may also see a generalized gray haziness overlying the whole abdomen (Fig. 6–45). Small amounts of ascites can easily be visualized on a CT scan along the edge of the liver and in the pericolic gutters. If your only interest is in determining whether the patient has ascites or in locating a suitable area to tap the ascites, ultrasound is a very efficient and much cheaper modality (Fig. 6–46).

The liver can also be imaged by using a nuclear medicine liver-spleen scan. This is done by injecting radioactively labeled small particles that are phagocytized by the reticuloendothelial system of both organs. Occasionally, this test is

ordered on patients in whom there is liver disease of uncertain etiology. In patients with cirrhosis there is a relatively small right lobe of the liver and a spared or hypertrophied left lobe. If there is portal hypertension, the spleen will be enlarged. If there is hepatitis, the liver will be poorly functioning and usually large. With hepatic dysfunction due to metastatic disease, the liver is usually enlarged with focal defects or inhomogeneous activity.

Trauma

In penetrating abdominal injuries the liver is the most commonly injured intra-abdominal organ and it is the second most commonly injured organ in blunt abdominal trauma. Blunt abdominal trauma can cause hepatic lacerations, subcapsular hematomas, and intraparenchymal hemorrhage. Usually, in cases of blunt abdominal trauma, a CT scan is ordered to assess not only the liver but also the spleen, kidneys, and other organs. Hepatic laceration and hemorrhage usually manifest as an area of low density compared with the liver, although very acute hemorrhage can be denser (whiter) than the liver (Fig. 6–47). Hepatic lacerations are often treated conservatively if possible, since removal of a large portion of liver carries a high risk of mortality. Intraparenchymal liver hemorrhages may ultimately resorb.

Hepatic Tumors

The most common benign hepatic tumor is a hemangioma. This is often discovered incidentally on ultrasound examination, where it appears as an area of increased or bright echo within the liver. Hemangiomas are also discovered incidentally on noncontrasted CT scans of the abdomen. On this type of scan, the lesion appears as a rounded area of low density within the liver. A hemangioma can look like a malignant primary tumor or even a metastatic lesion. One way to differentiate a benign hemangioma from other lesions is to do serial CT scans as intravenous contrast is administered. Usually, over 10 to 15 minutes the hemangioma will fill in with contrast and look like normal liver,

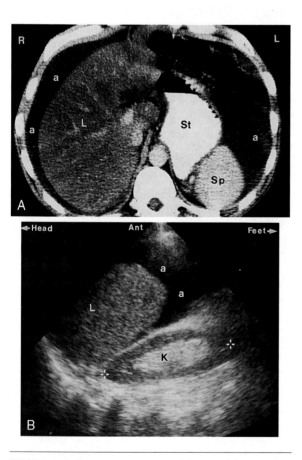

FIGURE 6–46. Ascites. A transverse CT scan of the upper abdomen (A) done without intravenous contrast shows fatty infiltration of most of the liver (L). Normally, without intravenous contrast, the liver should be the same density at the spleen (SP). Ascites (a) can also be seen around the edge of the liver and in the left paracolic gutter. A longitudinal ultrasound image (B) shows ascitic fluid (a) along the inferior aspect of the right lobe of the liver. The kidney is also seen.

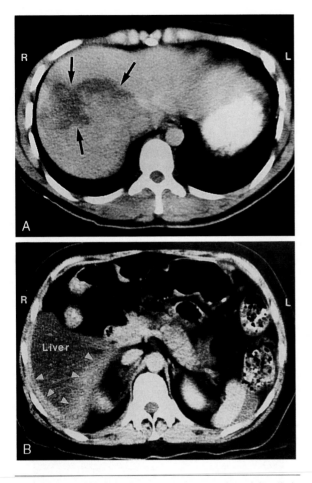

from cancer of the colon, 25 per cent from stomach, 20 per cent from pancreas, 15 per cent from breast, and 15 per cent from lung. Metastatic lesions may be small or large and single or multiple. You should be aware that the visibility of hepatic metastases on a CT scan varies greatly, depending upon the technical factors utilized when the filming is done from the computerized data. If a CT scan is done with very wide windows (wide-contrast scale) and without using intravenous contrast, it may be difficult to see the lesions. The best detectability is achieved by using intravenous contrast and narrow window

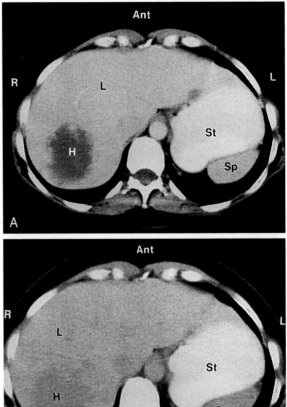

FIGURE 6–47. Hepatic laceration. *A,* A CT scan was obtained through the upper abdomen in this patient following a motor vehicle accident. An irregular area of low density *(arrows)* due to hemorrhage within the parenchyma of the liver is seen. A CT scan in another patient *(B),* who was drunk and in a motor vehicle accident, shows fatty infiltration of the liver and acute hemorrhage around the edge of the liver as an area of increased density *(arrowheads).*

whereas most malignancies will not do this (Fig. 6–48).

The most common primary malignant hepatic tumor is a hepatoma. On CT scans, this also appears as an irregular dark area within the liver (Fig. 6–49). You should remember that hepatomas can be multifocal. Five per cent of patients with cirrhosis and 10 per cent of patients with chronic hepatitis B will develop hepatocellular carcinoma. Hepatocellular carcinomas are solitary 25 per cent of the time, multiple 25 per cent of the time, and diffuse 50 per cent of the time.

Metastatic lesions of the liver are very common. Forty per cent of hepatic metastases are

FIGURE 6–48. *A and B,* **Hepatic hemangioma.** On an initial image of the contrast-enhanced CT scan of the upper abdomen, hemangioma (H) appears as a low-density area with irregular margins in the posterior aspect of the liver. This was an unexpected and incidental finding in this young woman. A scan through exactly the same level obtained 20 minutes later shows that the lesion has almost completely disappeared. In this particular patient, no further work-up is indicated.

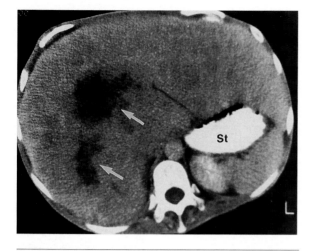

FIGURE 6–49. Hepatoma. In this patient with chronic hepatitis, two low-density lesions are easily visible *(arrows)* within the liver. The liver, however, is also markedly enlarged, displacing the stomach (ST) posteriorly. The low density lesions did not fill in with contrast; this patient has a multifocal hepatoma.

settings (Fig. 6–50). Technologists will often produce both types of images. The less useful images for this purpose are more pleasing to the eye. You should be sure that you are looking at the ones with narrow window settings. Normally these images are coarser or have more grain than those done with wide windows.

Abscess

Most hepatic abscesses are visualized with CT scanning. They are low density, or darker than the liver. Unless they have gas within them, their differentiation from neoplasm can be very difficult. Usually, the clinical presentation of a very sick, febrile patient is enough to suggest the correct diagnosis. If not, CT scanning can be used to help in the diagnosis and also to direct a needle aspiration and place a drainage catheter. Abscesses suspected anywhere in the abdomen are best imaged by CT with both intravenous and oral contrast.

GALLBLADDER AND BILIARY SYSTEM

Anatomy and Imaging Techniques

There are two common ways of visualizing the gallbladder depending upon the clinical presen-

tation. If you suspect gallstones (cholelithiasis) or biliary duct obstruction, the quickest, cheapest, and most efficient imaging test is an ultrasound examination of the right upper quadrant (see Fig. 6–10B). If, on the other hand, you suspect acute cholecystitis, the examination of choice is a nuclear medicine hepatobiliary scan. In a normal hepatobiliary scan the liver will clear the radioactive tracer, and it should appear in the gallbladder, common bile duct, and proximal small bowel within 1 hour (Fig. 6–51). Failure to visualize the gallbladder when imaging is carried out to 4 hours has a very high specificity for acute cholecystitis. The reason is that in

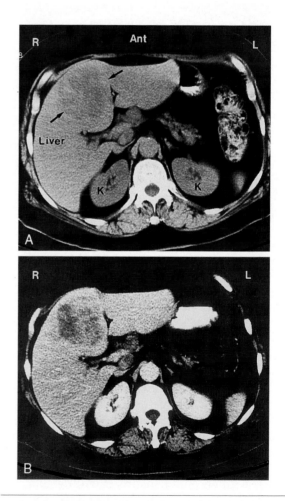

FIGURE 6–50. Effect of different CT techniques on detection of metastases. This patient has a fairly large metastatic deposit from colon carcinoma in the lateral segment of the left lobe of the liver. A CT scan performed without intravenous contrast (A) and filmed using wide windows makes it very difficult to see the metastasis *(arrows)*. By utilizing intravenous contrast and by filming the study with narrow windows (B), the image looks much coarser, but the metastatic deposit is much easier to see.

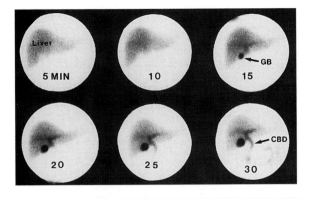

FIGURE 6–51. Normal nuclear medicine hepatobiliary study. Intravenous administration of a small amount of radioactively labeled material that is cleared by the biliary system allows visualization of the liver, the gallbladder by 15 minutes, and the common bile duct by 30 minutes.

acute cholecystitis there is usually blockage of the cystic duct, and the radioactive tracer cannot get into the gallbladder (Fig. 6–52). In chronic cholecystitis, the gallbladder fills with activity but later than normal. Some authors advocate the use of ultrasound for acute cholecystitis and look for gallbladder wall thickening and pain when the ultrasound transducer is pressed on the right upper quadrant. In fact, you should have noted the latter finding when you examined the patient before you ordered the test. Moreover, gallbladder wall thickening is nonspecific and can occur with other entities, such as hypoproteinemia.

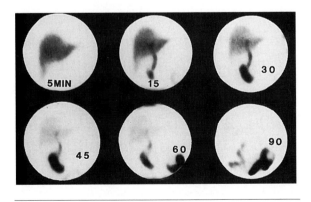

FIGURE 6–52. Acute cholecystitis. A nuclear medicine hepatobiliary study shows the liver, common bile duct, and activity in the jejunum by 60 and 90 minutes. The gallbladder was never visualized, even at 4 hours post injection. This is because with acute cholecystitis there is blockage of the cystic duct. If the gallbladder is visualized only 1 to 4 hours after injection, chronic (rather than acute) cholecystitis is likely.

When jaundice is present and there is a question of whether it is due to parenchymal liver disease, such as hepatitis, or to an obstructive lesion of the common bile duct, the initial imaging examination should be ultrasound. When complete ductal obstruction has been present for more than 24 hours, dilatation of the common and intrahepatic ducts is relatively easy to see with ultrasound. The upper portion of the common duct (which is what is normally measured at ultrasound) is usually less than 4 mm in diameter. It becomes slightly dilated with age and can be up to 7 mm in some patients less than 60 years of age. In normal persons who are over 60 years of age, the common duct diameter should be less than 10 mm. The common duct diameter also can be larger than 4 mm (up to 6 to 7 mm) if the patient has had a cholecystectomy.

Although a CT scan provides information on ductal dilatation, the fact that it uses ionizing radiation and is much more expensive usually limits its role to a follow-up examination (Fig. 6–53) (for example, when you suspect a pancreatic head neoplasm and are trying to assess the size and extent of tumor).

The fine architecture of both the biliary and the pancreatic ducts can be visualized by use of an endoscopic retrograde cholangiogram (ERCP). To do this, a large tube is passed down the esophagus and through the stomach to the duodenum. The ampulla of Vater is then cannulated. Contrast is injected into the pancreatic and common bile ducts (Fig. 6–54). An ERCP is a very useful way to assess the diameter of a stricture as well as its length (Fig. 6–55). During an ERCP, it is also possible to do a papillotomy and remove stones from the common duct.

Intrahepatic obstruction of the common duct is usually due to cholangitis, Caroli's disease, or an intrahepatic neoplasm (hepatoma compressing the ducts or a rare biliary neoplasm). Extrahepatic biliary obstruction usually occurs distally in the intrapancreatic portion of the duct. Common causes are gallstone, pancreatic cancer, and pancreatitis.

Sometimes, after a cholecystectomy and removal of stones from the common duct, a T tube is left in place. This is done to allow bile drainage through the abdominal wall while edema related to surgery and prior stones resolves. Be-

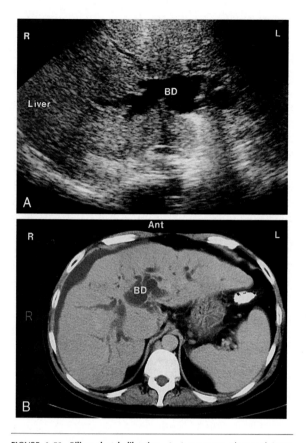

FIGURE 6–53. Biliary ductal dilatation. *A*, A transverse ultrasound image through the liver shows a central branching area without echoes that represents dilated bile ducts. A CT scan of the same patient *(B)* also demonstrates the intrahepatic dilated biliary system. As a screening test, ultrasound is cheaper and just as effective. CT scanning is more useful to localize the cause of obstruction, such as a pancreatic carcinoma.

fore the tube is pulled, contrast is injected into the T tube to look for possible retained stones.

Occasionally, as a result of surgery, air from the gastrointestinal tract will reflux into the biliary system. This may be visualized on a plain film of the abdomen (KUB). Air in the biliary tract is usually centrally located in the region of the porta hepatis, and the air is prevented from going very distally into the smaller bile ducts by flow of bile toward the porta hepatis. You must be able to differentiate this relatively benign finding from that of air in the portal venous system. Air in the portal venous system is usually seen as branching air collections near the periphery of the liver (within 2 mm). The air goes peripherally because that is the direction of the flow of blood in the portal veins. Visualization of branching lucencies in the outermost

2 cm of the liver is considered presumptive evidence of portal venous air. This is seen in diabetic patients and is associated with a high mortality (Fig. 6–56).

PANCREAS

Pancreatitis

Seventy per cent of cases of pancreatitis are caused either by alcoholic pancreatitis or by obstruction due to a gallstone in the distal common duct. The diagnosis is usually made by clinical findings of epigastric or lower abdominal pain and hyperamylasemia. Unfortunately, about 30 per cent of patients with pancreatitis have a normal serum amylase level, and about 35 per cent of persons with hyperamylasemia have a disease other than pancreatitis. The most useful imaging method for a patient with pancreatitis is CT scanning. In rare patients who have very sudden onset pancreatitis, the pan-

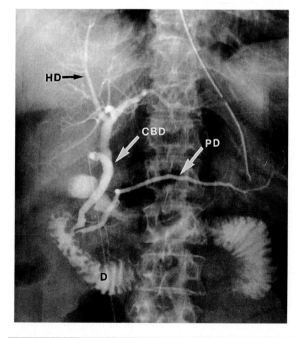

FIGURE 6–54. Normal ERCP. Placement of a fiberoptic gastroscope allows cannulation of the common bile duct and pancreatic duct at the level of the ampulla of Vater. Retrograde injection of contrast also allows visualization of intrahepatic ducts. Contrast is also seen spilling around the cannulation site into the duodenal sweep and proximal jejunum.

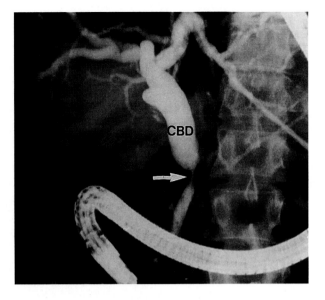

creas may be of normal size but the serum amylase value may be elevated. Most patients with acute pancreatitis have an enlarged pancreas with peripancreatic inflammation, thickening of the perirenal fascia, and peripancreatic fluid collections (Fig. 6–57). Occasionally, there may be one or a few dilated loops of small bowel over the central abdomen caused by a focal ileus from the underlying inflammation in the pancreas.

With fulminant pancreatitis, there may be formation of an abscess. This is seen on CT scan as a large soft tissue mass in the region of the pancreas that contains air bubbles. This condition has a very high mortality rate, and usually a percutaneous drain will be placed to try to drain the abscess. Another complication is progressive pancreatic necrosis due to digestion of tissue (a phlegmon); it is seen on CT as multiple areas of lucency within the pancreas. This condition also has a high mortality rate (Fig. 6–58*A*).

Late complications of acute pancreatitis are pancreatic duct obstruction and pseudocyst formation. A pseudocyst usually takes approximately 6 weeks to fully mature. At this time a CT scan shows a well-defined cystic area (Fig. 6–58*B*), and CT can be used to perform percutaneous drainage. You should be aware that pseudocysts do not necessarily need to be in the pancreas itself. They can present as focal fluid collections anywhere in the abdomen and occasionally even in the pelvis or thorax.

Tumor

Adenocarcinoma accounts for 95 per cent of all pancreatic cancer. It has a very poor prognosis, with a 1-year survival rate of 10 per cent or less. Clinically, the patients present with jaundice, weight loss, and occasionally a dilated, nontender gallbladder. CT scanning is the imaging modality of choice to assess not only the tumor size and location but also the possibility of hepatic and nodal metastases.

SPLEEN

Imaging of the spleen is sometimes done to assess splenic size, although this really should be done clinically by palpation and percussion. The spleen is usually about 10 cm in length, and up to 13 cm may be normal. Causes of splenomegaly are leukemia (especially chronic lymphocytic leukemia [CLL]), lymphoma, infection (mononucleosis), storage diseases (amyloid and Gaucher's diseases), portal hypertension, and hematologic abnormalities (anemias, thalassemia, myelofibrosis).

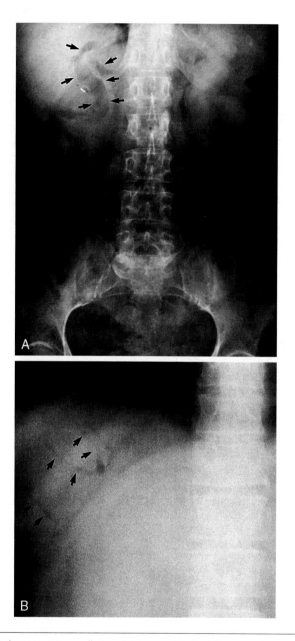

FIGURE 6–56. Air within the liver. A branching or serpiginous collection of air is seen within the right upper quadrant on a KUB examination *(A)*. This air is in the region of the porta hepatis and represents air within the biliary system. This is a common finding following gallbladder surgery and has little clinical significance. In contrast, branching collections of air seen peripherally in the liver *(B)* in a different patient represent air within the portal venous system, and this has a high associated mortality.

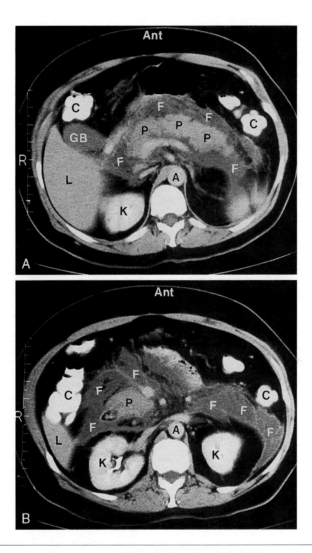

FIGURE 6–57. Acute pancreatitis. *A,* A CT scan in this young woman with hyperlipidemia shows the body of the pancreas (p) and surrounding fluid (f). The liver (l), kidney (k), gallbladder (gb), and colon (c) are also identified. Another image in the same patient obtained slightly more inferiorly *(B)* shows a marked amount of fluid (f) around the uncinate portion of the pancreas (p) and fluid extending around into the left paracolic gutter with associated thickening of Gerota's fascia.

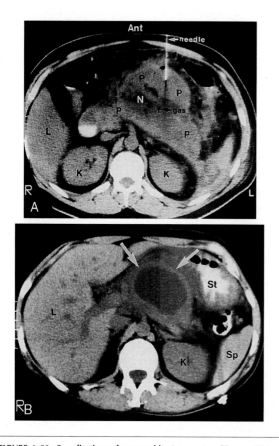

In addition to trauma, focal splenic lesions can easily be seen on a CT scan. These can be due to splenic abcesses, infarcts, tumor, and occasionally cysts. The sensitivity of CT for detection of these is high, but the specificity is poor, and often the clinical history is necessary to narrow the differential diagnosis.

SMALL BOWEL

You should be able to recognize some small bowel abnormalities by examining the gas pattern on plain film of the abdomen. Small bowel can be identified by its central location and by

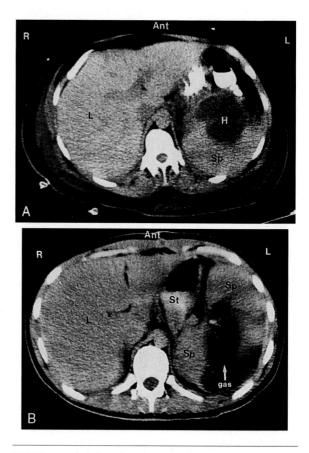

FIGURE 6–58. Complications of pancreatitis. A transverse CT scan *(A)* in a patient with pancreatitis and a persistent fever shows a very enlarged pancreas (p) with a low-density area within it representing necrosis of the pancreas. Also noted is a small gas bubble due to formation of a pancreatic abscess. A needle has been inserted under CT guidance to obtain material for culture and to place a percutaneous drain. In a different patient who is a chronic alcoholic, the CT scan *(B)* demonstrates a well-defined low-density area within the pancreas *(arrows)*. This represents a pancreatic pseudocyst.

Following blunt trauma, the spleen is the most commonly injured intra-abdominal organ, and there can be a splenic fracture or hematoma. Although surgeons usually try to manage these injuries conservatively, there can be splenic rupture even a week to 10 days after the initial injury. If you suspect splenic trauma, a CT scan is the test of choice. Hemorrhage and hematoma usually appear as areas of lower density than the spleen (Fig. 6–59). Dark areas that are round or irregular represent intrasplenic hematomas or lacerations, and abnormal crescentic areas at the edge of the spleen represent subcapsular hematomas. Occasionally, with conservative management an abscess may subsequently form and can be identified as such on a CT scan because it contains gas.

FIGURE 6–59. Splenic laceration. The CT scan done without intravenous contrast *(A)* through the upper abdomen in a patient who was involved in a motor vehicle accident demonstrates an intrasplenic low-density area from hemorrhage (H). Surgery was not performed, and the patient returned in about 2 weeks with right upper quadrant pain and fever. A CT scan at this time *(B)* showed an expanding mass within the spleen, which contained gas. This represented a splenic abscess, which required surgery. Also note the medial displacement of the stomach (ST).

its rather thin mucosal markings that extend across the entire lumen. One of the most common remarks that you hear made when a physician is examining a small bowel film is that air-fluid levels are present. The implication is that this is abnormal. In fact, it is quite normal, since small bowel contents are mostly fluid, and any air or carbon dioxide that is swallowed and passes through the stomach will cause an air-fluid level in the small bowel.

Obstruction vs. Ileus

A standard question in reference to a patient with abdominal pain is whether he or she has either a small bowel obstruction or paralytic ileus. This question can be resolved with a stethoscope rather than an x-ray, since if bowel sounds are present and relatively frequent, a paralytic ileus is unlikely. On a plain film x-ray of the abdomen, the diameter of the small bowel should not exceed 3 cm; if it does, you need to try to determine whether there is an obstruction or an ileus.

If the small bowel dilatation is greater than 4 cm, you are almost certainly looking at an obstruction, since in a paralytic ileus there is only mild dilatation. The upright film is used to look at the nature of the air-fluid levels. As mentioned earlier, air-fluid levels can be normal, but if you find them in bowel and the small bowel is dilated, you should look on an upright film for a single loop of small bowel to see whether the air-fluid levels at either end of the loop are at the same level or at differential levels. If they are at different levels in a given loop of small bowel, there is an obstruction. This is because there is muscle tone within the small bowel causing the differential levels, and this would not be present with a paralytic ileus (Fig. 6–60). You should remember that a long-standing bowel obstruction can ultimately result in a paralytic ileus. The common causes of a paralytic ileus are a postoperative state, vascular ischemia, nearby inflammatory processes (such as pancreatitis and appendicitis), electrolyte imbalance, and drugs (morphine and its derivatives). Small bowel obstructions are mostly due to adhesions, tumors, hernias, and inflammatory strictures.

With a very dilated diameter of the small bowel (i.e., obstruction), you should look to see how far bowel gas extends. If dilated small bowel extends to the lower portion of the abdomen, you are looking at an obstruction that is at least in the distal small bowel or perhaps in the proximal colon. If you see air distally in the colon or in the rectum, you may be looking at either a partial small bowel obstruction or a very acute complete small bowel obstruction (the distal air not yet having been expelled). Sometimes, as the lumen of obstructed small bowel fills with fluid, small bubbles of air are trapped in the most superior part of the lumen between the valvulae conniventes. This leads to the appearance of a "string of pearls."

The cause of a small bowel obstruction is often difficult to identify on a plain radiograph. You should look carefully for gas in the inguinal region to exclude a strangulated hernia (Fig. 6–61). Dilatation of the small bowel in a child over a few years of age should raise the suspicion of appendicitis (Fig. 6–62). When you see this, you should look carefully over the region of the sacrum and right ileum to see if an appendicolith may be present. Remember, the cause of appendicitis is obstruction of the appendiceal lumen. This is due to lymphoid hyperplasia about two thirds of the time and to an appendicolith one third of the time. The diagnosis of appendicitis really is a clinical one. At the present time, some authors recommend appendiceal ultrasound, but this is a difficult procedure to perform. A positive ultrasound finding is a total outer wall to outer wall appendiceal thickness of greater than 6 mm. Unfortunately, much of the time an overlying ileus with bowel gas makes it difficult or impossible to diagnose appendicitis using ultrasound.

Benign Diseases

There are a wide variety of diseases that can affect the small bowel and can be visualized on a barium study of the small bowel. The finer points of radiologic differential diagnosis of small bowel disease are beyond the scope of this text, but in general you are looking for mucosal thickening, nodules, dilatation, and areas of stricturing. Fold thickening is assessed by look-

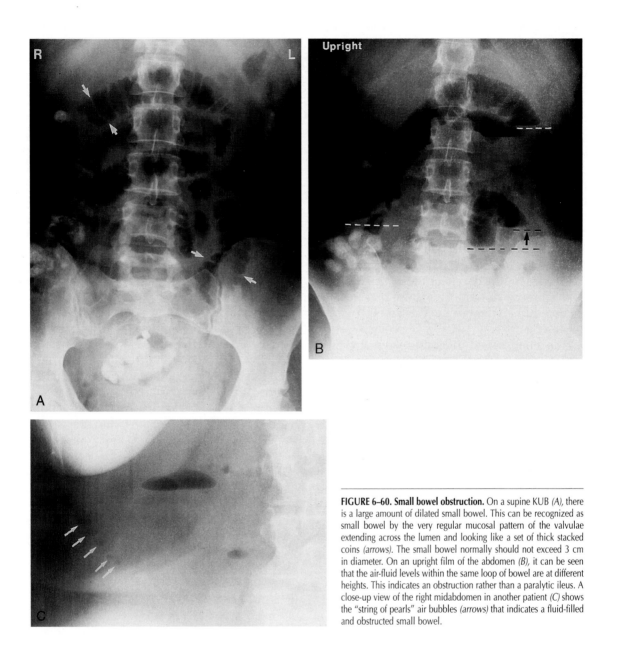

FIGURE 6–60. Small bowel obstruction. On a supine KUB *(A)*, there is a large amount of dilated small bowel. This can be recognized as small bowel by the very regular mucosal pattern of the valvulae extending across the lumen and looking like a set of thick stacked coins *(arrows)*. The small bowel normally should not exceed 3 cm in diameter. On an upright film of the abdomen *(B)*, it can be seen that the air-fluid levels within the same loop of bowel are at different heights. This indicates an obstruction rather than a paralytic ileus. A close-up view of the right midabdomen in another patient *(C)* shows the "string of pearls" air bubbles *(arrows)* that indicates a fluid-filled and obstructed small bowel.

FIGURE 6–61. Strangulated inguinal hernia. A film of the pelvis demonstrates some dilated loops of small bowel in the upper abdomen. Over the left groin, two air collections are seen (A), which represent loops of small bowel descending into the scrotum.

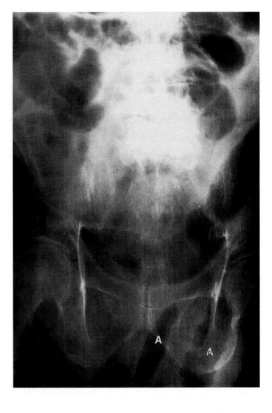

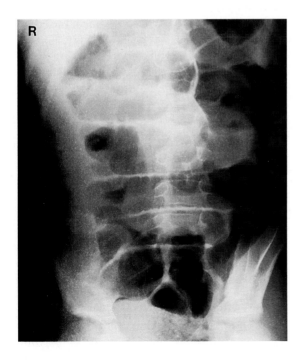

FIGURE 6–62. Acute appendicitis. In this supine film of the abdomen of a young child, dilated small bowel loops are seen centrally. No definite gas is seen in the colon. Dilated small bowel loops in a young child should raise the consideration of appendicitis as well as intestinal obstruction.

ing at the mucosal pattern. The valvulae conniventes should not measure more than 2 to 3 mm in thickness. The mnemonic for the differential diagnosis of small bowel fold thickening is WAG CLEM, which refers to Whipple's disease, amyloid, giardiasis, cryptosporidiosis, lymphoma, eosinophilic gastroenteritis, and Mycobacterium avium complex. The mnemonic for dilatation without fold thickening is SOSO, which stands for sprue, obstruction (or ileus), scleroderma, and other (medicines and vagotomy). Personally, I find it easier to remember the diseases than to figure out what these mnemonics stand for, but perhaps they will be useful to you.

There are some diseases and conditions that result in areas of stricturing. The most common are prior surgery, tumor, and Crohn's disease (regional enteritis). Lesions of regional enteritis are most common in the terminal ileum, and about half the patients will also have involvement of the colon. Patients have weight loss, recurrent abdominal pain, and diarrhea. Extraintestinal manifestations include skin, eye, joint, and liver abnormalities. Characteristic features are areas of relatively fixed narrowing in the terminal ileum (the string sign) (Fig. 6–63), sinus tracts, and fistulas. In the colon, there are areas of stricture and ulceration with skip areas that have normal mucosa in between.

Occasionally, there can be collections of air or gas in subserosal portions of the small bowel (pneumatosis intestinalis) (Fig. 6–64). In adults, this is often a benign finding, whereas in children it may be associated with necrotizing enterocolitis or ischemia. In adults, the benign form can occur in patients with COPD who have air dissecting down from the chest into the abdomen and along the mesentery of the bowel. This may also be associated with asymptomatic pneumoperitoneum. Gastrointestinal bleeding can occur as a result of a Meckel's diverticulum in the small bowel. Since this is most common in children, it is discussed in Chapter 9.

Tumors

Tumors of any sort in the small bowel are rare. Tumor incidence in the colon is about 40 times higher. The most common benign growths of the small bowel are leiomyomas, lipomas, adeno-

mas, and polyps. Malignant tumors tend to be adenocarcinomas and to a lesser extent carcinoids and lymphomas. Symptoms of any tumor in the small bowel can cause obstruction and bleeding.

COLON

All of the colon can be directly visualized with an endoscope. This procedure allows biopsy of lesions but it requires sedation and is expensive.

Radiographic examination of the colon is begun by examining the plain film but it is best performed by barium or water-soluble contrast enema. It is imperative that the colon be cleansed prior to the examination; otherwise, residual fecal material can be mistaken for polyps or malignant lesions. The diagnostic enema can be done either by filling the colon completely with barium (single-contrast examination) or by putting in a small amount of barium and then using air (double-contrast examination). The double-contrast examination is generally believed to have a higher sensitivity than the single-contrast examination. On a barium enema, a number of different views and projections are obtained. This is essential, because otherwise one loop of bowel would overlie another and lesions would be obscured. The ascending, transverse, and descending colon as well as portions of the sigmoid can be appreciated on the AP or PA views of the abdomen (Fig. 6–65). Lateral views are usually obtained of the rectum (Fig. 6–66) as well as steep oblique views of the hepatic and splenic flexures (Fig. 6–67).

It is important to be sure that patients are well hydrated after a barium enema. If the barium remains in the colon for several days, water will be reabsorbed, and the patient will have difficulty in excreting the barium. Occasionally, barium gets into the appendix during a barium enema. This is a normal finding. It may, however, stay there for months after the remainder of the barium is excreted. This can present a somewhat unusual and confusing appearance on a plain film of the abdomen (Fig. 6–68).

It is important to understand what the appearance of different lesions is on a barium

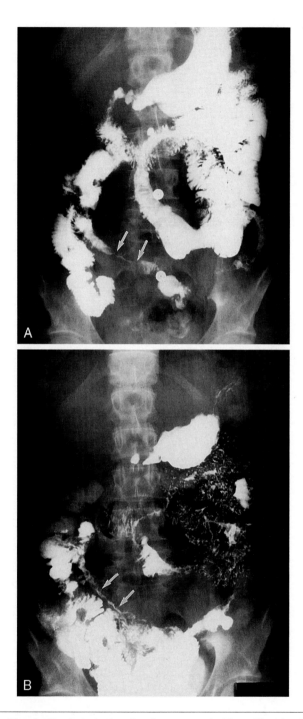

FIGURE 6–63. Crohn's disease of the small bowel. A film obtained midway through a contrast study of the small bowel *(A)* demonstrates a narrowed segment of distal ileum *(arrows)*. Another film obtained at the end of the study *(B)* shows that most of the barium has passed into the colon, but the previously identified area of narrowing remains and, therefore, represents a stricture rather than peristalsis.

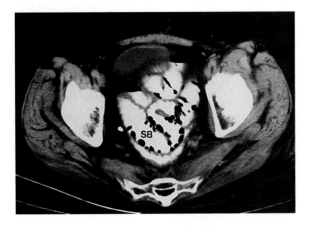

FIGURE 6–64. Pneumatosis of the small bowel. A transverse CT scan of the lower pelvis shows contrast-filled small bowel (SB). Small dark collections of gas in the wall of the small bowel are seen indenting the contrast-filled lumen.

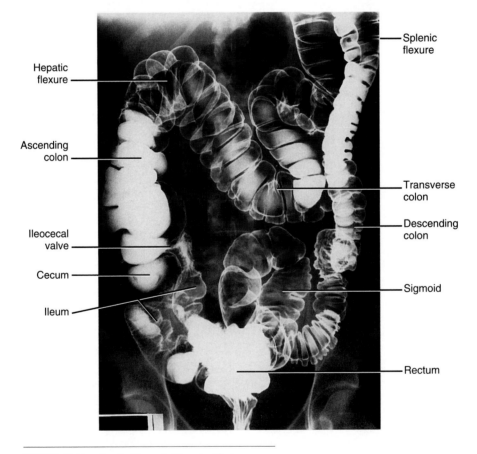

FIGURE 6–65. Normal supine film on double-contrast barium enema.

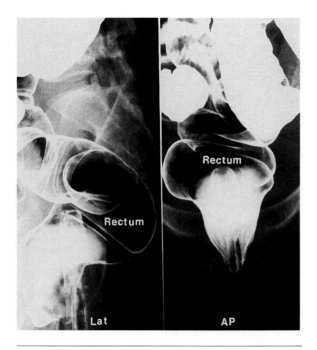

FIGURE 6–66. AP and lateral views of the normal rectum on a double-contrast barium enema.

study. These are shown graphically in Figure 6–69. These appearances apply to all types of contrast studies.

Colonic Obstruction vs. Paralytic Ileus

The key to the differentiation of colonic obstruction and paralytic ileus on a plain abdominal film is whether there is dilatation of the cecum. The cecum is most dilated in colonic obstruction compared with the rest of the colon. Colonic obstruction is most frequently due to a cancer (65 per cent), but it can also be due to diverticulitis (20 per cent) or a volvulus (5 per cent). If the transverse colon is more dilated than the cecum, you should consider a diagnosis of ileus. The term for an abnormally distended transverse colon is a megacolon, and this refers to dilatation greater than 6 cm in diameter. A toxic megacolon can result from ulcerative colitis, Crohn's disease, or infectious causes.

When there is an acute colonic distention (cecum >9 cm), there is a risk of perforation, and the likely causes are tumor obstruction, volvulus, and paralytic ileus. A number of patients have a chronically distended colon, and they have only a small risk of perforation. In such cases, chronic distention may be a result of chronic laxative abuse, neuromuscular disorders (including diabetes), psychogenic problems, or metabolic problems (electrolyte imbalance, hypothyroidism, morphine derivatives).

Diverticulosis and Diverticulitis

Chronic lack of fiber in the diet causes herniation of mucosa outward through the bowel wall (diverticula). Fifty per cent of individuals over the age of 50 years have acquired diverticula. Of this group, 15 to 30 per cent will present with rectal bleeding and pain. Ninety-five per cent of diverticula are located in the region of the sigmoid and descending colon (Fig. 6–70). Diverticulosis simply refers to the presence of multiple diverticula.

Diverticulitis is an inflammatory process often caused by extravasation of bowel contents from the tip of the diverticulum. It is confined to the sigmoid colon in 90 per cent of patients, and there usually is significant resultant bowel wall thickening or formation of intramural abscesses (Fig. 6–71). Patients present with left lower quadrant pain 70 per cent of the time, and they may also have diarrhea or constipation, fever, and leukocytosis. Diverticulitis can sometimes be seen on a contrast enema as a small longitudinal track of barium within the wall of the colon. If the diagnosis of diverticulitis is suspected, however, it is better to order a CT scan, since it is possible to have diverticulitis without diverticula being identified on the barium enema.

Ulcerative Colitis

Ulcerative colitis is associated with arthritis and arthralgia, and the patients have diarrhea and rectal bleeding. The disease is confined to the mucosa and submucosa. It begins in the rectum and then spreads from the distal to the proximal colon. There may also be backwash ileitis with involvement of the terminal ileum. Patients are at a 5- to 30-fold higher risk for malignancy than the general population. The barium enema

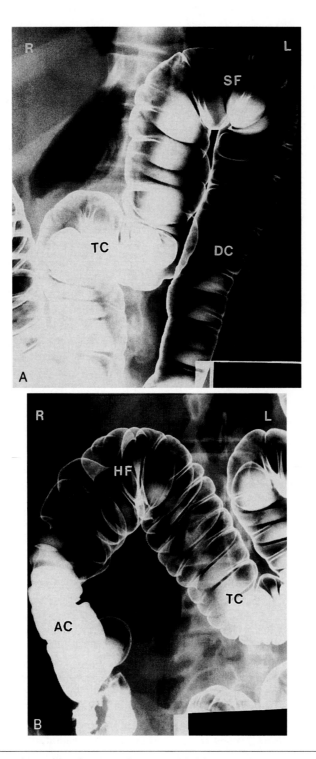

FIGURE 6–67. Normal splenic and hepatic flexure of the colon. A steep oblique view of the left upper quadrant *(A)* shows the splenic flexure and the transverse and descending colon while an oblique view of the right upper quadrant *(B)* shows the hepatic flexure and transverse and ascending colon.

FIGURE 6–68. Residual barium in the appendix. A view of the pelvis obtained on a patient who had a barium enema several months earlier reveals residual barium within the wormlike appendix *(arrow)*. Residual barium can also be seen in diverticula, but these appear round.

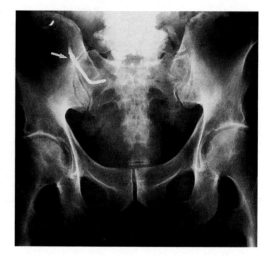

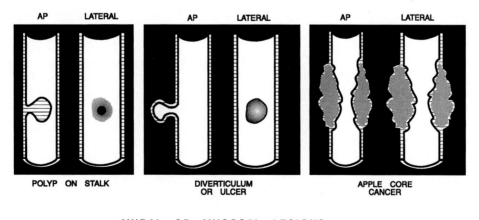

MURAL   OR   MUCOSAL   LESIONS

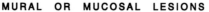

FIGURE 6–69. Schematic appearance of various gastrointestinal lesions on contrast examinations. A polyp seen in profile will show a stalk. Seen end-on it will be darkest in the center, with an ill-defined fading edge. A diverticulum seen in tangent will project outside the lumen and when seen end-on it will have very sharp edges. A cancer can be in one wall or, if circumferential, can leave contrast in the lumen that resembles an apple core.

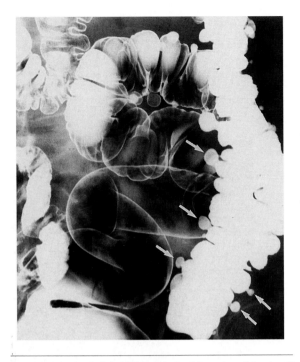

FIGURE 6–70. Diverticulosis of the colon. An oblique view of the sigmoid colon during a double-contrast barium enema shows multiple outpouching *(arrows)* that represent diverticula.

features of this disease are a short colon with granular mucosa and shallow, confluent ulcers (Fig. 6–72).

Crohn's Disease

Crohn's disease can affect the colon as well as the small bowel. In contrast to ulcerative colitis, it is transmural and rarely involves the rectum. On a barium enema there can be visualization of aphthous erosions, ulcers, cobblestone fissures, fistula, and strictures. Characteristically, the disease is noncontiguous and skips areas of the colon. Thus there are diseased areas of the colon with segments of normal colon in between.

Infectious Colitis

Pseudomembranous colitis and a number of other infections caused by *Campylobacter, Shigella,* and *Salmonella* can produce a radiographic pattern similar to that of ulcerative colitis. Cytomegalic virus colitis usually occurs in

immunocompromised persons and has variable radiographic features, including ulceration, which can be either localized or pancolonic (Fig. 6–73).

Ulcerative colitis and, less commonly, other colitises, can result in a toxic megacolon. A barium enema should not be ordered on a patient in whom a toxic megacolon is suspected, and proctoscopy should be performed. The radiographic features of toxic megacolon are a dilated colon with a deformed bowel wall, most evident in the transverse portion of the colon. The wall may be nodular, irregular, or haustral or even show what looks like thumbprints of soft tissue extending into the colonic lumen. This thickened fold appearance can also be due to ischemia of the colon, but it is usually limited

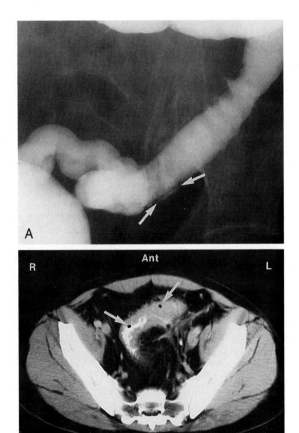

FIGURE 6–71. Diverticulitis. *A,* A view of the sigmoid colon obtained during a single-contrast barium enema shows tracking of the barium within the wall of the colon *(arrows).* A transverse CT scan *(B)* in the same patient shows the sigmoid colon with a markedly thickened wall. Several gas bubbles *(arrows)* are seen within the wall of the colon, representing abscess formation.

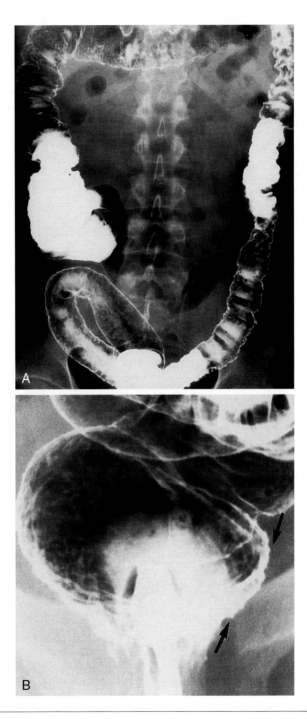

FIGURE 6–72. Ulcerative colitis. A double-contrast barium enema *(A)* shows very small irregular ulcers extending back from the rectum to at least the hepatic flexure. A spot view of the rectum *(B)* shows the tiny ulcers in better detail. (Case courtesy of Michael Davis, M.D.)

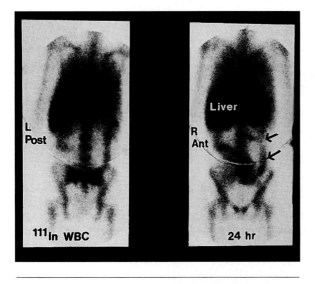

FIGURE 6–73. **Infectious colitis.** A nuclear medicine abscess localization study done with radioactively labeled white blood cells shows the front and back views of the torso of an immunosuppressed patient with a fever. Activity in the marrow and liver is normal. The abnormal activity in the lungs and colon (arrows) is due to infection by cytomegalic inclusion virus.

to the appropriate vascular distribution, that is, proximal to the splenic flexure for the superior mesenteric artery and distal to the splenic flexure for the inferior mesenteric artery distribution.

Polyps

About 90 per cent of polyps are hyperplastic and are non-neoplastic. Of those that are neoplastic, adenomas are the most common. Of the adenomatous polyps, 50 per cent are multiple, and although many are asymptomatic, they can cause diarrhea, pain, and bleeding. Seventy per cent of polyps occur in the rectum and sigmoid, and 10 per cent each in the ascending, transverse, and descending colon.

The larger the polyp is, the more likely it is to be malignant. Of polyps less than 1 cm, only 1 per cent are malignant; between 1 and 2 cm, 25 per cent are malignant; and over 2 cm, 40 per cent are malignant. A benign polyp is usually less than 2 cm in diameter, has a thin stalk and a smooth contour, is single, and has a smooth underlying colonic wall. Malignant polyps usually are over 2 cm, have no definite

stalk, can be multiple, and are often irregular or lobulated (Fig. 6–74A).

There are a number of syndromes with multiple polyps, including familial polyposis, Gardner's syndrome, Peutz-Jeghers syndrome, and juvenile polyposis. Most of the polyposis syndromes have adenomas as the underlying histology, but the familial type and Gardner's and Turcot's syndromes have an extremely high rate of malignancy. In familial polyposis, the rate of malignancy is so high that screening of family members begins at puberty (Fig. 6–74B), and treatment often involves a prophylactic total proctocolectomy.

Colon Carcinoma

Colon cancer is the second most common cancer in men and women. The most common cancer in men is lung, and in women it is breast cancer. Fifty per cent of colon cancers occur in the rectum or sigmoid, and about 10 per cent each in the cecum, ascending colon, transverse colon, and descending colon. The clinical presentation is most commonly colonic obstruction or rectal bleeding. There is a debate as to whether colonoscopy or barium enema is the appropriate method of work-up. Barium enema is relatively inexpensive compared with colonoscopy, and it has about the same accuracy rate. The advantage of colonoscopy is that if a lesion is identified, it can be biopsied immediately. The radiographic appearance of a colon cancer may be a polypoid lesion extending into the lumen of the colon or a mass on one wall of the colon; if more advanced, the lesion may be circumferential, resulting in an "apple core" (Fig. 6–75). You should not be so filled with gratification when you see a colon cancer that you stop looking. Remember that in about 5 per cent of patients there is a second colon cancer present at the same time. The radiologist will not usually put a lot of barium retrograde past a high-grade obstructing lesion because the barium will stay there; the colon will absorb the water, and it will almost turn to concrete. At surgery, however, one must look for second tumors.

CT scanning is usually done to assess the extent of disease locally and in lymph nodes and the liver. Accuracy for detection of lymph

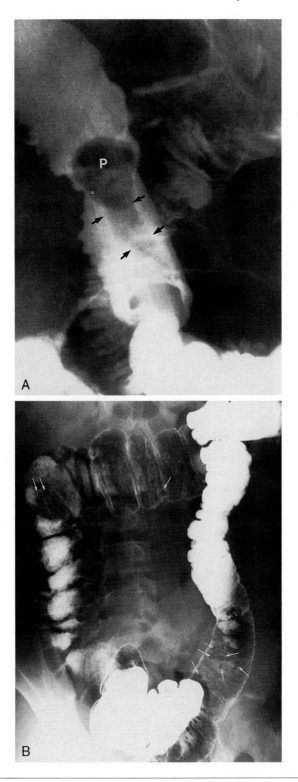

FIGURE 6–74. Colonic polyps. A magnified spot view of the sigmoid during a barium enema *(A)* outlines a single polyp (P) as well as its stalk. In a different patient, a barium enema *(B)* reveals multiple tiny polyps extending throughout the colon.

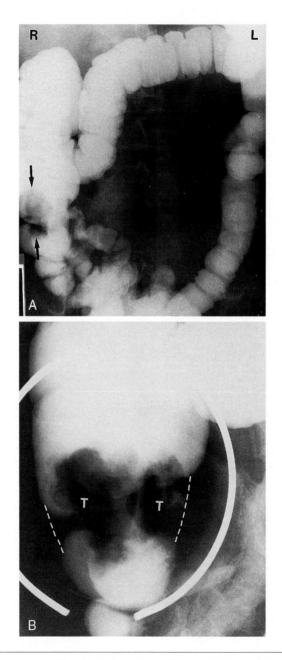

FIGURE 6–75. Colon carcinoma. A single-contrast view of the colon *(A)* demonstrates a filling defect in the cecum *(arrows)*. A compression ring was applied, and a spot view *(B)* was taken of the cecum. This shows that the tumor (T) has encircled the lumen, producing a typical "apple-core" lesion with overhanging edges. This is characteristic of a cancer.

FIGURE 6–76. Colonic bleeding from a diverticulum. A nuclear medicine gastrointestinal bleeding study done by tagging red cells with a small amount of radioactive material has images of the abdomen obtained at 5, 10, and 20 minutes. The aorta, inferior vena cava, and a transplanted kidney (k) are visible. In the left lower quadrant, there is increasing activity *(black arrow)* on the sequential images as a result of bleeding into the colon from a diverticulum.

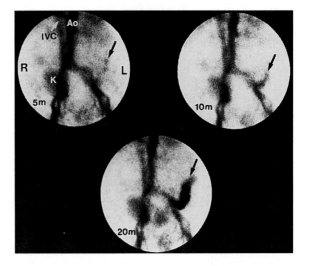

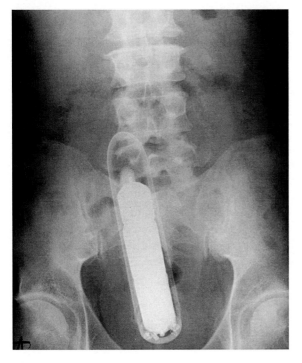

FIGURE 6–77. Vibrator in the rectum. This plain film shows the vibrator in this patient who "accidentally fell on it while gardening in the nude."

node metastases is poor (approximately 60 per cent). If the nodes are enlarged, they probably have tumor within them, but nodes can be of normal size and still contain tumor. A CT scan with intravenous contrast of the liver often will show multiple low-density metastases (see Fig. 6–50).

Gastrointestinal Bleeding

Bleeding is a common presentation of gastrointestinal pathology. Although bright red blood from the rectum implies a rectal or colonic lesion (98 per cent of the time), this is not necessarily the case; distal small bowel lesions can rarely present this way. When the source of gastrointestinal bleeding cannot be found by colonoscopy, it is often valuable to perform a nuclear medicine gastrointestinal bleeding study. This is done by labeling the red blood cells with radioactive material and then doing sequential imaging over the abdomen to look for abnormal pooling (Fig. 6–76). This examination should be ordered prior to an angiogram or barium enema. A nuclear medicine study should be ordered only when the patient is having active bleeding, and it is capable of localizing the bleeding site with bleeding rates as low as 0.5 ml per minute. In contrast, an angiogram needs approximately 4 ml per minute for the bleeding site to be identified. A nuclear medicine scan also is helpful to direct the radiologist as to which vessels to catheterize if an angiogram is needed. Occasionally bleeding and other symptoms may be due to a foreign body (Fig. 6–77). Most patients with these have very imaginative stories.

Volvulus

Twisting of the colon can cause either a sigmoid or a cecal volvulus. This obstruction causes severe colicky pain, nausea, abdominal distention, and vomiting. Sigmoid volvulus is about three times more common than a cecal volvulus. A sigmoid volvulus is seen on the KUB film as a massively dilated loop of colon that looks like

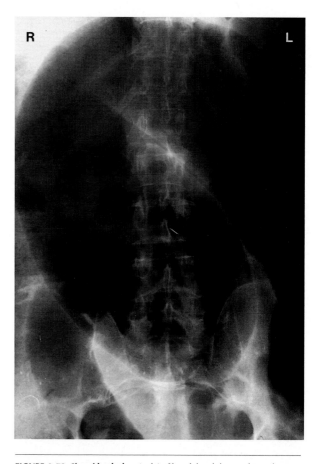

FIGURE 6–78. Sigmoid volvulus. A plain film of the abdomen shows the massively dilated "inverted U" of colon pointing toward the right upper quadrant. (Case courtesy of Michael Davis, M.D.)

an inverted U projecting up out of the pelvis toward the right upper quadrant (this is also called the "omega loop" sign; Fig. 6–78). There usually is air seen in the proximal colon. With a cecal volvulus, there is a dilated loop of colon pointing toward the left upper quadrant, and there usually is associated small bowel dilatation. The diagnostic study of choice for both these entities is a barium enema.

General Suggested Readings

Gore R, Levine M, Laufer I: Textbook of Gastrointestinal Radiology. Philadelphia, WB Saunders, 1994.
Margulis A, Burhenne H: Alimentary Tract Radiology, 4th ed. St. Louis, CV Mosby, 1989.

Chapter 7

Genitourinary System

ANATOMY AND IMAGING TECHNIQUES

There are a number of ways to image the urinary system. The initial study of choice for many suspected clinical problems is shown in Table 7–1. The most common radiographic method is by intravenous injection of an iodine-based contrast agent, which is rapidly cleared by the kidneys. This is called an intravenous pyelogram (IVP). The normal anatomy is shown in Figure 7–1. Initially, a plain film of the abdomen (KUB) is obtained. You should examine this carefully, looking for abnormalities in the skeleton, soft tissue margins of the liver, spleen and psoas regions, and the gas pattern in the bowel as well as for calcifications (Table 7–2). Of particular interest are those calcifications that project or overlie the region where you expect to find kidneys, ureters, and bladder. After injection of a contrast material, a tomogram may be obtained as part of the procedure. The tomogram essentially blurs structures in front of and behind the kidneys, leaving only the kidneys and part of the spine in focus.

The kidneys should be examined for size, shape, position, and axis. The length of kidneys on a radiographic study is typically about 13 cm. On an ultrasound examination they are smaller, being only about 10 to 11 cm in length. The reason is that there is magnification on the radiographic images, and the intravenous contrast being excreted during an IVP causes the kidneys to enlarge 1 to 2 cm in length. Normally, the left kidney is somewhat higher than the right; the long axis of the kidneys should be tilted slightly inward, with the superior pole of the kidney being more medial than the lower pole. You should look for uniform thickness of the cortex relative to the calyces of the collecting system. The shape of the kidneys should be relatively smooth in outline, although occasionally there is a slight lump on the lateral margin of the kidneys. The lateral lump is sometimes referred to as a dromedary hump, or column of Bertin (Fig. 7–2). Although this is a common variant, you cannot exclude a cyst or neoplasm if there is a major difference between the thick-

TABLE 7–1. Initial Imaging Studies for Common Clinical Problems

Clinical Problem	Imaging Study
Ureteral calculus	KUB
	IVP
Hematuria	IVP
	CT
	Cystoscopy
Infection (recurrent)	IVP
Abscess	CT
Renal trauma	CT
Hydronephrosis	IVP initially
	US for follow-up
Probable cyst on IVP	US
Probable mass on IVP	CT
Bladder rupture	Cystogram
Urethral obstruction or tear	Retrograde urethrogram
Bladder cancer	Cystoscopy
	CT
Hypertension	Nuclear medicine Captopril renogram
Testicular torsion	Nuclear medicine testicular scan or Doppler US
Testicular or scrotal mass	US
Pelvic mass (female)	US
Cervical cancer	CT
Ovarian cancer	CT
Uterine cancer	CT
Uterine fibroids	Pelvic US
Prostate cancer	Bone scan (to exclude metastases)

ness of the cortex between the calyces and the outer margin of the kidney or if one portion of the cortex is focally thicker than another. Often a renal ultrasound is the most cost efficient and innocuous way of resolving this problem.

On the IVP there is normally a dark area surrounding the collecting system of the kidneys, and this represents fat in the hilum of the kidney. You should look carefully at the calyces to make sure that they are very sharp and pointed—not blunted—at their outer corners, and you should examine the renal pelvis and ureters for any intrinsic or extrinsic defects that might be apparent. The ureters should course inferiorly and medially from the kidneys and anterior to the psoas muscles at the L3–L5 level. On the AP projection, the ureters typically are most medial and project over the lateral aspect of the transverse processes at L3, L4, and L5. As the ureters pass over the sacrum, they deviate laterally and then enter the bladder from the posterolateral aspect.

Renal ultrasound is a simple noninvasive examination (Fig. 7–3). Remember that all ultra-

sound images are "slices" and that the easiest view of the kidney to understand is the longitudinal view. The right kidney is easily visualized by transmitting sound through the right lobe of the liver. Since bowel and stomach gas prevents ultrasound transmission, the left kidney is usually visualized from the patient's back. The kidney is bean shaped and has bright central echoes owing to the fat surrounding the collecting system.

Although the bladder is seen on the IVP, you should remember that the contrast medium is heavier than urine and layers posteriorly in the bladder. What you are really looking at when you think you see the bladder on IVP films often

TABLE 7–2. Things to Look For on an Intravenous Pyelogram

Plain Film of the Abdomen
(often called a KUB or scout film)

- Label (for patient identification and age/sex)

- Skeleton

- Gas patterns of bowel

- Soft tissue margins (psoas, liver, spleen, kidneys), pelvic soft tissue masses

- Calcifications in expected areas of kidneys, ureters, bladder, and elsewhere

Contrasted Films

Kidneys

- Size (11–14 cm normally in adult)

- Shape and contour

- Thickness of cortex (uniform distance from the calyces to renal margin)

- Axis (upper poles medial to lower poles)

- Distortion of calyces by a mass

Collecting System

- Sharp calyceal corners or blunting

- Size of renal pelvis

- Filling defects in renal pelvis or ureters

- Course of ureters

Bladder

- Filling defects

- Extrinsic masses

- Large postvoid residual volume

- Trabeculation of wall or diverticula

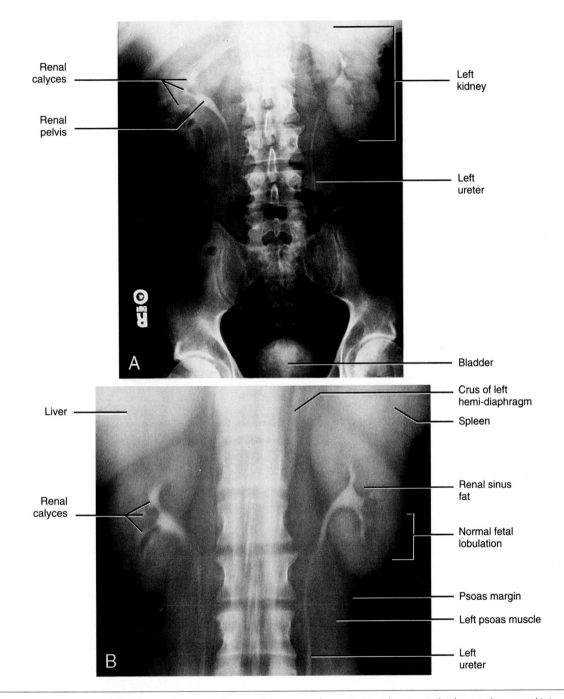

Renal
calyces

Renal
pelvis

Left
kidney

Left
ureter

Bladder

A

Liver

Crus of left
hemi-diaphragm

Spleen

Renal sinus
fat

Renal
calyces

Normal fetal
lobulation

Psoas margin

Left psoas muscle

Left
ureter

B

FIGURE 7–1. Normal anatomy of the kidneys, ureters, and bladder on an intravenous pyelogram *(A)*. Normal anatomy is also shown on the tomographic image *(B)* taken during an intravenous pyelogram.

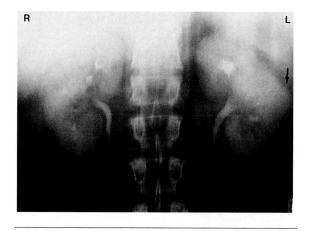

FIGURE 7–2. Dromedary hump. A tomogram obtained during an intravenous pyelogram shows a bulge on the lateral aspect of the left kidney *(arrows)*. This is a congenital variation that is quite commonly seen. There should be no underlying displacement of the renal calyces.

is only the lateral margins of the back of the bladder (Fig. 7–4). The anterior portion of the bladder is usually not well seen. Consequently, if you wish to see the entire bladder, a Foley catheter can be placed directly into the bladder, the urine drained, and the bladder refilled with contrast material. This is called a cystogram. On a cystogram, images of the bladder are obtained in several different projections. When the catheter is removed, the patient may be asked to void. In males, this gives a very good demonstration of the urethra (Fig. 7–5). The male urethra can also be studied in a retrograde fashion by inserting a small tube in the tip of the penis and injecting the contrast material. This is usually done only in cases of suspected urethral trauma or stricture.

KIDNEYS

Congenital Abnormalities

Congenital abnormalities of the urinary tract occur quite frequently, and you should be aware of the most common variants. Embryologically, the ureter buds and grows superiorly from the bladder in order to meet and connect with the renal parenchyma. The ureter can divide as it ascends, causing a person to have two, partially duplicated or completely separate, collecting systems for one kidney. If there is complete ure-

teral duplication, the ureter that supplies the upper half of the kidney often becomes obstructed. If the obstruction is not too bad, this can be seen filling with contrast on an IVP (Fig. 7–6). If the upper pole of the kidney is completely obstructed, all that is visualized is the normally draining lower pole collecting system, and it looks like a drooping lily. You should also be aware that the duplicated ureter that supplies the upper pole may often have an ectopic insertion into the bladder, urethra, or vagina.

A number of other anomalies occur in the course of the normal embryologic ascent of the kidneys out of the bony pelvis. These anomalies include one kidney rising normally and the other kidney remaining in the pelvis. Remember that it is very rare to have a unilateral kidney, and thus if you see only one kidney in normal position, you should look elsewhere for an ectopic kidney (Fig. 7–7). Another common variant is fusion of the inferior aspect of both kidneys (a horseshoe kidney). This is relatively easy to identify, since the axis of the kidneys is

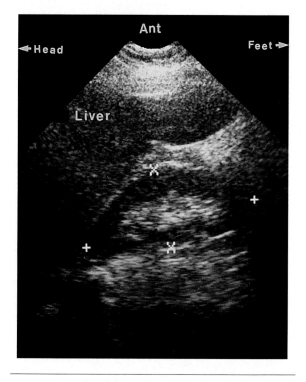

FIGURE 7–3. Normal renal ultrasound. A longitudinal view of the right kidney was obtained by passing the sound beam through the right lobe of the liver. The kidney is seen behind this, outlined by the markers. The central bright echoes in the kidney are due to fat around the collecting system.

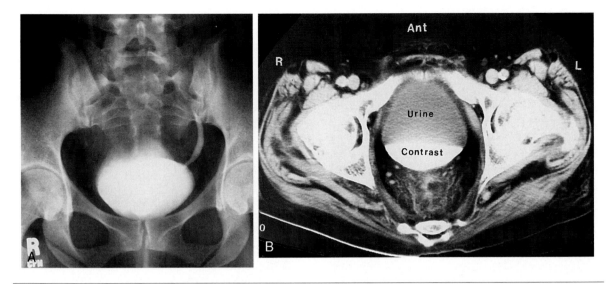

FIGURE 7–4. Distal ureters and bladder on an intravenous pyelogram. A single supine view of the pelvis during an intravenous pyelogram *(A)* shows the distal left ureter and what appears to be the bladder. A CT scan obtained on this patient at the same time at the level of the bladder *(B)* shows that the contrast from the intravenous pyelogram is layering only in the dependent portion of the bladder. Thus, on an intravenous pyelogram, when you think you are looking at the bladder, you are simply seeing a puddle of contrast in the back of the bladder.

abnormal, with the superior aspect of the kidneys tilted outward instead of inward (Fig. 7–8).

Renal Cysts

Renal cysts are quite common, and their incidence increases with age. Most persons over the age of 60 years have one or more simple renal cysts. These are often found incidentally on an IVP, and they are frequently seen on CT scans ordered for other reasons. Ultrasound is a good, inexpensive initial test to characterize a suspected renal cyst found on an IVP. The margins of a benign simple cyst should be well defined, and there should be increased echoes on the

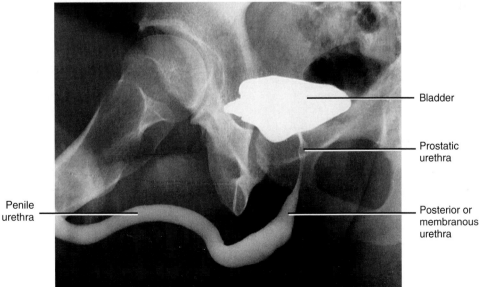

Penile urethra

Bladder

Prostatic urethra

Posterior or membranous urethra

FIGURE 7–5. Normal voiding urethrogram.

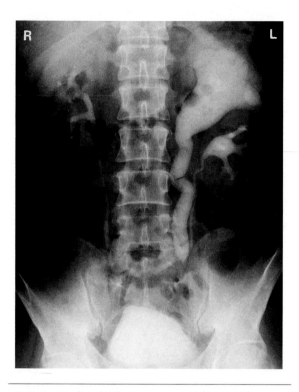

FIGURE 7–6. Duplicated collecting system of left kidney. A film from an intravenous pyelogram shows a normal right collecting system and ureter. On the left, there is a completely duplicated collecting system. As happens frequently with duplicated systems, the collecting system to the upper pole is dilated and obstructed.

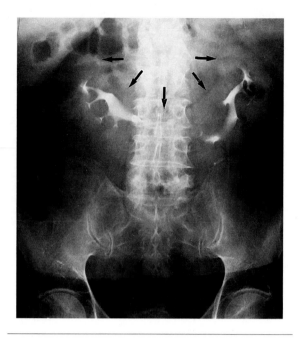

FIGURE 7–8. Horseshoe kidney. On this intravenous pyelogram, the inferior aspects of the right and left kidneys are seen to be joined. Note the abnormal axis of both the right and the left collecting systems, with the upper portion tipping outward from the spine instead of slightly inward.

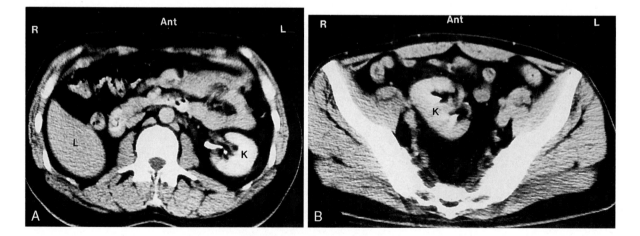

FIGURE 7–7. Pelvic kidney. In this young female a questionable mass was felt in the pelvis during a routine gynecologic examination. A transverse contrast-enhanced CT scan of the upper abdomen (A) reveals only the left kidney. The liver is seen, but no right kidney is identified. Continuing the scan down into the pelvis (B) shows that the right kidney is ectopic. This could have been demonstrated much more cheaply by ultrasound.

posterior aspect of the cyst owing to good transmission of sound through the fluid in the cyst (Fig. 7–9). If a cyst has septa or internal echoes, a CT scan is ordered to further evaluate for a possible cystic neoplasm.

Polycystic renal disease presents a difficult imaging problem. In the adult form of this heritable disorder, there often is progressive renal failure. A CT scan will demonstrate very lumpy kidneys, but the cysts may not be well defined, because there often is hemorrhage within the cyst. Cysts are also usually identified in the liver and sometimes in the pancreas (Fig. 7–10).

Renal Stone Disease

Calcification can occur within the substance of the kidney or within the collecting system. Calcification within the substance of the kidney (nephrocalcinosis) may be cortical (near the periphery of the kidney) or medullary (near the ends of the calyces). Cortical calcification can be due to chronic glomerulonephritis, cortical necrosis, or AIDS-related nephropathy. Medullary calcification may be idiopathic or caused by papillary necrosis, medullary sponge kid-

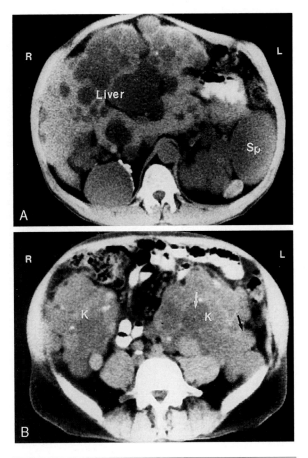

FIGURE 7–10. Adult polycystic disease of the liver and kidneys. A CT scan through the upper abdomen (A) shows the liver, with multiple low-density areas throughout it due to cysts within the liver. A transverse scan obtained slightly lower down (B) shows markedly deformed kidneys bilaterally. Notice that some of the cystic areas within the left kidney are of low density (white arrow) and some of the cysts are of higher density (black arrow). This makes it very difficult to exclude a malignancy in this patient.

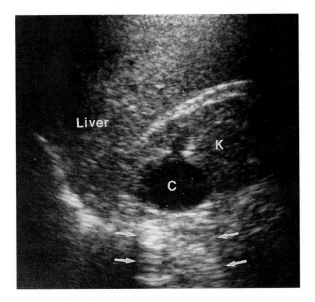

FIGURE 7–9. Simple renal cyst. A longitudinal ultrasound image shows the normal liver and renal parenchyma with a cyst (C) in the upper and posterior aspect of the right kidney (K). Notice that there are no (white) echoes within the cyst and that there is increased transmission of sound through the fluid of the cyst, producing a posterior enhanced echo pattern (arrows).

ney, or other hypercalcemic states (including hyperparathyroidism and osteoporosis) (Fig. 7–11).

At least 80 per cent (and perhaps up to 90 per cent) of renal calculi are radiopaque and appear dense (or white) on a routine x-ray (Fig. 7–12A). Occasionally, renal stones become very large and essentially fill the collecting system of the kidney. These are referred to as staghorn calculi (Fig. 7–12B). If calculi are smaller and are overlying the kidneys or within the course of a ureter, they are usually fairly easy to see. Sometimes it can be difficult to visualize a small stone in the region where the ureter passes anterior to the sacrum. Remember that there are a

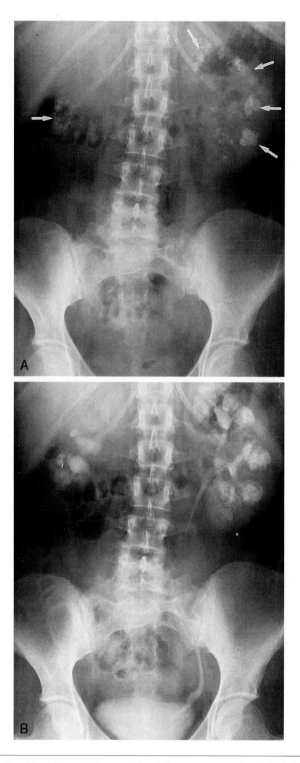

FIGURE 7–11. Nephrocalcinosis. A plain film of the abdomen *(A)* shows multiple calcifications *(arrows)* within the left kidney. On an intravenous pyelogram *(B)* the calcifications are located near the ends of the calyces (medullary) rather than in the cortex. This particular patient had medullary sponge kidneys.

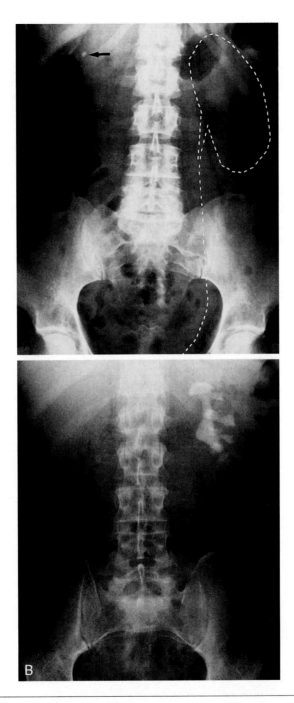

FIGURE 7–12. Renal calculi. On a plain film of the abdomen *(A),* a single calcification is seen in the right upper quadrant *(arrow).* This is a right renal calculus. Renal calculi should be suspected any time a calcification is seen within the renal outline or along the expected course of the ureter *(dotted lines).* In a different patient, a plain film of the abdomen *(B)* shows a calcification conforming perfectly to the collecting system of the left kidney. This is referred to as a staghorn calculus.

large number of vascular calcifications that occur low within the bony pelvis and to the sides of the bladder. These phleboliths typically can be recognized because they are round, have a lucent (dark) center, and are more lateral and lower in the pelvis than the normal course of the ureter.

The most common clinical and radiographic presentation of stone disease is intense flank pain with hematuria. On an IVP, the obstruction of the ureter by a stone may cause delayed visualization of the affected kidney and ureter. When it does visualize, the ureter is usually dilated, and the renal calyces are blunted (Fig. 7–13). On delayed radiographs, while the normal kidney is completely clear of contrast the affected kidney and ureter will be seen retaining contrast. Delayed images are often necessary to determine the exact level of the ureteral obstruction.

Occasionally, the back pressure caused by

an obstructing ureteral stone can rupture a renal calyx or renal pelvis. When this occurs, there is extravasation of urine and contrast outside the kidney into the perirenal space (Fig. 7–14).

When there is an obstructing lesion of the ureter, the urologist may perform cystoscopy and then put a little tube into the distal ureter and inject contrast (a retrograde pyelogram). The ureter, renal pelvis, and calyces are usually visualized. Since there is pressure being exerted during the injection, there can be minimal blunting of the calyces, which is normal under these circumstances. A retrograde pyelogram is useful for looking at small lesions within the collecting system, such as a transitional cell carcinoma. Occasionally, air bubbles will be inadvertently injected along with the contrast, and this may give the appearance of filling defects. The key to differentiation of these entities is that tumors will not move around on different views; also,

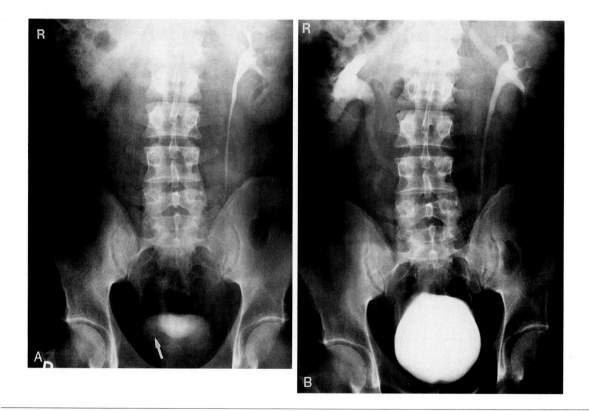

FIGURE 7–13. Ureteral calculus. This young male had intense right flank pain and hematuria. An x-ray taken at 5 minutes during an intravenous pyelogram shows good function of the left kidney, and the left ureter is well seen. The right kidney is faintly seen, and a small calcification is seen at the ureterovesicular junction *(arrow)*. A delayed image 20 minutes later *(B)* now shows a dilated right renal collecting system and right ureter due to obstruction by the distal ureteral calculus.

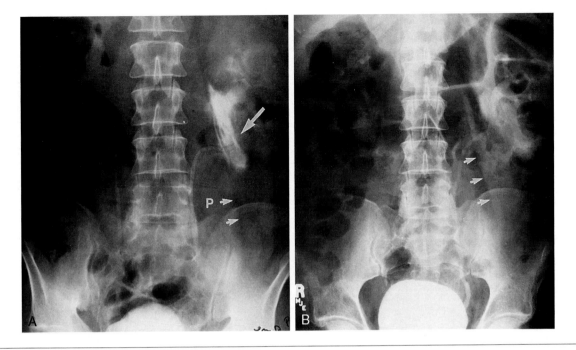

FIGURE 7–14. Urine extravasation. Occasionally, back pressure caused by an obstructing stone or trauma can rupture the urinary collecting system, causing extravasation. On an early film from an intravenous pyelogram *(A)*, a large amount of contrast is seen outside the left renal pelvis *(arrow)*. Note that the left psoas (p) margin is well seen and is darker along the lateral edge owing to fat in the retroperitoneum. On the later image *(B)*, the lateral aspect of the psoas margin has become white owing to contrast dissecting down along the lateral aspect of the psoas margin.

many calculi have sharp or geometric borders (Fig. 7–15). Air bubbles move and are completely round.

Renal Failure

Most imaging studies of the kidneys rely on normal function. The most common clinical question is whether renal failure is due to obstruction or medical renal disease. The imaging examination of choice in these circumstances is ultrasound. Normally, the cortex of the kidney has the same ultrasound echo density as the liver or has fewer echoes than the substance of the liver. In cases of medical renal disease, there are more echoes within the renal cortex than within the liver. This is probably the result of fibrosis and scarring (Fig. 7–16).

Renal Infections

Most patients with pyelonephritis have no findings that are discernible on imaging studies. Im-

aging studies are usually not warranted unless there are repetitive episodes. Sometimes, in patients who have severe acute pyelonephritis, there is enough edema of the renal parenchyma that the swelling causes compression of the calyces or renal pelvis, and there is not good collecting system visualization on an IVP (Fig. 7–17). Occasionally with acute pyelonephritis, focal areas of edema can be seen on CT scans, although this is usually incidental. The real purpose of ordering CT scans in these cases should be to look for a renal parenchymal or perirenal abscess.

In patients with chronic pyelonephritis, the kidney is usually shrunken and has an irregular outer margin. The cortex is also typically thinned. The irregularities of the outer cortical margin are fairly characteristic, with dimpling or scarring directly over a calyx. If there is dimpling or a defect in the margin of the kidney between two calyces, this is more likely to be the result of a focal infarct.

Diabetics are particularly prone to an unusual form of acute pyelonephritis, which is called emphysematous pyelonephritis. In these

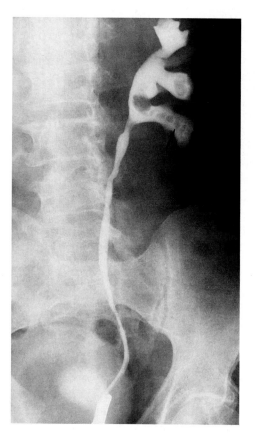

FIGURE 7-15. Ureteral calculi on a retrograde pyelogram. A cystoscope has been put in the bladder and the orifice of the left ureter catheterized. Contrast is then injected retrograde. Multiple lucencies can be seen within the collecting system of the left kidney *(arrow)*. The fact that these defects are not round but rather have sharp corners indicates that they are calculi and not inadvertently injected air bubbles.

FIGURE 7-16. Medical renal disease. Ultrasound is often performed in patients with renal failure to differentiate between hydronephrosis and renal parenchymal disease. Patients with renal parenchymal disease usually have smaller than normal kidneys. In this longitudinal ultrasound image of the right kidney, note that the parenchyma of the kidney has more echoes or is whiter than that of the liver at the same depth. Normal renal parenchyma will have an equal or lower number of echoes than the liver (see Fig. 7-26 for an ultrasound image of hydronephrosis).

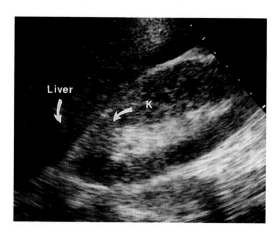

FIGURE 7–17. Acute pyelonephritis. An intravenous pyelogram done on a patient with infection clearly shows the renal pelvis and collecting system of the right kidney. On the left, although the ureter is seen, the renal pelvis and calyces are not. This is because of compression secondary to edema resulting from left-sided acute pyelonephritis.

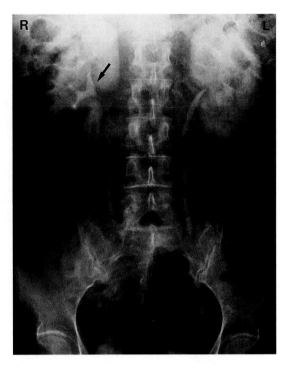

patients, there is actually gas generated by the bacteria within the parenchyma of the kidney. Usually, the kidney is nonfunctional, and a dark radiating striated gas pattern is seen where you would normally expect to find a kidney (Fig. 7–18).

Occasionally, inflammatory abnormalities can cause enlargement of both kidneys. This is particularly true in acute glomerulonephritis. The differential diagnosis for bilaterally enlarged kidneys includes bilateral obstruction, leukemia, glycogen storage diseases, lymphoma, and polycystic disease as well as a number of other entities (Fig. 7–19).

Infections of the kidney can progress to the stage at which the kidney is essentially nonfunctional. There is an entity known as xanthogranulomatous pyelonephritis in which there is a nonfunctional kidney with some calcification visible within the kidney (Fig. 7–20). The kidney is removed surgically. On the basis of any imaging study, it is difficult to differentiate xanthogranulomatous pyelonephritis from a renal tumor.

Renal tuberculosis can affect the kidneys, ureter, and bladder; the infection typically begins in the kidneys, and you should look there

first. In the early stages, there is narrowing or amputation of the infundibulum between a renal calyx and the renal pelvis. In late stages, there is a nonfunctional shrunken kidney with clumps of calcification (Fig. 7–21). A number of fungal infections can affect the kidney in diabetic and immunosuppressed patients. Fungal infections often cause large fungal clumps or balls within the collecting system that can obstruct the kidney (Fig. 7–22).

Renal Trauma

Blunt trauma, particularly during motor vehicle accidents, can cause a number of renal abnormalities. Significant kidney trauma should be suspected when there is a fracture of the twelfth rib or fractures of the transverse processes of the lumbar vertebrae. Another useful sign on the plain film is nonvisualization of the psoas margin on one side. In a renal contusion the kidney is intact, but there is interstitial edema that may lead to reduced blood flow. Lacerations and intrarenal hematomas can be incomplete (not extending into the calyceal system), whereas complete lacerations are usually accompanied by a

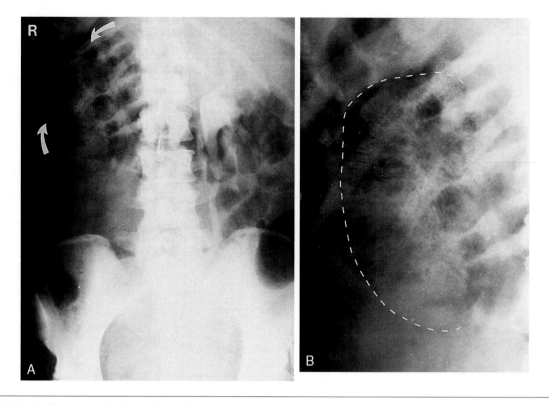

FIGURE 7–18. Emphysematous pyelonephritis. This condition most commonly occurs in diabetics. On an intravenous pyelogram *(A)*, there will be nonfunction of the affected kidney, in this case on the right *(arrows)*. A more detailed view of the right upper quadrant *(B)* shows radiating dark thin lines of gas within the parenchyma of the right kidney.

significant hemorrhage and urine extravasation (Fig. 7–23). Minor renal injuries are usually treated conservatively, and even kidneys that have large lacerations may ultimately heal. Surgical intervention may not be required unless there is major blood loss. Occasionally there may be avulsion of the renal vascular pedicle with disruption of the blood supply.

The advantage of CT scanning in cases of renal trauma is that you can assess other organs, such as the liver and spleen, for concomitant injuries and the peritoneal and retroperitoneal areas for hematomas. Although it is not generally appreciated, lithotripsy (ultrasound used to fragment renal stones) can cause significant renal trauma. Postlithotripsy hemorrhage generally resolves without intervention, and imaging studies are not usually ordered.

Renal Tumors

Renal cell carcinoma constitutes about 85 per cent of all primary renal malignancies. It usually occurs in the sixth decade, and males are affected twice as often as females. The classic clinical triad consists of gross hematuria, flank pain, and a flank mass, although this triad is seen in only approximately 10 per cent of patients. Typically, gross or microscopic hematuria is what raises the suspicion of a urinary malignancy. Large mass lesions within the kidney will displace the collecting system and produce an irregular contour of the kidney on an IVP, but very small tumors or pedunculated neoplasms can be difficult to appreciate. At the present time, CT scanning with and without intravenous contrast (with thin cuts through the kidneys) is the imaging procedure of choice in an older patient with persistent painless hematuria and a normal IVP and normal cystoscopy.

Most renal cell carcinomas are relatively solid, but some are very cystic, and you may have some difficulty differentiating a cystic neoplasm from a benign renal cyst. On a CT scan, the finding of a thickened wall or a mural mass within a cystic abnormality is a criterion for

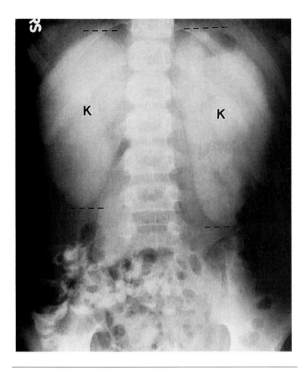

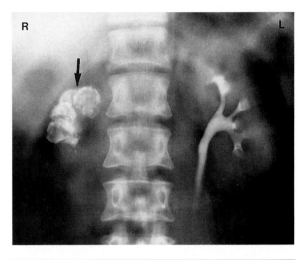

FIGURE 7–21. End-stage renal tuberculosis. A tomogram obtained during an intravenous pyelogram shows a normally functioning left kidney, but a completely nonfunctional shrunken right kidney replaced by mottled calcification (*arrow*).

FIGURE 7–19. Acute glomerulonephritis. An intravenous pyelogram in this child demonstrates markedly enlarged kidneys bilaterally. The injected contrast has made the kidneys visible, but the kidneys are unable to excrete the contrast.

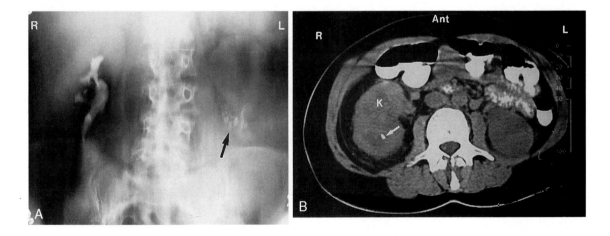

FIGURE 7–20. Xanthogranulomatous pyelonephritis. On an intravenous pyelogram (*A*), no function is seen in the left kidney, although there is some evidence of calcification (*arrow*). In a different patient with the same condition in the right kidney, a CT scan (*B*) again shows nonfunction, with areas of low density and calcification (*arrow*). With any imaging modality it is very difficult to differentiate this condition from a neoplasm.

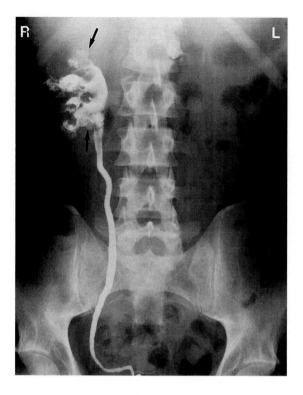

FIGURE 7–22. Aspergillosis. In this immunocompromised patient, there was no function identified of the right kidney on an intravenous pyelogram. Therefore, a right retrograde pyelogram was performed and is shown here. There is marked irregularity of the renal pelvis and collecting system, with intraluminal irregular defects *(arrows).* These are due to fungus balls and debris within the collecting system.

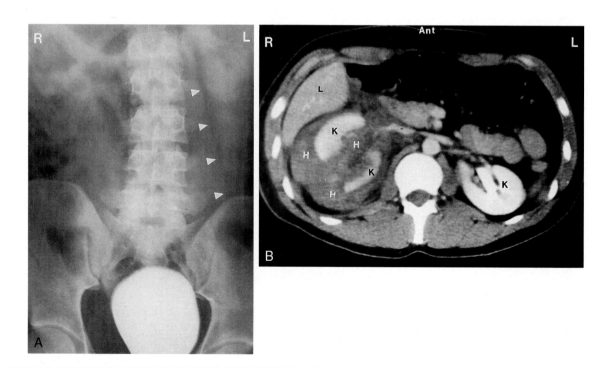

FIGURE 7–23. Renal laceration. An x-ray of the abdomen *(A)* in a young male involved in an automobile accident shows a well-defined left psoas margin *(arrowheads).* The right psoas margin is not identified, and a contrast-enhanced CT scan *(B)* at the level of the kidneys shows a fracture through the midportion of the right kidney. The kidney can be seen in two separate pieces with intervening and surrounding hemorrhage (h).

malignancy (Fig. 7–24). On the CT scan you should also look for potential extension into the renal vein and inferior vena cava as well as into the nearby nodes. Metastases from renal cell carcinoma tend to go either to the lung or to the bone. On the chest x-ray, the metastases are usually nodules ranging from 0.5 cm to several centimeters in size. When the metastases are in bone, they tend to be very aggressive, expansile, and lytic (destructive) (Fig. 7–25).

Obstruction of the Renal Collecting System

Obstruction of the ureter of the kidney is easily visualized by an IVP, which affords a detailed

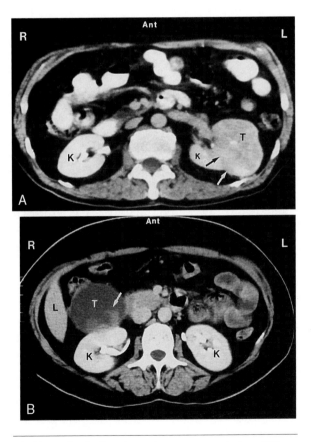

FIGURE 7–24. Renal cell carcinoma. A transverse contrast-enhanced CT scan (A) in a patient with hematuria shows that there has been significant replacement of the left kidney by tumor (t). The left renal vein exiting the kidney is also very thick, indicating tumor extension into the renal vein. A cystic renal cell carcinoma is shown in a CT scan on a different patient (B). In this patient, a pedunculated cystic lesion is seen projecting off the anterior aspect of the right kidney. The fact that there is a mass projecting within the generally cystic lesion (arrow) as well as an irregularly thickened wall makes this highly suspicious for a cancer.

view of the anatomy. For other clinical indications, however, ultrasound may be more useful. Although it is difficult or impossible to visualize the full length of the ureter by ultrasound, it is very easy to determine whether there is dilatation of the collecting system within the kidney itself (Fig. 7–26). This is seen as an area with relatively few echoes splaying the high-intensity echoes (caused by fat) around the renal collecting system. If you are following a patient with known hydronephrosis, ultrasound is the test that you should order. Ultrasound is also the test of choice when you are trying to differentiate hydronephrosis from medical renal disease in a patient who has presented with renal failure.

Occasionally, there is dilatation of the renal pelvis that is not caused by obstruction. This may have a congenital basis or may be the result of a flaccid collecting system. A simple way of differentiating the two is to order a nuclear medicine Lasix renogram (Fig. 7–27). The patient is injected with a radioactive material that is rapidly cleared by glomerular filtration. This will give you a picture of both kidneys that looks like a poor man's IVP. The advantage of this study, however, is that you can inject the patient with Lasix approximately 15 minutes into the study. If there is rapid clearance of activity from the kidney and renal pelvis, you know that you are dealing with a flaccid system rather than an obstructed one.

THE URETER

You should be able to recognize frequent and characteristic lesions that occur in the ureter. Duplication of the ureter and collecting system has already been discussed. Sometimes the ureter has an abnormal entrance into the bladder, with dilatation of the ureter as it passes through the bladder wall (ureterocele) causing a "cobra head" deformity (Fig. 7–28). Ureteroceles are not of much clinical importance and generally do not require treatment.

The ureter normally has peristaltic waves, and, therefore, on any single film there usually will be visualization of some portions of the ureter and not others. You should not be fooled into diagnosing a stricture unless you see con-

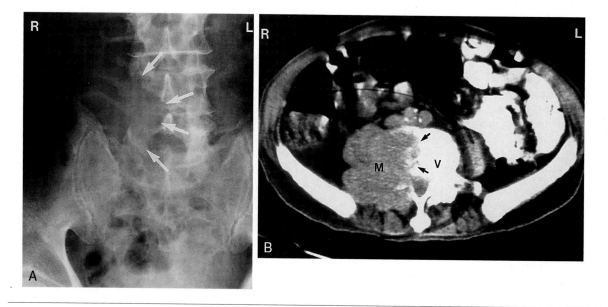

FIGURE 7–25. Bone metastasis from renal cell carcinoma. An AP view of the lower lumbar spine *(A)* shows destruction of the right lateral aspects of L4 and L5 *(arrows)*. A transverse CT scan at the same level *(B)* shows that not only has the vertebral body been destroyed but also there is a significant soft tissue mass (m) extending laterally.

trast above, below, and at the level of the lesion and are able to confirm it on several different films. Since an IVP is done with the patient supine and contrast is heavier than urine, the most anterior portions of the ureters (as they pass over the sacroiliac [SI] joints into the pelvis) are usually very difficult to see. Sometimes the radiologist will order a prone film to rectify this situation.

Dilatation of a ureter is diagnosed only

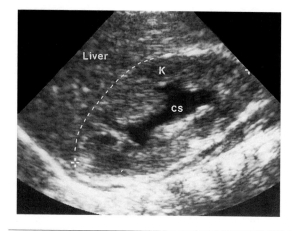

FIGURE 7–26. Hydronephrosis. Ultrasound is the simplest and most cost-effective way of determining whether hydronephrosis is present. Here, a longitudinal image of the right kidney demonstrates a dilated collecting system (cs).

when the ureter is seen to be greater than 8 mm in diameter and contrast is backed up in the ureter without peristaltic waves. When there is an acute obstruction there is almost always calyceal blunting as well. Dilatation of a ureter usually elicits a reflex response from students, who immediately say "hydronephrosis" and then "obstruction." Dilatation can be due to a number of other causes, including ureterovesicular reflux, infection, and congenital megaureter.

Common intraluminal abnormalities of the ureter are renal calculi (see earlier), blood clots, transitional cell carcinomas, and, occasionally, fungal lesions. A clot within the ureter is not visible on a plain film, and on an IVP it will be a filling defect that can look like a nonopaque stone (Fig. 7–29). Remember that most renal calculi (80 per cent) are radiopaque and should be visible on plain films. A clot should be suspected following trauma and in patients who are taking anticoagulants.

Transitional cell carcinomas can occur either in the renal collecting system or in the bladder. In the renal collecting system, they can form a mass that spreads the renal sinus fat and can cause obstruction (Fig. 7–30A). In the ureter, a renal cell carcinoma may look like a lesion in the wall of the ureter, or it may cause an "apple core" deformity with encirclement of the lumen.

FIGURE 7-27. Differentiation of causes of a dilated collecting system. A nuclear medicine renogram is performed by administering a small amount of radioactivity that is cleared by the kidney. Two-minute sequential images are obtained in a posterior projection. At 14 minutes, activity is seen in both the right and the left dilated collecting systems, and furosemide is given intravenously. The right kidney excretes its activity into the bladder (b), but the left kidney (k) remains essentially unchanged, indicating a flaccid dilated collecting system on the right but an obstructed left collecting system.

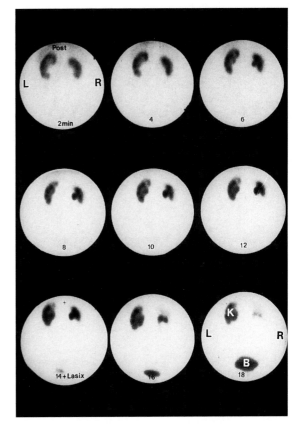

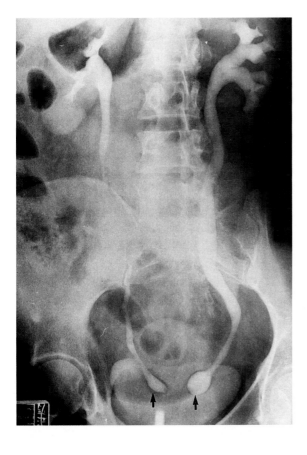

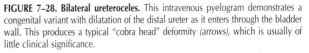

FIGURE 7-28. Bilateral ureteroceles. This intravenous pyelogram demonstrates a congenital variant with dilatation of the distal ureter as it enters through the bladder wall. This produces a typical "cobra head" deformity (arrows), which is usually of little clinical significance.

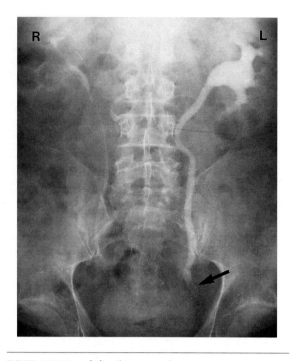

FIGURE 7–29. Ureteral clot. This patient, who was on anticoagulant therapy, developed hematuria and left flank pain. The intravenous pyelogram demonstrates a filling defect in the distal left ureter *(arrow)* caused by a clot that has partially obstructed the left collecting system, causing it to be dilated compared with the right ureter.

Occasionally, on an IVP an intraluminal transitional cell carcinoma causes an appearance that looks like an upside-down goblet (Bergman's sign) (Fig. 7–30*B*).

In addition to lesions that are entirely contained within the lumen, there may be lesions that project into the lumen or are the result of extrinsic pressure. In some patients, there are indentations across the upper one third of the collecting system caused by vascular impressions of blood vessels as they cross over the ureter. Collateral vessels may cause ureteral notching (Fig. 7–31). In patients who have an infection, there may be small fluid-filled cysts in the ureteral wall that project into the lumen (pyelitis cystica). Occasionally, even metastases can indent the ureter at multiple locations. This most often is the result of metastatic melanoma. If you think that there is a ureteral lesion on an IVP, this is almost always confirmed by the urologist, who will perform a retrograde ureterogram prior to any sort of surgery.

Deviation of the ureter can signal nearby pathology. In the region between the lower pole of the kidney and the sacrum, the normal course of the ureters on an AP or a PA film is over the transverse processes of the spine. Lateral deviation of a ureter can be the result of retroperitoneal adenopathy, retroperitoneal tumors, abdominal aortic aneurysms, and, occasionally, large psoas muscles (in young men or horse riders). Medial deviation can be due to traction caused by fibrosis from chronic leakage of an aneurysm, by methysergide use, or, if only on the right side, by a congenital retrocaval ureter.

BLADDER

Anatomy and Imaging Techniques

As the bladder fills with urine it has a water or soft tissue density. The bladder can often be seen on a plain x-ray, since it is frequently outlined by perivesicular fat. As the bladder enlarges with urine, it pushes the small bowel superiorly and laterally. An enlarged bladder can be very striking (Fig. 7–32), and without having contrast material in the bladder it is often difficult to tell whether you are looking at an enlarged fluid-filled bladder or some other soft tissue mass arising from the pelvis or an abdominal mass. One of the rules that I use is that it is unusual for abdominal masses or tumors to grow down into the pelvis but that it is very common for pelvic masses to grow up out of the pelvis into the lower abdomen. Thus, if you see a soft tissue mass that involves both the lower abdomen and the pelvis, the mass probably arose in the pelvis. The differential diagnosis of a pelvic mass includes uterine enlargement, ovarian cysts, and tumor or pelvic sarcomas. If the patient is female and the bladder is displaced to one side, you should expect an ovarian etiology. Usually the bladder is visualized by using water-soluble contrast from an IVP, CT, or cystogram.

Trauma

Fractures of the pelvis are accompanied by hematomas. These may displace the bladder to one

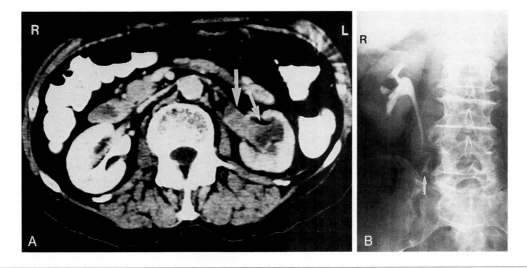

FIGURE 7–30. Transitional cell carcinoma. A transverse contrast-enhanced CT scan at the level of the kidneys *(A)* shows expansion of the left renal pelvis *(arrows)*. This is due to a transitional cell carcinoma within the renal pelvis. In a different patient, an intravenous pyelogram *(B)* demonstrates an upside-down goblet deformity in the right midureter *(arrow)*. This is a sign of a ureteral transitional cell carcinoma.

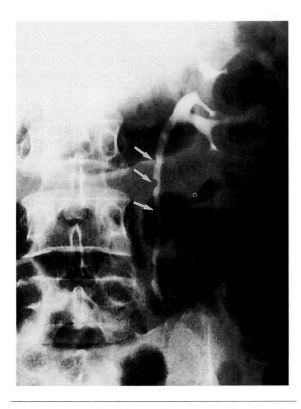

FIGURE 7–31. Ureteral notching. On this intravenous pyelogram, notching along the medial aspect of the proximal left ureter is easily seen *(arrows)*. This can be due to a number of abnormalities, but in this case it was due to impression on the lumen of the ureter by collateral vessels.

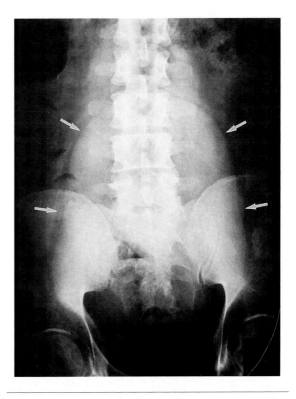

FIGURE 7–32. Distended bladder. On this plain film of the abdomen, a large soft tissue mass is seen arising from the pelvis *(arrows)*. It has pushed small bowel out of the way. The differential diagnosis includes a pelvic tumor, distended bladder, or cystic abnormality arising from the pelvis.

side if they are unilateral, but more often pelvic hematomas are bilateral, and they will compress and elevate the inferior portion of the bladder (Fig. 7–33) so that it looks like an upside-down teardrop. This shape of the bladder can also be caused by pelvic adenopathy, pelvic lipomatosis (mostly in black males with hypertension), and by very prominent iliopsoas muscles.

With pelvic fractures or as a result of direct compression of a fluid-filled distended bladder, there can be bladder rupture. This is almost always accompanied by hematuria. About 10 per cent of patients who have a pelvic fracture will have bladder rupture. The bladder can rupture either extraperitoneally (80%) or intraperitoneally (20%). Intraperitoneal rupture of the bladder is recognized on an IVP or a cystogram because there is contrast extravasation into the peritoneal cavity that outlines loops of bowel, and the contrast will also layer in the paracolic gutters.

The vast majority of patients with an extraperitoneal bladder rupture will have associated pelvic fractures. With extraperitoneal rupture, the extravasated contrast material will be in a streaky or sunburst pattern (Fig. 7–34). About 10 per cent of patients with ruptured bladders will have both an intraperitoneal and an extraperitoneal component.

Pelvic trauma can also result in injury to the urethra. Since the female urethra is so short,

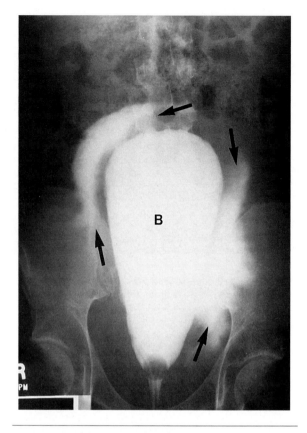

FIGURE 7–34. Bladder rupture. A cystogram done in a patient following a motor vehicle accident shows extravasation of contrast *(arrows)* into the tissues surrounding the bladder. This is an extraperitoneal bladder rupture. With an intraperitoneal bladder rupture, contrast would be seen outlining loops of bowel.

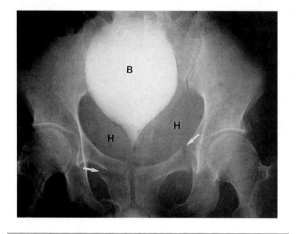

FIGURE 7–33. Pelvic fractures with hematoma. This cystogram demonstrates multiple pelvic fractures *(arrows).* The associated bilateral hematomas (H) have elevated and compressed the bladder.

this is rarely, if ever, injured in an accident. In the male, urethral injuries are more common than bladder injuries. Since the urethra is fixed at the prostatomembranous junction, tears in this area are secondary to shearing. In a patient with pelvic trauma who has blood at the urethral meatus and who is unable to void or can void only with difficulty, a posterior urethral tear should be suspected. In these cases, a retrograde urethrogram should be done before any attempt is made to catheterize the bladder. The reason is that a small initial tear may be significantly enlarged by any attempt at catheterization (Fig. 7–35). Injuries to the anterior portion of the urethra are much less common. Injuries to the bulbous portion of the urethra are most commonly due to a straddle injury in which the patient falls astride a solid object, such as a beam.

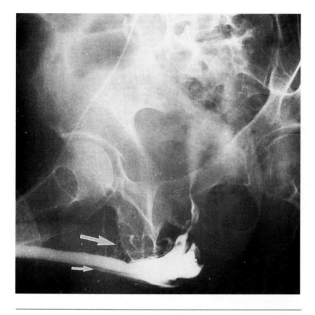

FIGURE 7–35. Urethral rupture. Following a straddle type injury, this young male patient had hematuria and was unable to void. A retrograde urethrogram was performed, and there was extravasation of contrast into the soft tissues *(small arrow)* as well as into nearby venous structures *(large arrow).*

Neurologic Abnormalities

If trauma compromises the spinal cord, the bladder may become either flaccid or spastic. On a contrasted study, a spastic bladder has the shape of a Christmas tree, with little outpouchings along the lateral margins (Fig. 7–36). These areas of outpouching of contrast or urine are pseudo-

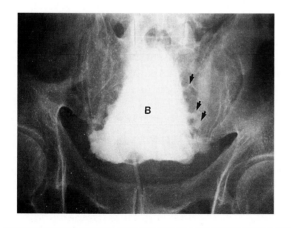

FIGURE 7–36. Spastic bladder. In this patient with a spinal cord injury, there is the typical "Christmas tree" deformity of the bladder with lateral diverticula *(arrows).*

diverticula caused by hypertrophy of the bladder musculature. A hyper-reflexive bladder usually occurs when the spinal cord lesion is at the level of T5 or higher. These patients are prime candidates for urinary infection, calculi, and bilateral collecting system dilatation. Hyporeflexive bladders are usually the result of a herniated disk, multiple sclerosis, diabetic neuropathy, or lower spinal cord tumor. Although these patients may demonstrate a large bladder, the upper urinary collecting systems are usually within normal limits, and vesicoureteral reflux is rare.

Infections

There is little reason to do imaging studies in female patients with uncomplicated cystitis. If there are repeated bouts of infection, an IVP may be indicated to exclude anatomic abnormalities. Since cystitis is rare in males, an IVP may be indicated after an initial infection. With severe cystitis, there may be mucosal thickening; however, this should not be evaluated on a study that has a nondistended bladder. Once the bladder is fully distended, it may be possible to image thickened mucosa, although this finding rarely changes treatment.

There are a number of unusual bladder infections in which imaging findings are fairly characteristic. Diabetic patients may develop emphysematous cystitis, in which gas is present in either the wall or the lumen of the bladder (Fig. 7–37A). In contrast to emphysematous pyelonephritis, morbidity is not increased with emphysematous cystitis. This condition usually responds well to antibiotic therapy. Air within the bladder itself is more likely due to instrumentation or a bladder-bowel fistula.

Tuberculosis can affect the bladder, but this is extremely rare without strictures and stenosis of the ureters and stenosis of the calyces of the renal collecting system. Schistosomiasis, although very rare, can produce characteristic bladder wall calcification (Fig. 7–37B). A number of inflammatory conditions can cause a small bladder, including interstitial cystitis, cyclophosphamide cystitis, and radiation therapy. These can also cause calcification within the bladder wall. With the exception of the small

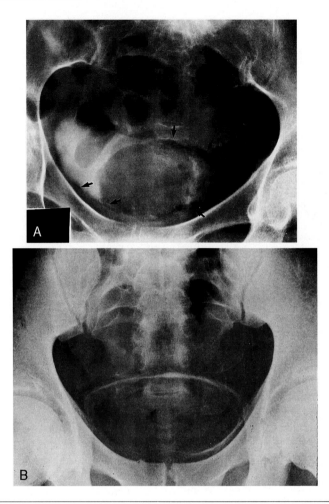

FIGURE 7–37. Unusual forms of cystitis. A view of the pelvis obtained during an intravenous pyelogram *(A)* in a diabetic patient shows air within the wall of the bladder as well as within the bladder *(arrows)*. This is called emphysematous cystitis. In a different patient, calcification of the bladder wall is seen on a plain x-ray of the pelvis *(B)*. This is due to schistosomiasis.

capacity, very little is characteristic or disease specific about the imaging findings.

Tumors

Ninety-five per cent of bladder tumors are transitional cell carcinomas. Transitional cell carcinoma is four times more common in men than in women, and a significantly increased incidence has been associated with cigarette smoking. Patients frequently present with hematuria and occasionally with urinary frequency and dysuria. Pelvic lymph node extension is relatively common. Hematogenous metastases tend to go to liver and lungs and, to a much lesser extent, bone. When bone lesions are seen, they are typically lytic. Transitional cell carcinoma of the bladder is associated with upper tract transitional cell tumors, and close follow-up of these patients is essential.

Tumors of the bladder rarely calcify, and the diagnosis of tumors is not obvious on plain films. An IVP may show a filling defect within the lumen of the bladder (Fig. 7–38). You should be very cautious about saying that there is no cancer on the basis of an IVP. As pointed out earlier, intravenously administered contrast is heavier than urine and layers dependently in the bladder. A tumor will not be visualized unless it is located in the dependent portion of the bladder. CT scanning is useful only to evaluate

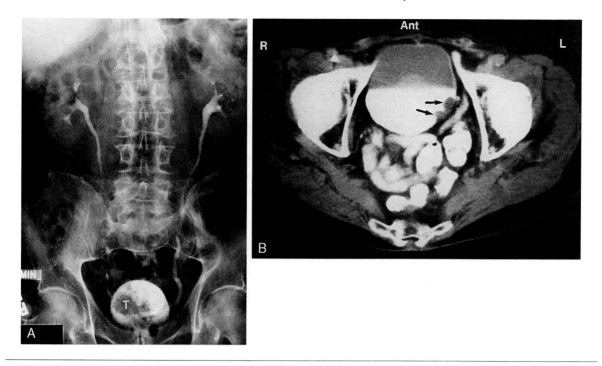

FIGURE 7–38. Bladder carcinoma. An intravenous pyelogram (A) in a patient with hematuria clearly shows a large irregular filling defect within the bladder caused by a tumor (t). A CT scan (B) in a different patient shows a small bladder carcinoma (arrows). This is visible only because the tumor happens to be in the dependent portion of the bladder with the contrast. Had this lesion been on the anterior surface of the bladder, it probably would not have been visualized on either a CT scan or an intravenous pyelogram.

invasion of adjacent organs and pelvic lymph-adenopathy. If a bladder carcinoma is suspected, the initial study of choice should be direct visualization utilizing cystoscopy.

PROSTATE AND SCROTUM

Anatomy and Imaging Techniques

Enlargement of the prostate causes elevation of the base of the bladder (Fig. 7–39). Prostate enlargement is most often the result of benign prostatic hypertrophy rather than prostatic carcinoma. If the prostate is big enough, there can be outlet obstruction of the bladder. Recently, there has been a lot of interest in transrectal ultrasound of the prostate as a screening test for prostate cancer. At the present time, this is not a useful test by itself. The initial investigation for prostate carcinoma should be by digital rectal examination and evaluation of the serum level of prostate-specific antigen (PSA). If the

serum value is elevated, ultrasound may be helpful in locating a suspicious area that can be biopsied transrectally.

The most common lesions of the scrotum

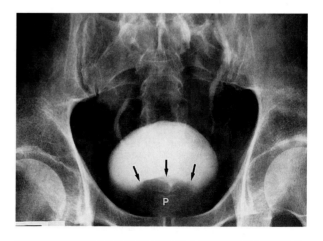

FIGURE 7–39. Benign prostatic hyperplasia. A view of the bladder obtained during an intravenous pyelogram shows a smooth defect impressing upon the inferior aspect of the bladder (arrows) caused by a benign enlargement of the prostate (p).

that may require imaging are epididymitis, testicular torsion, and hydrocele in addition to evaluation for testicular tumors. In cases in which testicular torsion needs to be differentiated from epididymitis, a radionuclide testicular scan is widely used (Fig. 7–40). Epididymitis will be seen as a lesion with hyperemia on the affected side. In acute torsion, there will be an area of decreased blood flow on the side in which there is pain. In a torsion that has been present for a day or more (missed torsion), there will be a lesion without much blood flow centrally but with a hypervascular rim. Occasionally, Doppler ultrasound can be used to exclude a testicular torsion, although this is quite operator dependent and difficult to do.

Imaging evaluation of the testicle for either a hydrocele or a tumor should be done utilizing ultrasound. In general, any mass within the testicle itself should be considered malignant, whereas those lesions outside the testicle but within the scrotum are usually benign. Ninety-five per cent of solid testicular masses are germ cell tumors (seminoma, embryonal carcinoma, choriocarcinoma, and teratoma).

FEMALE PELVIS

Anatomy and Imaging Techniques

The most common and fruitful imaging methods are pelvic ultrasound and CT. Ultrasound is un-

doubtedly the most widely used method, since it can easily image the uterus and adnexal regions. Because it does not use ionizing radiation it can even be used during pregnancy. Imaging of the female pelvis with a plain x-ray is usually of low yield, since most significant pathology associated with female pelvic organs is not calcified. Sometimes a large soft tissue mass can be seen displacing bowel.

Female pelvic ultrasound is done either transabdominally (by having the transducer on the lower anterior abdominal wall and using the bladder as a window) or transvaginally. Transvaginal ultrasound has a much smaller field of view, and it is often very difficult to orient yourself with respect to the images unless you were actually there when they were taken. With transabdominal ultrasound, orientation is much easier. Remember that ultrasound imaging gives you a "slice" picture. The slices are typically either longitudinal or transverse. In the longitudinal plane, you can easily see the vagina, cervix, uterus, and bladder (Fig. 7–41). Areas of high-intensity echoes can be seen in the vagina and sometimes in the center of the uterus as a result of mucus production, hemorrhage, or decidual reaction. Fluid in the bladder, uterus, or cul-de-sac appears as an area without echoes. A small amount of fluid within the cul-de-sac can be a normal finding in the middle of the menstrual period, but in patients in whom an ectopic pregnancy is suspected this may represent hemorrhage (Fig. 7–42).

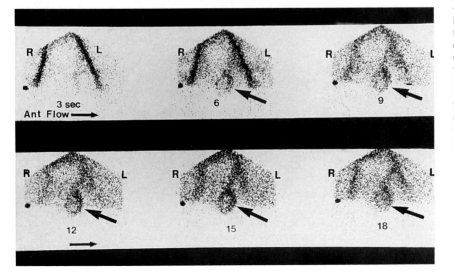

FIGURE 7–40. Testicular torsion. Evaluation of blood flow to the testicle has been done by giving an intravenous bolus of radioactive material. The right and left iliac vessels are clearly identified, and sequential images are obtained every 3 seconds. Here, increased flow is seen to the rim of the left testicle (arrow), and there is no blood flow centrally. This is the appearance of a testicular torsion in which the torsion has been present for more than approximately 24 hours.

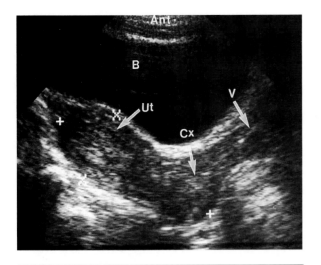

FIGURE 7-41. Normal female pelvic ultrasound. On this longitudinal image obtained in the midportion of the pelvis, the bladder, uterus, cervix, and vagina are easily visualized.

Evaluation of the uterus by ultrasound does not allow determination of patency of the fallopian tubes. A hysterosalpingogram is typically done to assess tubal patency. This is done by putting a cannula in the cervical os and injecting a water-based contrast material. After the uterus is filled, the contrast goes out the fallopian tubes and spills into the peritoneal cavity. In cases in which there is obstruction of the fallopian tubes (hydrosalpinx), the contrast

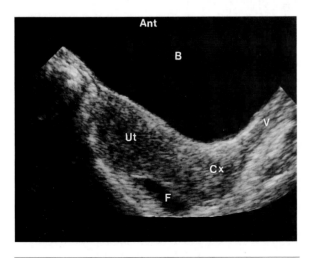

FIGURE 7-42. Free fluid in the cul-de-sac. This longitudinal image of the pelvis demonstrates a collection of fluid (F) behind the uterus. This can be a normal finding during the middle of the menstrual cycle or may represent bleeding from entities such as an ectopic pregnancy.

proceeds to the point of obstruction in the fallopian tubes and then collects in a dilated portion of the fallopian tube without free spill into the pelvis (Fig. 7–43).

Pregnancy

Ultrasound is the imaging method of choice to evaluate the status of a pregnancy. In very early pregnancy, transvaginal, rather than transabdominal, ultrasound is the most sensitive. By measuring the fetal crown-rump length as well as a number of other parameters, the gestational age of the fetus can be determined. The age that

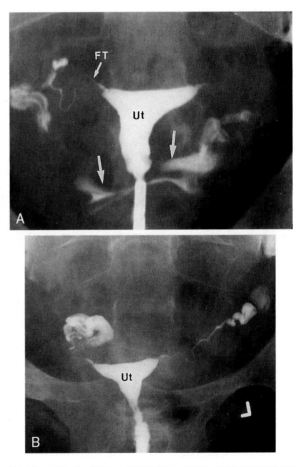

FIGURE 7-43. Normal and abnormal hysterosalpingogram. In a normal patient (A), the uterine cervix is cannulated and contrast is injected to visualize the uterus. Contrast then goes out the fallopian tubes and has free spill into the pelvis (arrows). In a different patient complaining of infertility, a hysterosalpingogram (B) demonstrates the uterus and dilated fallopian tubes with no spill into the pelvis. This is known as hydrosalpinx.

is usually quoted refers to menstrual age rather than conceptual age. Thus, a report that indicates a 5-week pregnancy (gestational age) really corresponds to a 3-week pregnancy (conception dates).

The first ultrasound sign of pregnancy is the appearance of the gestational sac at 28 to 30 days. A yolk sac can be seen at 5 to 6 weeks, and this is the first reliable sign of an intrauterine pregnancy. A heartbeat is also typically seen at approximately 5 weeks (gestational age) (Fig. 7–44). As the fetus becomes more advanced, it is possible to see decidual thickening and formation of the placenta. A low-lying placenta early in pregnancy will not necessarily result in a placenta previa, since there is significant growth of the lower uterine segment later in pregnancy.

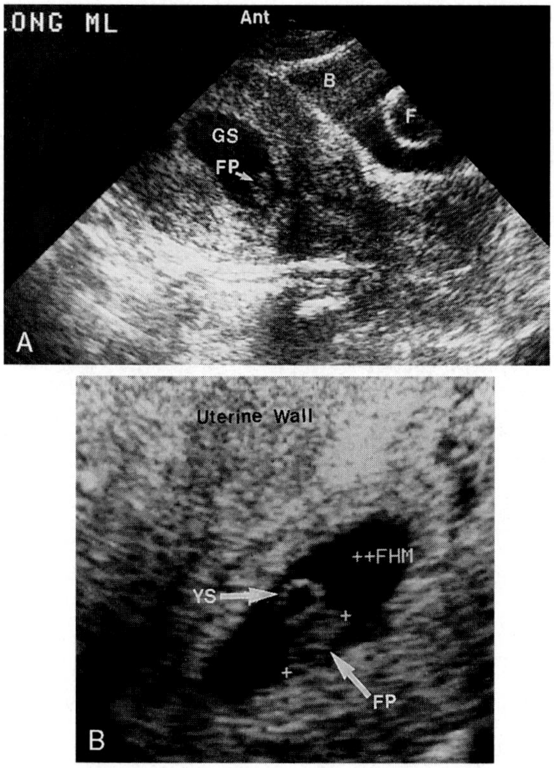

FIGURE 7–44. Early normal obstetric ultrasound. A longitudinal transabdominal ultrasound image (A) demonstrates the bladder (b) and a Foley catheter (f) within it. Superior and behind the bladder is the uterus with a gestational sac (gs) centrally and a fetal pole (fp) within it. More detail can be obtained using transvaginal ultrasound (B). In this case, the fetal pole can be measured; a yolk sac (ys) is also seen; and the technician has indicated that fetal heart motion was seen (+ +FHM).

The very common emergent clinical question is whether a patient with pelvic pain and a missed menstrual period has an intrauterine pregnancy, an ectopic pregnancy, or an incomplete or missed abortion. An imaging study is not appropriate until the results of a pregnancy test are available. As mentioned earlier, if suspected gestational age is greater than 5 weeks, an intrauterine gestational sac should be identified. In addition, fetal components should be seen within this gestational sac, particularly if transvaginal ultrasound is used.

Patients with an ectopic pregnancy almost always have pain and bleeding, but only 40 per cent will have a palpable adnexal mass. On ultrasound, a normal-looking uterus and normal adnexal areas do not exclude an ectopic pregnancy. Under these circumstances, a repeat examination in 7 to 10 days may be necessary. If the uterus appears normal and there is a complex adnexal mass, the likelihood of an ectopic pregnancy should be considered high. Sometimes, a gestational sac and fetal heart motion can be seen outside the uterus. In these circumstances, there is certain diagnosis of an ectopic pregnancy (Fig. 7–45).

If an empty gestational sac is seen within the uterus, it may represent a very early intrauterine pregnancy, particularly if the diameter of the sac is 10 to 20 mm. It may also represent a blighted ovum or a pseudogestational sac in a patient with an ectopic pregnancy. A pseudogestational sac is seen in approximately 20 per cent of patients with ectopic pregnancies.

In the second and third trimesters of pregnancy, there can be quite complete ultrasonic evaluation of the fetus. The most common reason for an ultrasound at this stage is to determine placental location, fetal growth, and gestational age. The earlier in pregnancy that gestational age is determined, the more accurate it will be. Dating is done by measuring the biparietal diameter of the head (Fig. 7–46) as well as the length of the femur and other structures. At the same time there should be evaluation of the intracranial structures, the heart (to see that it has four chambers), and the abdominal organs to look for abnormalities such as duodenal atresia, obstructed kidneys, and defects in the spine and anterior abdominal wall.

X-rays may be done during pregnancy but

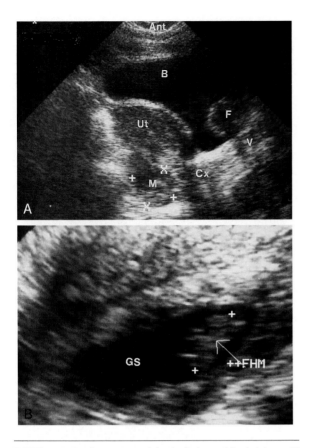

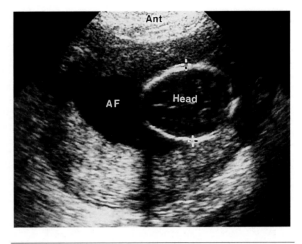

FIGURE 7–46. **Measurement of biparietal diameter.** A transabdominal ultrasound image is done to find and measure the greatest biparietal diameter. This is one of the measurements utilized for estimating fetal age. Amniotic fluid (AF) is clearly seen.

FIGURE 7–45. **Ectopic pregnancy.** A longitudinal transabdominal image (A) clearly shows the bladder, uterus, and cervix. There is a Foley catheter within the bladder. A mass (M) is noted and marked behind the uterus. A transvaginal ultrasound (B) was performed to get better detail of this abnormality. A gestational sac, a fetal pole, and fetal heart motion were identified in this ectopic pregnancy.

Tumors

The most common benign uterine tumor is a fibroid. These are often calcified and are seen on x-ray in the central portion of the pelvis. The calcification is typically somewhat popcorn shaped (see Fig. 6–17). This finding is usually incidental, since x-rays should not be ordered to look for uterine fibroids. The most common method used to image uterine fibroids and other pelvic masses, as mentioned earlier, is ultrasound. Fibroids will enlarge the uterus in a lumpy fashion and make the internal echo pattern very inhomogeneous (Fig. 7–48). Although it is difficult to differentiate fibroids from endometrial carcinoma on ultrasound, this is easily done on clinical grounds, since most endometrial carcinomas are associated with bleeding. Dermoid tumors typically contain hair, teeth, and sebaceous secretions. Often a molar type tooth can be seen on an x-ray of the pelvis (Fig. 7–49).

Most ovarian tumors are cystadenomas or cystadenocarcinomas. Both benign and malignant tumors are bilateral in a fair number of cases. When an ovarian tumor is suspected, ultrasound imaging should optimally be done in the first 10 days of the menstrual cycle to minimize the presence of benign ovarian cysts. Cystadenomas and cystadenocarcinomas are usually large cystic adnexal lesions.

only after careful consideration. Historically, it was common to take radiographs of the pelvis and to make measurements prior to labor. Currently, there is little, if any, reason to use x-rays in the management of labor. Occasionally, x-rays may be taken to assess potential injuries of the spine, pelvis, or hips after an automobile accident involving a pregnant woman. Under these circumstances, you should first ensure that the same information cannot be obtained by using ultrasound. If x-rays are necessary, you should determine the information that is needed and whether the examination can be tailored or done with less than the normal number of views. For example, if your question is whether both kidneys are functional or whether there are pelvic or spine fractures, a single AP x-ray may be all that is needed (Fig. 7–47).

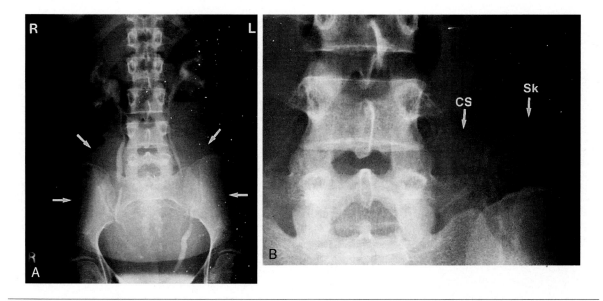

FIGURE 7–47. Tailored intravenous pyelogram during pregnancy. This young pregnant female was in a motor vehicle accident and had hematuria. Clinicians wished an assessment of bony structures as well as an assessment of renal function. Rather than do all the routine x-rays of an intravenous pyelogram only a single film was taken at 10 minutes after injection *(A)*. This showed the enlarged uterus *(arrows)* and bony structures, as well as both kidneys and ureters. A close-up view *(B)* clearly shows the fetal skull (Sk) as well as the fetal cervical spine (CS).

One of the most frequent clinical presentations of ovarian carcinoma is increasing weight and abdominal girth due to the presence of ascites. Pleural effusions are also common. CT scanning is often done for suspected pelvic malignancies to determine the size of the mass, possible involvement of pelvic side walls, and ureteral obstruction as well as to look for metastatic disease. The finding of a pelvic mass on CT or ultrasound is usually somewhat nonspecific, although if the mass can be traced down into the pelvis and into the adnexa, it is most likely of ovarian origin. Ovarian carcinoma may involve the bowel, particularly the serosa (Fig. 7–50).

Carcinoma of the cervix is usually found

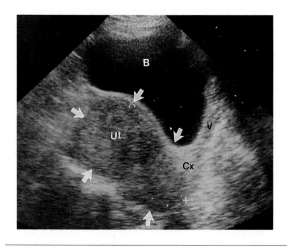

FIGURE 7–48. Ultrasound of uterine fibroids. A longitudinal transabdominal view of the pelvis shows that the uterus (Ut) is enlarged and lumpy *(arrows)*. The echo pattern within the uterus is inhomogeneous; this is the most common appearance of uterine fibroids.

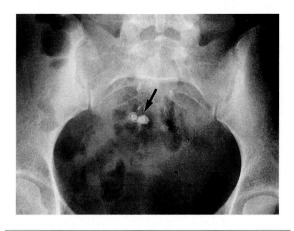

FIGURE 7–49. Ovarian teratoma. A plain film of the pelvis shows a relatively classic molar tooth calcification *(arrow)*.

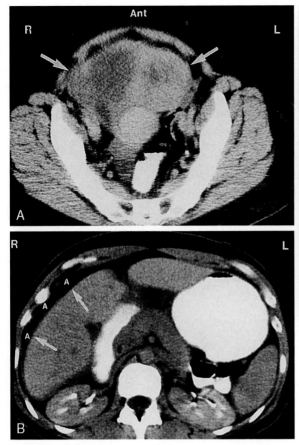

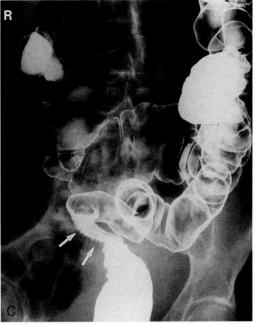

FIGURE 7–50. Ovarian carcinoma. A transverse CT scan through the pelvis *(A)* shows a large soft tissue mass *(arrows)*. There are some low-density areas within this, suggesting necrosis. A CT scan performed higher up in the abdomen *(B)* shows a small amount of ascites over the lateral aspect of the liver. A barium enema performed on the same patient *(C)* shows narrowing of the rectosigmoid with fine toothlike serrations *(arrows)*, indicating serosal involvement by the tumor.

during annual examination and with a Pap smear. Once a cervical carcinoma has been found, CT scanning can assess the overall size of the tumor and the potential presence of metastases. Often, this cancer will obstruct the cervical canal and cause buildup of fluid within the uterus. Cervical carcinomas tend to obstruct the distal ureters, and renal obstruction is the most frequent cause of death from this tumor. Evaluation can initially be done using an IVP (Fig. 7–51); however, in follow-up of these patients it is probably cheaper and safer to look for potentially obstructed kidneys by means of ultrasound. In contrast to ovarian carcinoma, cervical carcinomas often spread locally and involve lymph nodes (Fig. 7–52). Even though CT can detect metastases if the lymph nodes are enlarged, its accuracy for detection of metastases from cervical carcinoma is only 65 per cent, since the nodes may have small metastatic deposits and not be enlarged.

ADRENAL GLANDS AND RETROPERITONEUM

Retroperitoneum

The adrenal glands are not normally visualized on a plain film of the abdomen. They can be seen if prior hemorrhage or infection has produced calcification or if a tumor or mass large enough to displace the kidney is present in the adrenal.

Most anatomy texts would have you believe that the adrenal gland sits on top of the kidney like a little cap. This is not true. The right adrenal gland is located above and slightly anterior to the right kidney, and it is between the right lobe of the liver and the crus of the diaphragm. Often it can be seen on a CT scan as just a small line. The left adrenal gland likewise does not sit on top of the left kidney but actually sits just anterior and slightly medial to the upper pole of the left kidney. The left adrenal gland typi-

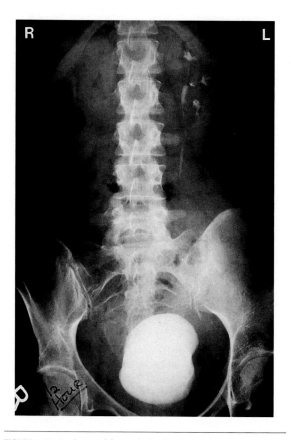

FIGURE 7–51. Carcinoma of the cervix. On this intravenous pyelogram, the left kidney is clearly identified and is functional. No contrast is seen in the collecting system of the right kidney owing to obstruction of the distal right ureter by the cervical carcinoma.

cally has an upside-down Y shape. If you suspect adrenal pathology, the imaging study of choice is a CT scan (Fig. 7–53).

The width of the adrenal gland should be less than 1 cm, and the limbs of the Y should be 3 to 6 mm thick. Masses in the adrenal glands are the result of adenomas (50 per cent), metastases (35 per cent), pheochromocytoma (10 per cent), lymphoma, and neuroblastoma (in children <2 years of age). Bilateral masses are usually the result of metastases, bilateral pheochromocytoma, lymphoma, and granulomatous diseases.

At autopsy, about 25 per cent of individuals who died of cancer have adrenal metastases. Lung, breast, stomach, colon, and kidney are the most common primary lesions to metastasize to the adrenal gland. In a patient with cancer and an adrenal mass, there is a high probability that

the latter is metastatic (particularly if the masses are bilateral) (Fig. 7–54).

An adrenal adenoma usually is low density (dark) on CT and occurs in about 3 per cent of persons. Usually, these are discovered incidentally. An adrenal lesion in excess of 2 to 3 cm in diameter that is not low density on CT should be considered a malignancy. A CT scan may be utilized to perform fine needle biopsy of these lesions.

Adrenal hyperplasia may be nodular in Cushing's syndrome or smooth, as in 25 per cent of patients with Conn's syndrome. Both these diseases are related to hormone overproduction (ACTH, cortisol, or aldosterone), which may be caused by an adenoma, tumor, or hyperplasia. The primary diagnosis for most of these lesions

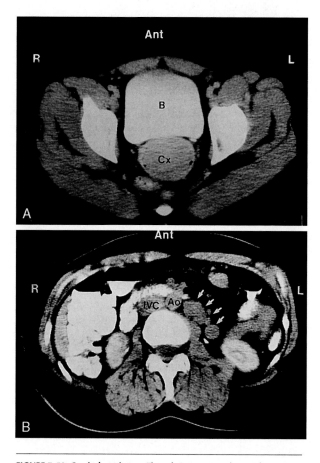

FIGURE 7–52. Cervical carcinoma. The soft tissue extent of cervical carcinoma (cx) is seen on a transverse CT scan of the lower pelvis (A). An image obtained higher up in the abdomen (B) shows the inferior vena cava and the aorta, but lateral to the aorta are multiple soft tissue structures representing nodes (arrows) enlarged with metastatic disease.

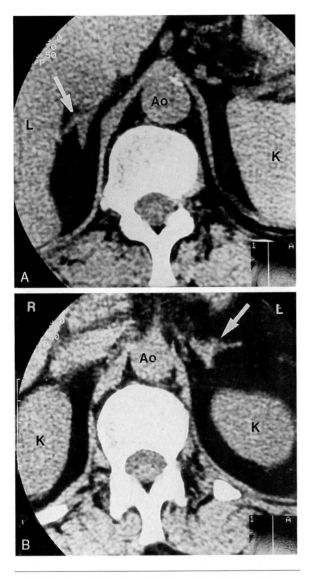

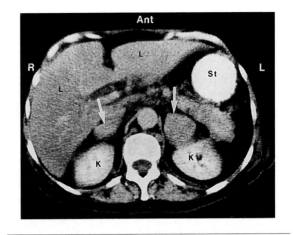

FIGURE 7–54. Bilateral adrenal metastases. A contrast-enhanced CT scan of the upper abdomen shows bilateral adrenal masses *(arrows)* due to metastases from lung carcinoma.

ally they occur elsewhere in the abdomen. Localization should be done using a nuclear medicine scan with a substance called MIBG (metaiodobenzylguanidine) or by MRI.

Retroperitoneal Adenopathy and Neoplasms

CT scanning is the only convenient and practical way to assess patients for retroperitoneal adenopathy. As mentioned earlier in this chapter, patients can have normal-sized lymph nodes that have microscopic metastases. Therefore,

FIGURE 7–53. Normal adrenal anatomy. A coned-down CT scan of the upper abdomen above the level of the right kidney *(A)* shows the right adrenal gland *(arrow)*. It is usually shaped like an upside down V or as a thin line. The left adrenal gland is seen on a slightly lower CT cut *(B)* and is a triangular structure anterior and slightly medial to the upper pole of the left kidney.

is made by evaluation of serum or urine hormone levels. Tumors and clinically significant functional adenomas can usually be localized by CT, but hyperplasia can be difficult to differentiate from normal glands. In these latter rare cases a nuclear medicine scan with a substance called NP-59 will demonstate increased activity of an adenoma or hyperplasia. Most pheochromocytomas (90 per cent) occur in the adrenal medulla, and 10 per cent are bilateral. Occasion-

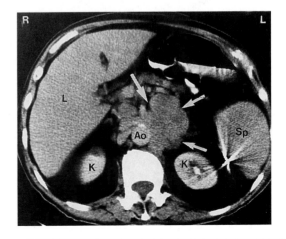

FIGURE 7–55. Retroperitoneal lymphoma. In this young patient with suspected Hodgkin's disease, a contrast-enhanced CT scan clearly shows the kidneys and the aorta. The aorta is surrounded by a lobular soft tissue mass *(arrows)* due to lymphoma.

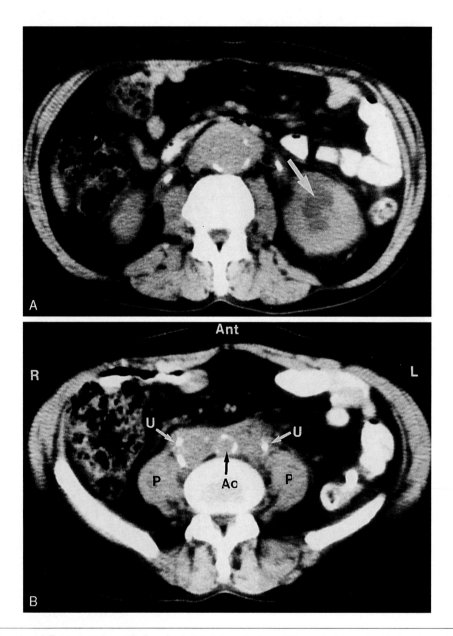

FIGURE 7–56. Retroperitoneal fibrosis. A CT scan at the lower level of the kidneys *(A)* shows dilation of the left renal pelvis *(arrow)* and, incidentally, a slightly dilated aorta. A scan obtained just below the iliac crest in the same patient *(B)* again shows the aortic wall outlined by calcium. The right and left ureters (U) are pulled medially and encased by a soft tissue mass caused by retroperitoneal fibrosis. The white densities in the ureters are from stents or tubes placed in the ureters to relieve obstruction. The psoas muscles (P) are also easily seen.

you should not automatically assume that if adenopathy is absent, there is no spread of tumor. When there is nodal enlargement in a patient with a known neoplasm, the chances of malignant involvement are high, although not certain, since some patients have hyperplastic lymph nodes without actual tumor involvement.

CT scanning not only can identify adenopathy but also can be used on a serial basis to assess the results of therapy. Unless intravenous contrast is given, it can be difficult to differentiate a large mass of lymphadenopathy about the aorta from an abdominal aortic aneurysm. Another major advantage of CT is that you can look at the abdominal organs and mesenteric regions for metastatic disease while you are searching for adenopathy (Fig. 7–55).

Retroperitoneal fibrosis can be confused with an aneurysm or retroperitoneal adenopathy. The distinction is not always easy to make on CT. One differentiating factor is that with retroperitoneal fibrosis, there usually is medial deviation of the ureters due to traction by the fibrotic process (Fig. 7–56). With adenopathy and aneurysms, there usually is lateral deviation of the ureters by a soft tissue mass.

General Suggested Readings

Dunnick N, McCallum R, Sandler C: Textbook of Uroradiology. Baltimore, Williams & Wilkins, 1991.
Pollack H: Clinical Urography. Philadelphia, WB Saunders, 1990.

Chapter 8

Skeletal System

Fractures and other abnormalities involving the skull and face were covered in Chapter 2. Initial imaging studies for a number of clinical problems are presented in Table 8–1. There are a few general comments that need to be made about the structure of bone. Most bones consist of a densely calcified cortex or shell that surrounds the medullary space. The medullary space con-

tains either active (red) marrow or fatty replaced (yellow) marrow. In the adult there is red marrow in the skull, ribs, spine, pelvis, and proximal portions of the femurs and humeri. Since this red marrow acts as a filter, most bone metastases begin in these locations and chew outward until they involve the cortex.

The midportion of the long bones is referred to as the diaphysis. Toward the ends of long bones is the metaphysis, which extends up to the epiphyseal plate. Beyond the epiphyseal plate is the epiphysis. An epiphysis by definition involves a joint space. Occasionally, there are growth centers on portions of long bones where the joint space is not involved (for example, along the greater trochanter of the femur). These centers are referred to as apophyses.

Growth of long bones occcurs primarily at the epiphyseal plate, where new bone is added to the metaphysis and the epiphyseal plate moves farther along. There is some growth occurring along the lateral periosteum as well, in order to allow the bones to become thicker with age. Some epiphyses are present at birth, and most are closed by the age of 20 years. The different parts of long bones are important, because some lesions will preferentially affect

TABLE 8–1. Imaging Studies of Choice For Various Clinical Problems

Clinical Problem	Imaging Study
Fracture	Plain radiographs
Occult fracture	Nuclear medicine bone scan or CT
Stress fracture	Nuclear medicine bone scan
Metastases	Nuclear medicine bone scan
	Plain radiograph in area of pain
Osteomyelitis	Plain radiograph
	Nuclear medicine three-phase bone scan
Low back pain	
without radiculopathy	Bed rest (for several weeks)
with radiculopathy	Noncontrasted CT; if persistent, MRI
Loose prosthesis	Plain radiographs
	Nuclear medicine bone scan
Arthritis	Plain radiographs
Knee or shoulder pain	Plain radiography, MRI

only certain parts of the bone. For example, it is very common for a Ewing tumor to affect the diaphysis of a long bone, but it will rarely, if ever, affect the epiphysis.

The cortex of bone has fine white lines, which are the trabecula. These are located predominantly along the lines of stress in the bone, as they provide little pillars of support. There will be occasional cross-linking trabecula. With disuse, old age, or states of increased blood flow, calcium is carried away from bone. This does not occur in a random fashion but preferentially removes the cross-linking trabecula first. As the process becomes more advanced the trabecula along the lines of stress are removed and the bone becomes weakened and may be subject to compression fractures. This process is seen in older women. Often in a female with osteoporosis, if you look at the lateral chest film you will see only the outline of the thoracic vertebral bodies (because the trabecula have been resorbed), and there will be many mid- and upper thoracic wedge compression fractures. As will be shown later, with disuse of an extremity or in hyperemic states, there will be initial resorption of calcium in a periarticular distribution because there is more blood flow here than along the shaft of bones.

A final word of caution before we begin: Most bone lesions will be relatively obvious to you as a result of the clinical history. Over 95 per cent of bone films are obtained for evaluation of trauma, arthritis, degenerative conditions, or metastases. There are a number of classic fractures that you should be able to recognize and a few that, if missed, can have dire consequences (especially cervical spine fractures). It is crucial that you spend time on these. Although some details of the various arthritic conditions are presented, these are relatively nonspecific and certainly not emergent or life threatening. Primary bone tumors are very rare, and you should not expect to develop competence regarding these. In clinical practice (other than orthopedics or oncology) you probably will see a primary bone tumor once every 5 or 10 years. Most radiologists are lucky if they see three or four bone tumors per year. The main point is to be able to discern the lesions and refer them to a radiologist for a reasonable differential diagnosis.

CERVICAL SPINE

Normal Anatomy

The lateral view of the cervical spine is the initial view obtained, particularly in trauma cases. Table 8–2 provides a summary of how to examine a cervical spine examination done for trauma. Initial inspection should be directed toward the various contour lines of the cervical spine, which are shown in Figure 8–1. These include the anterior soft tissues, the anterior and posterior spinal line, the spinal laminal line, and the posterior spinous process line. On the lateral view, the cervical spine should be bowed forward and have a relatively smooth curve. There should not be a sharp angulation at any level. If the patient was lying on a stretcher

---

TABLE 8–2. Items to Look For on a Trauma AP and Lateral Cervical Spine Examination

Lateral View

- Count vertebral bodies to assure that all seven are seen (if not, consider swimmer's view or shallow oblique view)

- Alignment of
  anterior vertebral body margins
  posterior vertebral body margins
  posterior spinal canal

- Cervical curvature, straightening, or sudden angulation

- Prevertebral soft tissue thickness (see text)

- Widening of vertical distance between posterior processes

- Common fractures
  C1 arch
  C2 odontoid
      arch (hangman's)
      widening between anterior arch of C1 and odontoid
  C3–C7 anterior avulsion
      wedge compression
  C6–C7 posterior process (clay shoveler's)

- Facets (to exclude unilateral locked facet)

Anterior View

- Odontoid view
  Widening of the lateral portion of C1 relative to C2 (Jefferson fracture)

- General alignment of lateral margins and spinous processes

- Lucent fracture lines

Oblique view (if no major trauma is suspected)

- Neural foraminal narrowing

- Alignment of facet joints

...

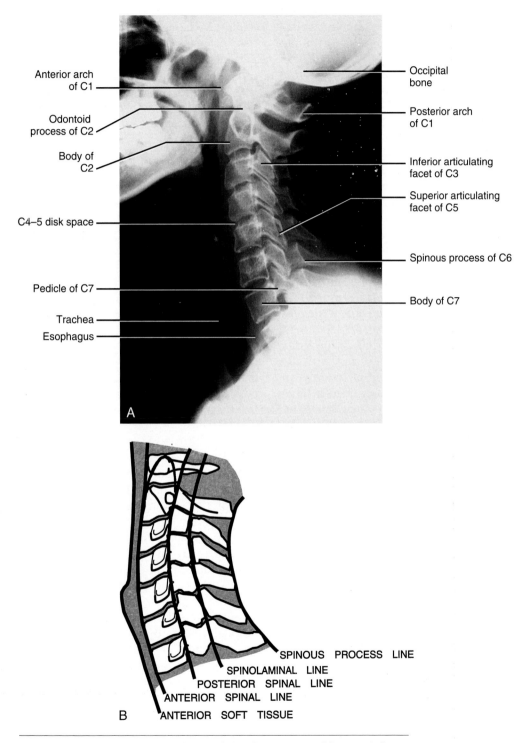

Anterior arch
of C1

Odontoid
process of C2

Body of
C2

C4–5 disk space

Pedicle of C7

Trachea

Esophagus

Occipital
bone

Posterior arch
of C1

Inferior articulating
facet of C3

Superior articulating
facet of C5

Spinous process of C6

Body of C7

A

SPINOUS PROCESS LINE
SPINOLAMINAL LINE
POSTERIOR SPINAL LINE
ANTERIOR SPINAL LINE
ANTERIOR SOFT TISSUE

B

FIGURE 8–1. Normal anatomy of the cervical spine in the lateral projection *(A)* and diagrammatically *(B)*.

when the lateral view was taken, the neck is often somewhat flexed, and the cervical spine is straight rather than curved. When you see this, you cannot be sure whether the straightening is due simply to the supine positioning of the patient or to muscular spasm. If the trauma was relatively minor, an upright lateral x-ray of the cervical spine usually will solve the problem. If major trauma is suspected, a CT (computed tomography) or MRI (magnetic resonance imaging) scan may be needed.

Examination of the anterior soft tissues and spaces should be done at several vertebral levels. Evaluation of soft tissue width is typically not a problem unless the patient has an endotracheal tube in place, in which case the normal air and soft tissue interface is obscured, and you will have to rely on other findings. The width of the soft tissue immediately anterior to the body of C3 typically should be between 4 and 5 mm, although occasionally it may normally be up to 7 mm. Actual width of the soft tissues as measured on an x-ray, of course, is dependent on the magnification that occurred as the x-ray was taken. On a portable trauma series (with the patient supine) the x-ray tube is often only 40 inches from the film cassette. As a result, there will be significant magnification, and a measurement of up to 7 mm may be normal in the prevertebral soft tissues at the C3 level. However, if the examination was done with the tube 72 inches, or 6 feet, from the film, the soft tissue normally should not exceed 4 to 5 mm.

Below the level of C4, the air column moves anteriorly in the region of the larynx; there is thickened soft tissue between the larynx and the vertebral bodies that is due to the esophagus. Soft tissue anterior to the lower cervical bodies averages about 15 mm, with a range of 10 to 20 mm. If the soft tissue in this region equals or exceeds the width of the vertebra at or below the level of C4, pathology should be suspected.

Another measurement that one should note on the lateral view is the distance from the posterior aspect of the anterior arch of C1 to the most anterior portion of the odontoid. In an adult, this should not exceed 3 mm; in a child, it should not exceed 5 mm.

Examination of the bony contour lines is done to exclude subluxations. Remember that on the lateral view you should be able to see down to at least the bottom of the C7 or the top of the T1 vertebral body. If there is difficulty in seeing this far down owing to the patient's shoulders being in the way, a swimmer's view can be ordered. For this view, one of the patient's arms is raised next to the head and the other arm placed down alongside the waist. This essentially raises one shoulder and lowers the other, allowing the x-ray beam to more easily penetrate the area of the cervicothoracic junction (Fig. 8–2).

There are typically two anterior views that are done after the lateral cervical spine view has been examined by a physician and found to be free of fracture or subluxation. These are, first, the anterior view of the lower cervical spine with the mouth closed; this view is used to examine alignment and to exclude lucent oblique fractures. Additionally, an open-mouth view of the odontoid is obtained (Fig. 8–3). This view shows the relationship of the inferior aspect and lateral margins of C1 to the superior aspect and lateral margins of C2, and it also shows the odontoid very well. It is important to have the mouth open wide enough that the front teeth do not overlie the odontoid. If this happens, you can see the air gap between the two front teeth and mistakenly call this a fracture (Fig. 8–4).

There are two relatively common normal variants that you should be aware of on the lateral view. The first of these looks like a calcified spike or nail and represents calcification of the stylohyoid ligament. It is actually quite lateral, but on the lateral cervical spine view it projects posterior to the mandible and anterior to C1 and C2 (Fig. 8–5). Another common variant is embryologic fusion of two or more vertebral bodies to create a "block" vertebra; this may be a complete or an incomplete fusion. Typically, it can be distinguished from a surgical fusion by the fact that the posterior processes may be fused and by the fact that the total height of the block vertebra is equal to the total height of two other vertebral bodies plus a disk space. In surgical fusions there is loss of the disk space, and the total height will be smaller. Often a block vertebral body will cause abnormal motion, and there may be associated early degenerative changes.

Oblique views of the cervical spine are ob-

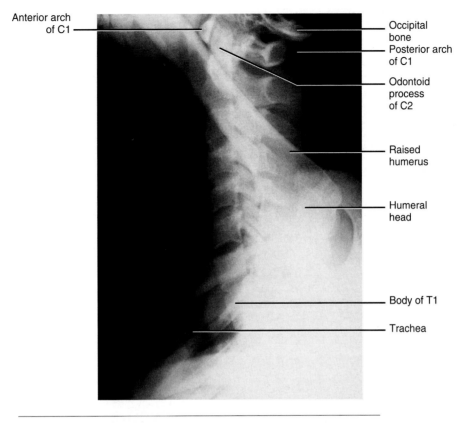

Anterior arch
of C1

Occipital
bone

Posterior arch
of C1

Odontoid
process
of C2

Raised
humerus

Humeral
head

Body of T1

Trachea

FIGURE 8-2. Normal anatomy of the cervical spine on the lateral swimmer's view.

tained only when you are quite sure that no major trauma, fracture, or dislocation is present. The value of the oblique views is mostly to see whether there is impingement and narrowing of the neural foramina by bony degenerative spurs. On a good oblique view you should be able to see the neural foramina very well from C2 down through T1 (Fig. 8–6). Additionally, you should look to see that the articular facets are lined up like shingles on a roof. This view may be helpful to see a unilateral perched, subluxed, or locked facet if CT is not available. Both CT and MRI are useful to image the cervical spine. CT is best suited to detecting subtle bony fractures, while MRI provides exquisite detail of soft tissues, such as the spinal cord, and cerebral spinal fluid (CSF) (Fig. 8–7).

Trauma

There are some general considerations about acute traumatic spinal fractures that you should

be aware of. Fifty per cent are due to motor vehicle accidents, about 25 per cent to falls, and about 10 per cent to sports injuries. The most common sites are the upper (C1–C2) and lower (C5–C7) cervical spine and the thoracolumbar junction (T9–L2). Twenty per cent of spinal fractures are multiple, and about 5 per cent occur at discontinuous levels.

Dislocation of the skull from the cervical spine (atlanto-occipital dislocation) is rare and usually fatal. Approximately 5 per cent of cervical spine fractures involve C1. Fractures of the atlas can involve any portion of the bony ring. Combination fractures, or burst fractures of the ring of C1, are called Jefferson fractures. This bursting is usually secondary to axial loading as a result of the skull being smashed down onto the cervical spine (as in diving into a shallow pool) (Fig. 8–8A).

Approximately 10 per cent of all cervical spine fractures involve the odontoid process of C2. The most common type of odontoid fracture occurs at the very base of the odontoid process.

Text continued on page 266

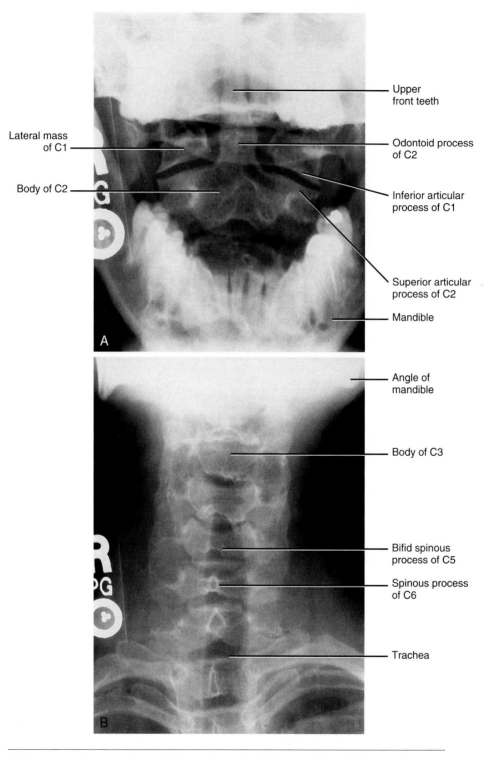

Upper
front teeth

Lateral mass
of C1

Odontoid process
of C2

Body of C2

Inferior articular
process of C1

Superior articular
process of C2

Mandible

A

Angle of
mandible

Body of C3

Bifid spinous
process of C5

Spinous process
of C6

Trachea

B

FIGURE 8–3. Normal anatomy of the cervical spine on the AP odontoid view *(A)* and the standard AP cervical view *(B)*.

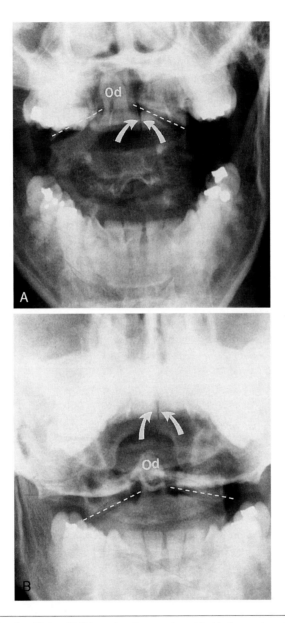

FIGURE 8–4. Pseudofracture of C2. On the odontoid view *(A)*, if the teeth project over the vertebral bodies, an air gap between the front teeth *(arrows)* can cause what appears to be a horizontal fracture through either the odontoid process or the body of C2. The junction between the articular surfaces of lateral masses of C1 and C2 is indicated by the dotted lines. If there is a question, the pseudofracture artifact can be corrected by raising the maxilla and repeating the view *(B)*.

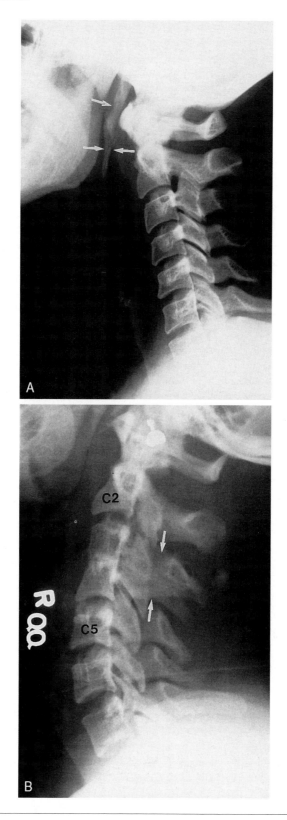

FIGURE 8–5. Normal variants of the cervical spine. On the lateral view *(A)*, there often is prominent calcification of the stylohyoid ligament, causing what looks like a long, calcified icicle. In a different patient, the lateral view demonstrates congenital fusion *(B)* of the bodies of C3 and C4. Note also that the posterior elements are fused.

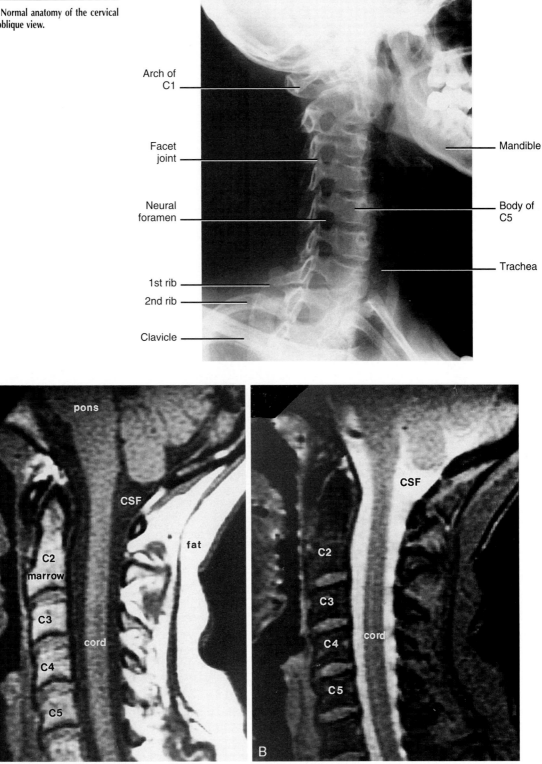

FIGURE 8–6. Normal anatomy of the cervical spine on the oblique view.

FIGURE 8–7. Normal appearance of the cervical spine and spinal cord on magnetic resonance imaging. A sagittal (lateral) view with a T1 weighted sequence *(A)* shows that the subcutaneous fat and marrow within the vertebral bodies have a high signal and appear white. The cerebrospinal fluid appears almost black, and the cerebellum, pons, and spinal cord appear gray. On the T2 weighted sequence *(B)*, the contrast is somewhat reversed, with fluid or CSF appearing white and the fat becoming dark. The spinal cord remains gray.

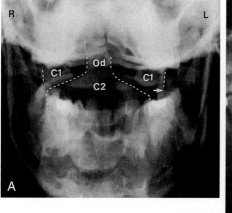

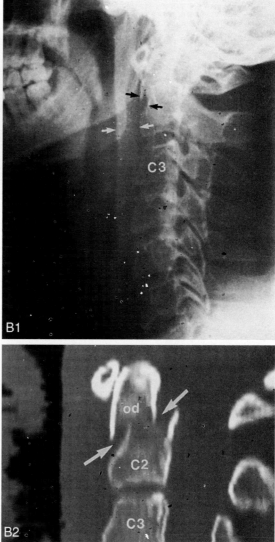

FIGURE 8–8. *A,* **Jefferson burst fracture of C1.** On this open-mouth AP view, there is widening of the space between the odontoid and the left lateral mass of C1. The lateral aspect also projects out past the lateral margin of C2 *(arrow).* *B,* **Fracture of the odontoid.** In a different patient the lateral view of the cervical spine *(B1)* shows marked soft tissue swelling in front of the body of C2 *(white arrows).* There is also discontinuity of the cortex along the anterior surface of C2 *(black arrows),* indicating an odontoid fracture. A sagittal reconstruction on a CT scan *(B2)* shows the fracture much more clearly.

You can identify the fracture on the lateral view by being very careful to trace the anterior and posterior cortex of the odontoid process. Often, there is associated soft tissue swelling (Fig. 8–8*B*). Note should be made that in young children the odontoid may not be completely fused to the body of C2, and this should not be mistaken for a fracture (see Fig. 8–166*A*).

Occasionally, there can be C1–C2 injury of the transverse ligament, causing traumatic atlantoaxial subluxation. Although this may occur with an associated odontoid fracture, it can also occur without it. If no fracture is present, the subluxation is often fatal, since the odontoid

process pushes posteriorly into the spinal cord that is contained within the arch of C1. On the lateral view the only sign of ligament injury may be some soft tissue swelling anterior to the vertebral bodies. Flexion views will sometimes demonstrate increased widening not only of the atlantoaxial space but also of the space between the posterior spinous processes. This type of subluxation also occurs as a complication of rheumatoid arthritis (Fig. 8–9).

A relatively classic fracture of C2 is the so-called hangman's fracture. This involves fracture of the posterior elements of C2, and there is often associated spinal cord compromise. This

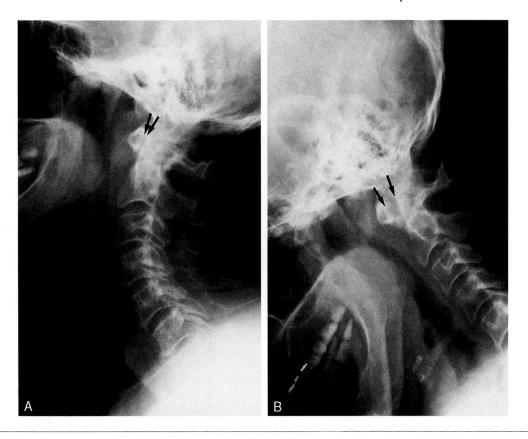

FIGURE 8–9. Instability of the transverse ligament of C1. In this patient with rheumatoid arthritis, a lateral view of the cervical spine with the neck extended *(A)* shows very little space (which is normal) between the posterior aspect of the arch of C1 and the anterior portion of the odontoid *(arrows)*. With flexion *(B)*, this space markedly widens, and the odontoid is free to compress the spinal cord, which is posterior to it.

fracture typically occurs secondary to hyperextension and compression of the upper cervical spine, and there is usually anterior subluxation of the body of C2 relative to C3 (Fig. 8–10). In spite of the name, this is not the usual fracture that occurs as a result of judicial hangings.

There are two, rather characteristic, fractures of the midcervical spine vertebral bodies. The first of these is caused by hyperextension, which typically tears off either a superior or an inferior anterior portion of the cortex from a vertebral body (Fig. 8–11). A second type of fracture that commonly occurs in the middle cervical spine is a hyperflexion injury. In this, there is compression of the vertebral body, usually with anterior wedging and sometimes with a posteriorly displaced disk fragment. Usually, there will be associated soft tissue swelling due to the hemorrhage. Evaluation with MRI may show compromise of the neural canal at the level of the fracture (Fig. 8–12).

In addition to fractures associated with subluxation, there can be ligamentous injury that has allowed the facets of one vertebral body to become slightly subluxated, perched, or locked. These represent a more anterior subluxation of a superior vertebral body on a lower one. Generally these injuries occur in the lower half of the cervical spine and are caused by extreme flexion of the head and neck without axial compression. Occasionally, there may be a fracture or ligamentous injury present that cannot be identified utilizing plain radiographs. If there is a high suspicion of clinical injury in spite of negative plain films, CT scanning (Fig. 8–13) or MRI may be useful. CT scanning is able to identify small cortical breaks, whereas the MR scan can show areas of increased signal where there is hematoma or edema, suggesting at least ligamentous injury.

There are three fractures of the lower portion of the cervical spine that are easily missed.

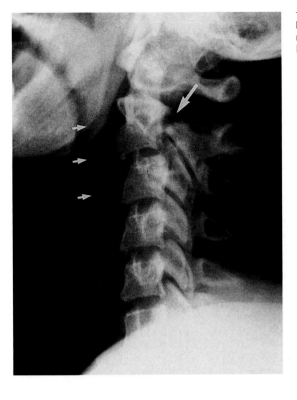

FIGURE 8–10. Hangman's fracture. The lateral view of the cervical spine demonstrates marked soft tissue swelling anterior to C1, C2, and C3 *(small white arrows)*. A fracture line is seen just posterior to the body of C2 *(large arrow)*.

FIGURE 8–11. Anterior avulsion fracture. A small avulsed fragment is seen along the superior and anterior aspect of C5 *(arrows)*.

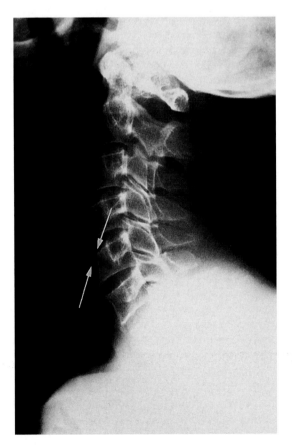

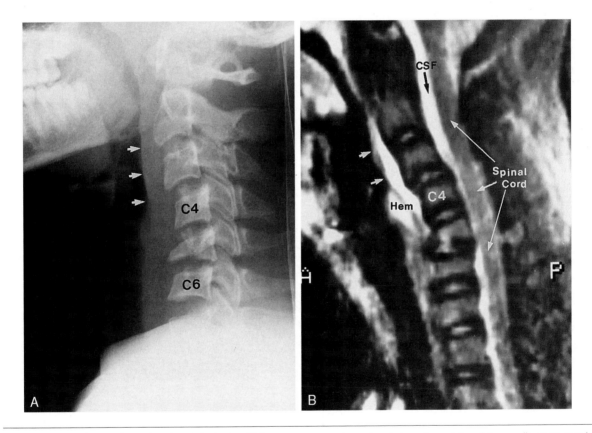

FIGURE 8–12. Wedge fracture of C5. A lateral cervical spine view *(A)* demonstrates a reversed normal cervical curvature, anterior soft tissue swelling *(arrows)*, and a wedge fracture of the body of C5. An MRI scan *(B)*, presented in the same projection, shows hemorrhage as an area of high signal anterior to the body of C4. The spinal cord is also identified, and the spinal canal is clearly narrowed at the level of the fracture.

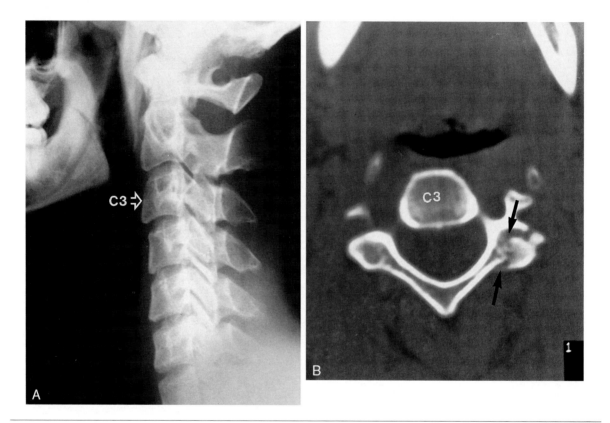

FIGURE 8–13. Occult cervical spine fracture. A lateral view of the cervical spine *(A)* shows normal-appearing structures at C3. There is no anterior soft tissue swelling. The AP view was also normal. Since the patient was complaining of severe pain and had been ejected during a motor vehicle accident, a CT scan was obtained *(B)*, and a transverse image showed a fracture through the lateral mass of C3 *(arrows)*.

Occasionally there are oblique fractures of the lower cervical spine that are seen only on the AP view (Fig. 8–14). The second fracture involves the posterior spinous process at the C6, C7, T1, or T2 level. This is called the clay-shoveler's fracture, and it is due predominantly to hyperflexion injury (Fig. 8–15). A third and most significant problem, relative to the lower cervical spine, is accepting a trauma lateral cervical spine film that does not include adequate evaluation of C6 and C7. Failure to visualize this region can result in your missing significant subluxations and fractures, and for purposes of complete evaluation, either a swimmer's view or shallow oblique views through the cervico-thoracic junction are necessary (Fig. 8–16).

Degenerative Changes

In terms of anatomic and mechanical design, the lower aspect of the cervical spine is less than optimal, and by the third or fourth decade of life there are almost always degenerative changes involving C4 through C7. Degenerative changes are visualized as decreased disk spaces, sclerosis (increased density) of the vertebral body end plates, and beaking or spurring of the anterior, lateral, and posterior margins of the vertebral bodies. Often patients present with arm pain, and an oblique cervical spine view can easily visualize hypertrophic osteophytes or spurs projecting into the neural foramen (Fig. 8–17).

Cervical Impingement Lesions

If a herniated cervical disk is suspected, the procedure of choice is an MRI scan. Metastatic disease can also involve the cervical spine with posterior or lateral extension and impingement upon the spinal cord or nerve roots. For these

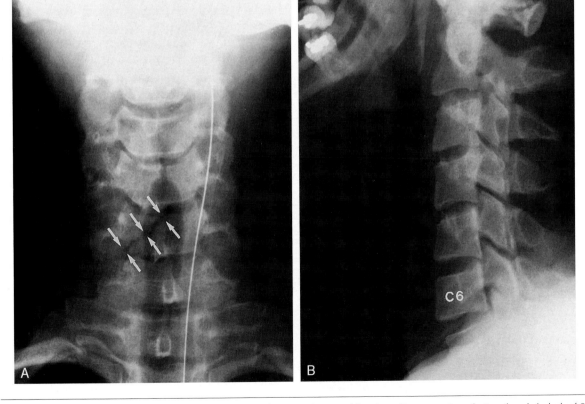

FIGURE 8–14. Oblique fracture of C6. The AP view of the lower cervical spine (A) shows an oblique lucent line, representing a fracture, through the body of C6. This is the only view on which this fracture was seen. The lateral view in the same patient (B) was completely normal.

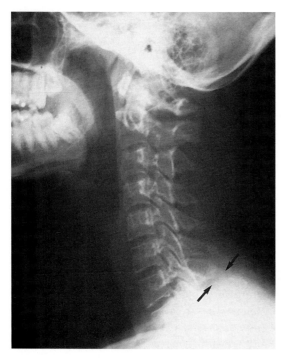

FIGURE 8–15. Fracture of the posterior spinous process of C7. This fracture is identified only on the lateral view (arrows) and is referred to as a clay shoveler's fracture.

types of lesions, MRI is the procedure of choice (Fig. 8–18).

THORACIC SPINE

Anatomy

Plain x-rays of the thoracic spine are taken in AP and lateral projections. The AP projection is useful for examining spinal alignment, the paraspinous soft tissues (to exclude hematomas or other masses), and the pedicles (Fig. 8–19). The lateral thoracic spine is usually a difficult film to assess. In the upper portion the vertebral bodies are obscured by the shoulders; as mentioned in the discussion of the cervical spine, if you suspect pathology in the T1–T5 region, often a swimmer's view or shallow oblique views are necessary. The mid- and lower thoracic spine is usually well seen on the lateral view. When pathology is identified on the lateral view, it is often not easy to tell exactly the level of the vertebral body involved. Once you have identified pathology on the lateral view, you can usually go back to the AP view, look at the ribs, and then count up from T12.

A common normal variant is seen on the lateral thoracic spine views in children. This is an apophysis that occurs along the superior and inferior anterior margins of the vertebral bodies. This should not be mistaken for a fracture (Fig. 8–20).

Trauma

Fractures of the thoracic spine typically are the result of motor vehicle accidents or of the normal aging process, with osteoporosis and resultant anterior wedging of vertebral bodies. Fractures due to significant acute trauma are sometimes seen well only on either the AP or the lateral view. On the AP view, you should examine the spine for malalignment of the posterior spinous processes (Fig. 8–21) as well as for paraspinous soft tissue swelling. These are both signs that a fracture may be present. If you suspect a spinal fracture, both AP and lateral views should be examined. Sometimes there can be significant subluxation of one vertebral body forward on another, and this will be difficult to see on the AP view (Fig. 8–22). This usually occurs when there is a hyperflexion injury resulting in a compression burst fracture. Often,

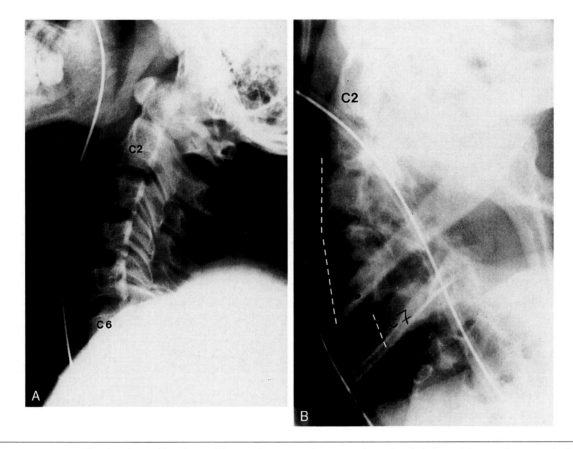

FIGURE 8–16. C6–C7 subluxation. The initial lateral view of the cervical spine *(A)* in this patient with paraplegia looked normal; however, C7 was not visualized. When a swimmer's lateral view *(B)* was obtained, it became clear that there was a complete subluxation of C6 forward on the body of C7.

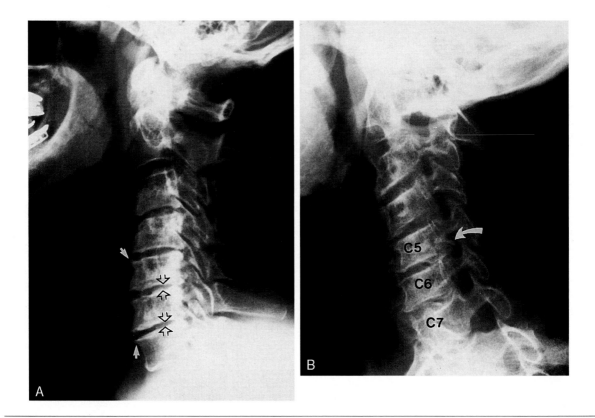

FIGURE 8–17. Degenerative changes of the cervical spine. The lateral view *(A)* shows decreased disk spaces *(black arrows)* and hypertrophic spurring along the anterior aspects of the vertebral bodies. These changes are most common at the C4–C7 level. An oblique view *(B)* in the same patient shows that bony spurs are projecting into the neural foramen *(arrow)*. This can cause pain down the arms.

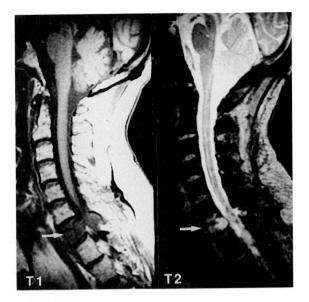

FIGURE 8–18. Tumor involvement of the cervical spine. In this patient with lymphoma and neurologic deficit, a sagittal MRI image of the cervical spine demonstrates complete replacement of the marrow of C7, seen as a dark area on the T1 image *(arrow)*. The T2 image also shows the tumor as a white area *(arrow)* narrowing the spinal canal and compressing the spinal cord.

there are retropulsed fragments of both disk and bony material that project into the spinal canal and can cause significant compromise of the spinal cord.

In older persons, compression fractures of the mid- and lower thoracic spine are common (Fig. 8–23*A*). These are noted as loss of height of the anterior portion of the vertebral bodies. It is almost impossible to tell whether any one of these fractures is new or old, but it usually does not make any difference clinically. If you suspect metastatic disease as a cause of back pain in an older patient, a plain x-ray and a nuclear medicine bone scan are usually satisfactory.

Degenerative Changes

Three relatively common degenerative findings are seen in the thoracic spine. The first are spurs or hypertrophic osteophytes, similar to those that are seen in the lower cervical spine. These are almost never a clinical issue and are not an interpretative problem unless they are very large, at which point they can cause confusing shadows on the AP or PA chest radiograph. These are pointed areas that project out to the side of the spine and are usually seen right over the proximal end of a rib. On the lateral view, these can look like lung nodules, but they always are seen to be projecting over the disk spaces (see Fig. 3–17).

A second relatively common degenerative change is calcification along the anterior ligament. This can cross over the length of several vertebral bodies (Fig. 8–23*B*) and is sometimes referred to by radiologists as DISH (diffuse idiopathic skeletal hyperostosis). This is of no clinical significance to the patient. The third, relatively common, degenerative change is calcification of an intervertebral disk (Fig. 8–24). This can occur at almost any level in the spine but is seen most frequently in the midthoracic region. A single calcified disk is usually the result of degenerative change or trauma. If there is calcification at multiple disk levels, one should consider diseases that cause hypercalcemia or rare entities such as ochronosis.

LUMBAR SPINE

Normal Anatomy and Imaging Techniques

The standard views obtained of the lumbar spine are AP, lateral, and a lateral spot view of the L5–S1 area (Fig. 8–25). The spot view is necessary because on the lateral view both iliac wings and a significant amount of additional soft tissue mean that more radiation exposure is necessary to adequately penetrate and visualize the L5–S1 area.

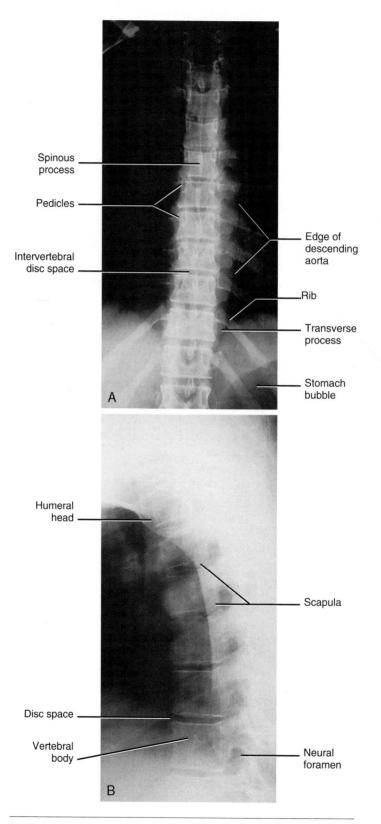

FIGURE 8–19. Normal anatomy of the thoracic spine in the AP *(A)* and lateral *(B)* projections.

FIGURE 8–20. Normal spinal apophyses. In children, a normal apophysis can occasionally be seen on the lateral projection along the anterior superior and inferior margins of the vertebral bodies. These are normal, will be seen on multiple vertebral bodies, and should not be mistaken for avulsion fractures.

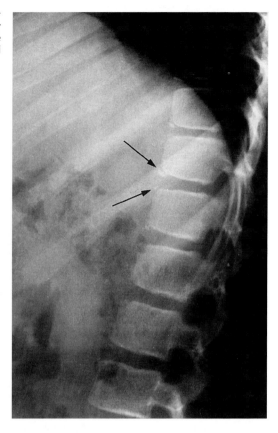

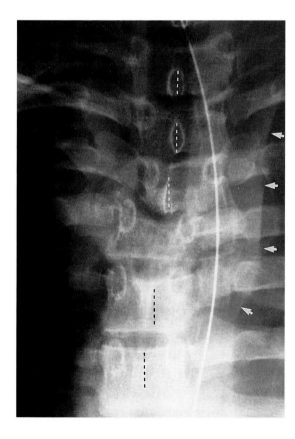

FIGURE 8–21. Laterally displaced thoracic spine fracture. An AP view of the upper thoracic spine in a paraplegic patient who was hit in the driver's side door during a motor vehicle accident shows lateral displacement of the upper thoracic vertebral bodies relative to the lower bodies. This can be assessed by looking at the line formed by the posterior spinous processes *(dotted lines)*. You should also note the lateral soft tissue swelling *(arrows)* due to the paraspinous hemorrhage resulting from the fracture. This sort of a fracture is difficult or impossible to visualize on the lateral view.

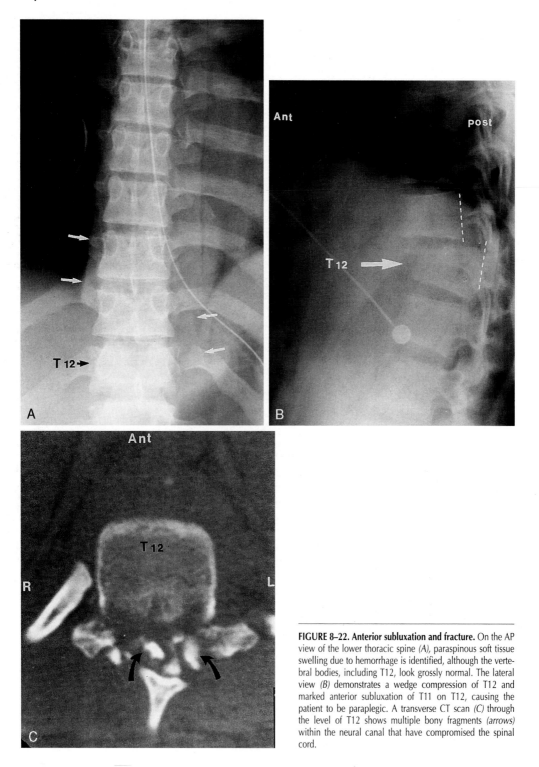

FIGURE 8–22. Anterior subluxation and fracture. On the AP view of the lower thoracic spine *(A)*, paraspinous soft tissue swelling due to hemorrhage is identified, although the verte-bral bodies, including T12, look grossly normal. The lateral view *(B)* demonstrates a wedge compression of T12 and marked anterior subluxation of T11 on T12, causing the patient to be paraplegic. A transverse CT scan *(C)* through the level of T12 shows multiple bony fragments *(arrows)* within the neural canal that have compromised the spinal cord.

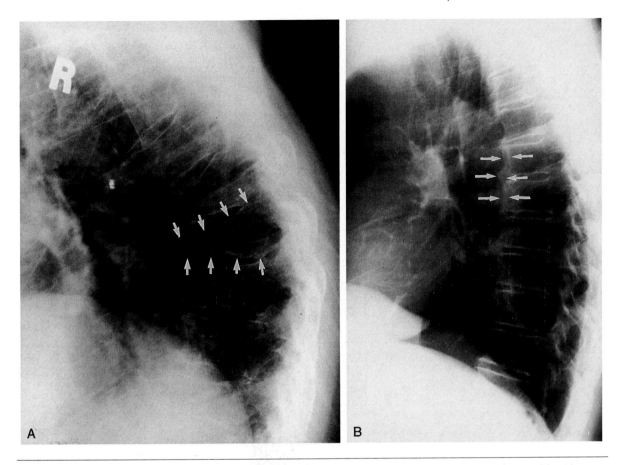

FIGURE 8–23. Degenerative changes of the thoracic spine. A, With aging and osteoporosis, there can be minimal wedge compression fractures of the mid- to upper thoracic spine. B, In a different patient there is development of calcification of the anterior ligament *(arrows)*.

On the AP view, you should examine the alignment of the spine as well as the visibility of the psoas margins bilaterally. It is often useful to count the number of vertebral bodies, since commonly there can be six, rather than five, non–rib bearing vertebrae. The transverse processes should be examined to exclude fracture, and the pedicles at each level should be examined to make sure that they have not been eroded by a pathologic process. Additionally, the sacrum and sacroiliac joints should be examined. The sacroiliac joints can become fused in various arthritic processes (such as ankylosing spondylitis) or can be widened by a pelvic fracture.

On the lateral view of the lumbar spine, an analysis is made to see if there is subluxation of the vertebral bodies; this is done by looking down the contour lines formed by the anterior and posterior margins of the vertebral bodies.

The height and shape of vertebral bodies and the disk spaces should be uniform. The posterior spinous processes also can be visualized.

Oblique views of the lumbar spine are useful for examining the facet joints. The typical anatomy on the oblique view is seen in the outline of a "Scottie dog" (see Figs. 8–25D and 8–29). In this oblique projection, the pedicle is the eye of the Scottie dog, and the transverse process represents the nose. The superior articular process forms the ears, and the inferior articular process forms the front legs.

A common normal variant of the lumbar spine is incomplete fusion of the posterior aspect of L5 or S1 (so-called spina bifida occulta), which is seen on the AP view (Fig. 8–26A). It is of no clinical significance and should be disregarded. A second common anomaly is sacralization or partial fusion of L5 with the sa-

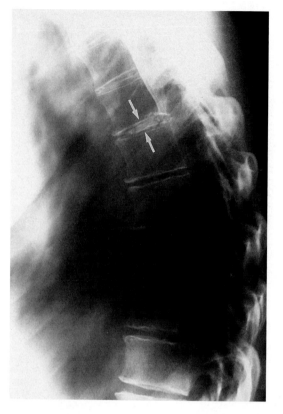

FIGURE 8–24. Calcified intervertebral disk. Calcification of a single disk can be identified on this lateral view *(arrows)*. This is most commonly due to trauma and is of little clinical significance. Calcification at multiple levels has a differential diagnosis, which includes hypercalcemic states as well as ochronosis.

crum (Fig. 8–26*B*). This can occur just on one side, or it can be bilateral.

On any given view of the lumbar spine or pelvis, you can see normal bowel gas projecting over bone. This looks dark and can easily mimic a destructive bone lesion. I have seen several instances in which physicians told patients that they had "cancer of the spine," which in reality was overlying bowel gas. Make sure that any bone lesion that you suspect is confined to the bone and stays within that bone on AP, lateral, and oblique views.

Postsurgical Changes

The most common postsurgical change involves either lower lumbar fusion or laminectomy. It is often not easy to appreciate laminectomy on the lateral film; however, on the frontal views, provided you look for it, you see that one or more posterior spinous processes are gone (Fig. 8–27). Noticing things that are gone is always harder than seeing abnormal objects that are present.

Fractures

The most common fractures of the lumbar spine are wedge compression fractures and compression burst fractures. These are very similar to those already described in the thoracic spine. Note should be made, again, that the compression burst fractures frequently have fragments that are retropulsed, and CT or MRI is often necessary to evaluate compromise of the spinal canal.

There is a somewhat unusual fracture that occurs in the lumbar spine, typically at L1, L2, or L3. This is a Chance fracture. It is most commonly the result of a motor vehicle accident when a lap seat belt is worn without the shoulder harness. Under these circumstances, there is rotation of the trunk of the body about the horizontal axis of the seat belt, resulting in a vertical distraction force along the lumbar spine. This essentially tears a vertebral body (horizontally) in half. On the AP view, this fracture is recognized by discontinuity of the outline of the pedicles, and on the lateral view by a lucency

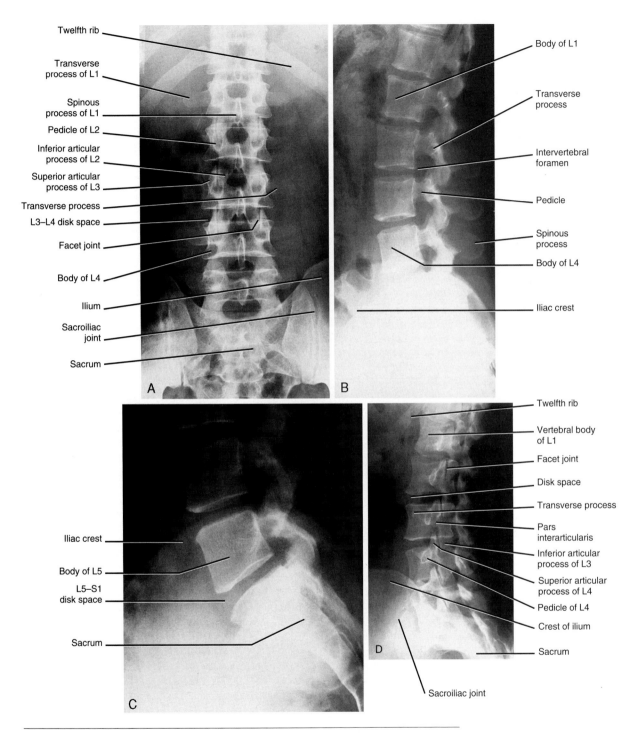

FIGURE 8–25. Normal anatomy of the lumbar spine in the AP *(A)*, lateral *(B)*, lateral sacral *(C)*, and oblique *(D)* views.

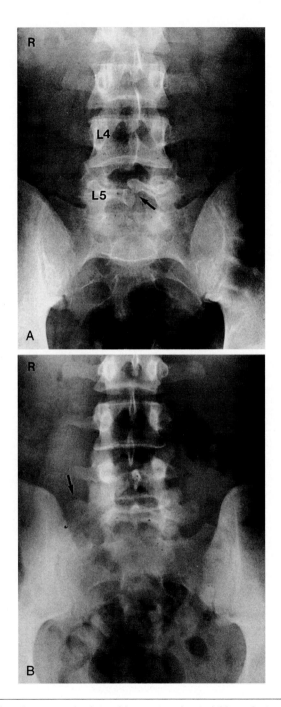

FIGURE 8–26. Normal variants of the lumbar spine. *A,* Incomplete fusion of the posterior arch (spina bifida occulta) is seen on the AP view as a defect at L5 *(arrow).* *B,* Sacralization of the right side of L5 *(arrow).*

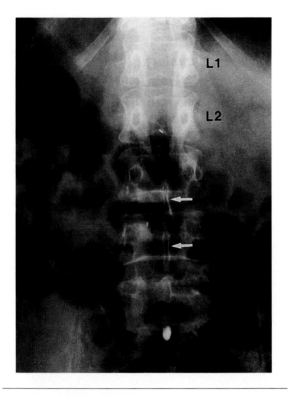

FIGURE 8–27. Postsurgical laminectomy. On the AP view of the lumbar spine, the posterior spinous processes of L3 and L4 are clearly seen *(arrows)*. Spinous processes are absent on L1 and L2 owing to a laminectomy.

extending through the posterior spinous process and lamina (Fig. 8–28).

The pars interarticularis of the vertebral body also can be fractured. This injury typically occurs at the L4 or L5 level. It can sometimes be seen on the lateral view as a lucency but more commonly is clearly identified as a break in the neck of the "Scottie dog" on the oblique view (Fig. 8–29). This finding was originally thought to be congenital, but most of the time it probably is the result of trauma in the early years of life. The term applied to a break in the pars interarticularis is spondylolysis. If there is bilateral spondylolysis, the vertebral body can slip forward on the vertebral body that is immediately below. When this happens, it is termed spondylolisthesis. The amount of offset caused by the slippage is used to grade the spondylolisthesis. If there is up to one fourth of the vertebral body offset, this is called grade 1. If it is between one fourth and one half, it is called grade 2, and so on (Fig. 8–30). In a young patient or athlete with low back pain and normal plain

x-rays, a bone scan with "slice" or SPECT technology may identify otherwise occult lesions (Fig. 8–31).

Degenerative Changes

As mentioned earlier, degenerative change can result in disk space narrowing, hypertrophic spurs (osteophytes) (Fig. 8–32), or calcification of a disk. In the lumbar spine, loss of the disk space is quite common, as is hypertrophic spurring. Occasionally you can see a thin dark line in a narrowed disk space (Fig. 8–33) that is referred to as a vacuum disk phenomenon. Actually, it is not a vacuum but actually nitrogen that is in the joint space. This can appear or be accentuated as a result of hyperextension of the spine, but it is a finding of no special clinical significance.

A very common degenerative change that occurs in the lower lumbar spine is a herniated disk or a protruded disk. A herniated disk often has a fragment that is asymmetric or loose in the neural canal, whereas a disk protrusion is a posterior central bulge of the disk. Both can be imaged by either CT or MR (Fig. 8–34). At the present time, MRI is commonly used to make this diagnosis, although it is more expensive than CT scanning, and many clinicians will simply order a noncontrasted CT scan. If you order CT, you should specify thin cuts through the disk space at which you suspect the pathology. You should not order thin cuts through every disk space in the lumbar spine.

Management of Low Back Pain

This is probably one of the areas of greatest controversy in medical imaging. Unless there is major acute trauma, plain films of the lumbar spine are not of much use. The reason is that a patient can have a herniated disk and totally normal plain films. Conversely, many people who have horrible-looking degenerative spurs and decreased disk spaces are totally asymptomatic. The most common cause of low back pain is a herniated or bulging disk. If a patient presents with a radiculopathy, an MR scan is probably most cost effective. The most cost-effective

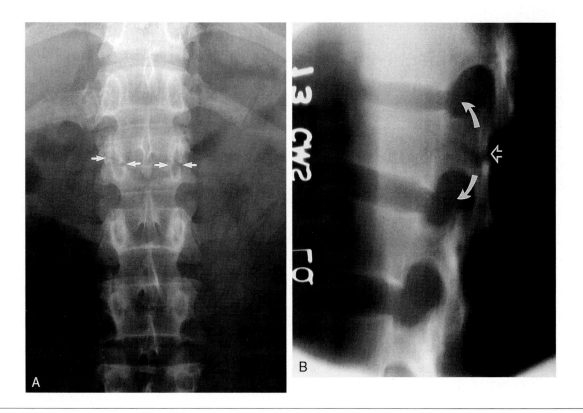

FIGURE 8–28. Chance fracture. This is a distraction fracture, which usually occurs between L1 and L3. On the AP view of the lumbar spine *(A)*, all that can be identified is a discontinuity *(arrows)* in the normal white oval ring of the pedicles. On the lateral view *(B)*, there is a lucent dark line in the posterior elements extending toward the vertebral body *(arrowhead)*. This is caused by tearing of the bone due to seat belt injury.

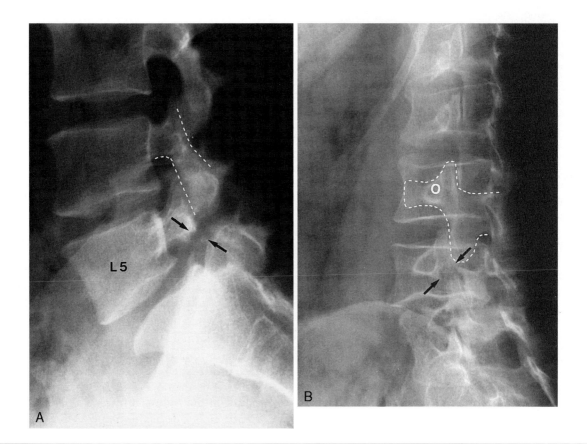

FIGURE 8–29. Spondylolysis. On the lateral view of the lower lumbar spine *(A)*, the normal contour of the posterior elements of L4 is outlined by the white dotted lines. At L5, lysis *(fracture)* of the posterior elements has occurred *(arrows)*. On the oblique view *(B)*, this is seen as a fracture through the neck of the "Scottie dog" *(arrows)*. The normal outline for the L4 level is shown.

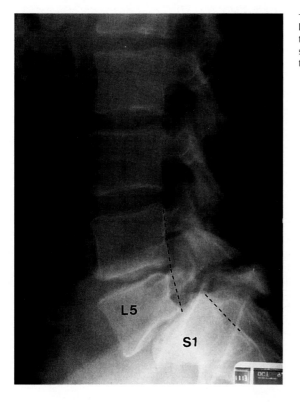

FIGURE 8–30. Spondylolysis with resulting grade 2 spondylolisthesis. Discontinuity of the posterior elements of L5 has allowed L5 to slip forward on S1. The degree of slippage is ascertained by looking at the relationship between the posterior portions of the vertebral bodies.

thing to do in a case of simple low back pain is to put the patient at bed rest, although most patients resist this and demand expensive imaging studies. After several weeks of bed rest, if pain persists, a noncontrasted CT scan is probably the procedure of choice.

Infections

Most infections in the spine involve a disk space and will cause destruction of the vertebral body above and below (Fig. 8–35). It is very rare for tumor to involve or cross a disk space. Tumors typically will destroy a single vertebral body and then may extend above and below. Thus, if you see a destructive process centered about a disk space, an infection should be your first choice. Evaluation of the bony destruction of a vertebral body is best visualized by CT scan, but if there is a neurologic deficit, MR is more appropriate.

Neoplasms

Although there can be primary bony neoplasms of the spine, they are very rare. The most com-

mon neoplastic involvement is from metastatic disease. The metastases may be destructive and cause holes (lytic lesions) in the bone, or they may be dense white (sclerotic lesions). Most neoplasms, including lung, renal, and breast cancer as well as multiple myeloma, will cause lytic lesions in bones. Most sclerotic metastases in men are due to prostate cancer, and in women, to breast cancer (Fig. 8–36).

Metastases do not begin in the bone cortex but rather in the red marrow, which has filtered the tumor cells out of the blood. After growing within the marrow space, the lesion becomes large enough to erode the bony cortex. The most sensitive method of finding metastatic disease in the spine is through utilization of MRI (Fig. 8–37). Unfortunately, MRI can look only at limited portions of the body at one time, and it is very expensive. Therefore, if you are thinking about metastatic disease to the skeleton, the most cost-effective imaging study is a nuclear medicine bone scan. If a patient has pain in a specific area, and you expect a very aggressive destructive lesion (such as from renal cell carcinoma), a plain x-ray of the area should be ordered. Multiple myeloma not only can produce

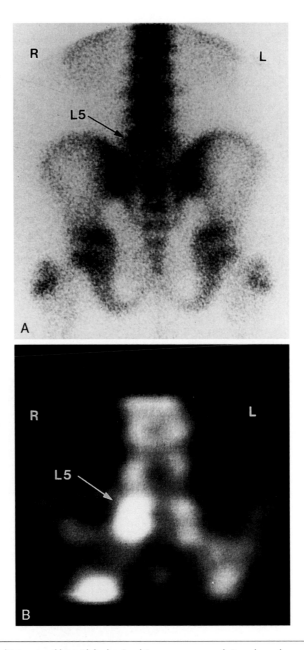

FIGURE 8–31. Occult spondylolysis. In this teenage athlete with back pain, plain x-rays were normal. A regular nuclear medicine bone scan *(A)* was obtained with images over the lower lumbar spine and pelvis. There may be a very minimal increase in activity seen on the right side of L5. An additional tomographic or coronal SPECT image *(B)* was obtained. It shows markedly increased activity on the right side of L5 due to a traumatic fracture of the pars interarticularis on that side.

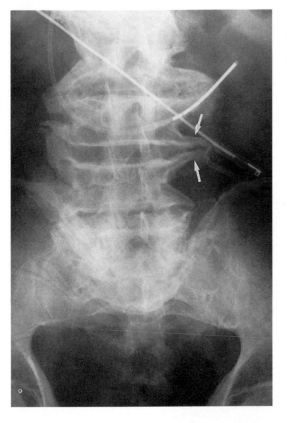

FIGURE 8–32. Degenerative changes of the lumbar spine. An AP view of the lower lumbar spine shows extensive and florid bone spur formation as a result of degenerative change. The extent of these changes does not correlate very well with the presence of back pain.

FIGURE 8–33. Degenerative disk disease of the lumbar spine. A lateral view of the lower lumbar spine shows spondylolisthesis and subluxation of L4 on L5. The degenerative changes noted are almost complete loss of the disk spaces at L4–L5 and L5–S1. The small dark area within the disk space *(arrows)* is nitrogen; this is referred to as a vacuum disk.

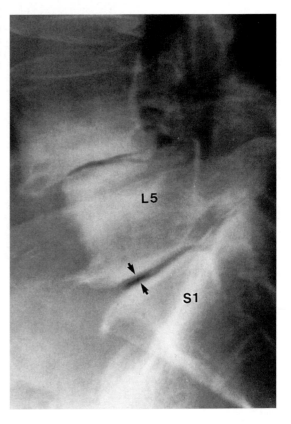

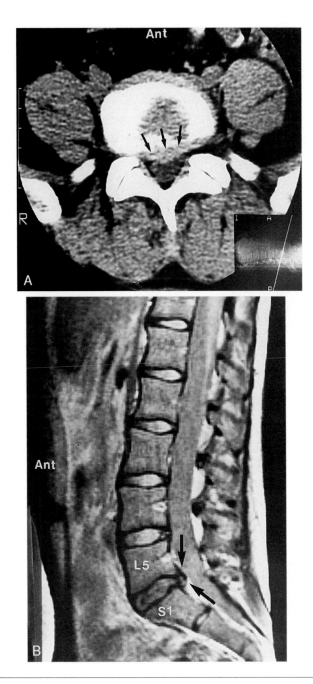

FIGURE 8–34. Disk herniation and protrusion. A transverse CT scan *(A)* obtained at the L5–S1 disk space shows posterior protrusion of disk material *(arrows)* into the spinal canal. In a different patient, the sagittal or lateral MRI view *(B)* of the lumbar spine shows a posterior L5–S1 disk *(arrows)* protruding into the spinal canal.

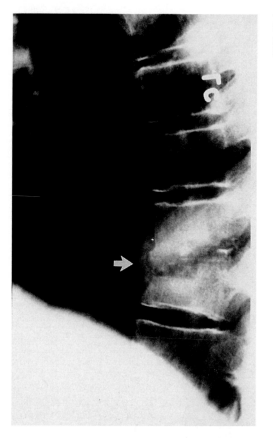

FIGURE 8–35. Osteomyelitis of the spine. A lateral view of the lower thoracic spine demonstrates destruction of the disk space *(arrow)* as well as destruction of the adjoining vertebral bodies.

focal lytic lesions but also can diffusely involve the bones, removing enough of the calcium so that all the bones become very difficult to see.

Unusual Lesions

A very characteristic, but unusual, lesion of the lumbar spine is ankylosing spondylitis. It occurs primarily in young males (onset about age 20 years) and sometimes is associated with ulcerative colitis. Ninety-five per cent of patients are positive for HLA-B27 antigen. In this disease, there is calcification bridging the disk spaces. This is easily seen on the lateral plain x-ray and is referred to as a bamboo spine. On the AP view, you will notice that there has been fusion of the sacroiliac joints (Fig. 8–38), and sometimes you can see "whiskering" (also called enthesopathy) of the ischial tuberosities and along the lateral ilium. About 30 per cent of the patients will have a peripheral arthritis that spares the hands but involves the feet.

SHOULDER AND HUMERUS

Normal Anatomy and Imaging

The standard view of the shoulder is obtained in an AP or a PA projection with the arm rotated internally and then externally. When the arm is in internal rotation, the humeral head looks generally smooth and spherical over the upper portion. In external rotation, there is a concavity of the bicipital groove seen in the lateral aspect of the humeral head. In children, the proximal humeral epiphysis and an epiphyseal plate are visualized. This can sometimes be confused with a fracture. If the epiphyseal plate is not parallel to the x-ray beam, several lucent lines traversing the proximal portion of the humerus can be seen, since the epiphyseal plate is tilted off axis relative to the x-ray beam (Fig. 8–39).

On a plain AP x-ray of the adult shoulder, the medial portion of the humeral head overlaps with the lateral aspect of the glenoid (Fig. 8–40). Sometimes the humeral head may project

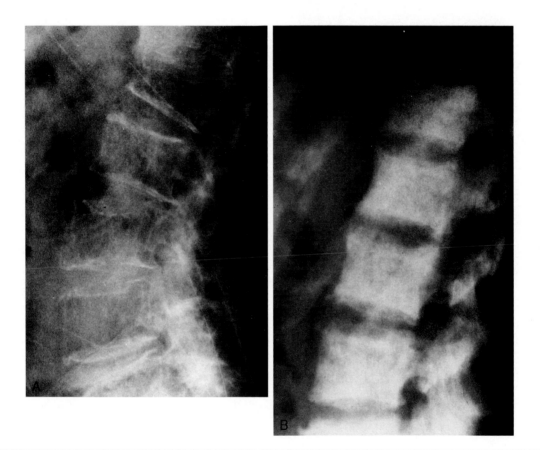

FIGURE 8–36. Diffuse neoplastic involvement of the lumbar spine. In a patient with multiple myeloma, a lateral view of the lumbar spine *(A)* demonstrates vertebral bodies that are difficult to see owing to diffuse loss of calcium. Also note vertebral body compression fracture. A lateral view of the spine *(B)* in a different patient with diffuse metastatic prostate cancer shows blastic or dense white metastases in most of the bones visualized.

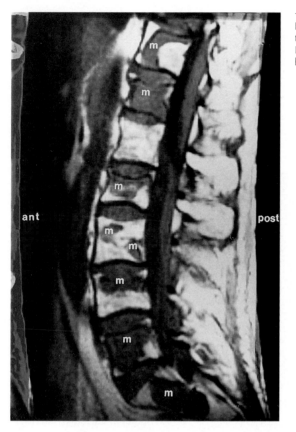

FIGURE 8–37. Focal spine metastases. A sagittal or lateral T1 weighted MR image of the lumbar spine shows the normal white or high signal in fat within the bone marrow. In many of the vertebral bodies, the high signal of normal marrow has been replaced by dark areas of metastatic deposits (M).

slightly lower or slightly higher than the center of the glenoid. Since the humerus is somewhat anterior to the glenoid, if the patient is tilted back when the x-ray is taken, the humeral head will project high relative to the glenoid; if the patient is tilted somewhat forward, it will appear slightly low. You should examine the relationship of the distal clavicle to the acromion to see whether there has been an acromioclavicular (AC) separation. In teenagers there is an apophysis that you should be aware of, both on the end of the coracoid process and on the acromion. This is seen as a thin crescentic white line and should not be mistaken for an avulsion fracture (Fig. 8–41). The clavicle, scapula, and ribs should be examined for fractures and other lesions. You should also look to see whether there is any pathology in the visualized portions of the lung.

There are two other commonly ordered views of the shoulder. The first is called the Y view. This is done with the patient rotated somewhat so that the scapular blade is seen on end and projects off the chest wall. The acromion, spine of the scapula, and blade of the scapula form a Y (Fig. 8–42). The humeral head should normally project at or near the intersection of the three lines. This view is usually obtained if a shoulder dislocation is suspected and is also useful to look for fractures of the scapular blade.

Another view that is often obtained is the axillary view, in which the elbow is elevated and the beam projection is directly up and down through the shoulder. This allows clear visualization of the relationship of the glenoid to the humeral head (Fig. 8–43). Unfortunately, this view is difficult to obtain on patients who have a true dislocation. You need to be careful about ordering this projection if you suspect a humeral head or humeral shaft fracture, since the technologists may make the situation worse by elevating the patient's elbow in an attempt to obtain the axillary view.

Radiographs of the shoulder are really useful only to define bony anatomy. There are many

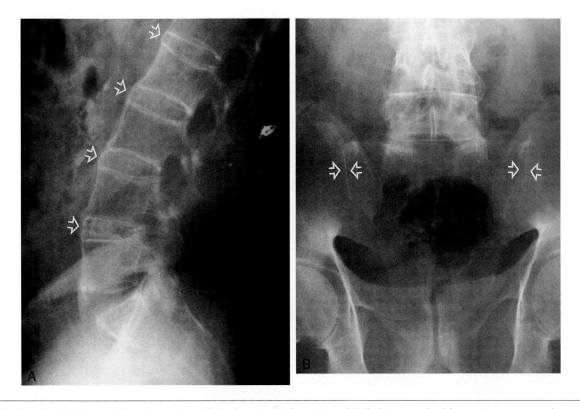

FIGURE 8–38. Ankylosing spondylitis. A lateral view of the lumbar spine *(A)* demonstrates calcific bridging across the disk spaces *(arrows)*, causing the typical "bamboo spine" appearance. *B*, AP view of the pelvis shows that the region of the sacroiliac joints *(arrows)* is not easily visualized owing to fusion of both sacroiliac joints.

shoulder injuries that involve soft tissues, and for evaluation of these the most useful imaging test is an MR scan. The joint and soft tissues can also be visualized by injecting contrast directly into the joint or by using ultrasound. These are difficult to interpret and give a limited view, so they are rarely done. MRI allows excellent visualization not only of the muscle but also of the joint space as well as the tendons (Fig. 8–44). Remember that what appears to be a white bone on an MR image is really fat within the marrow space, and the cortex of the bone is seen as a black line around the edge. Fat in the subcutaneous areas is also seen as white, and muscle is usually gray.

Trauma

Table 8–3 shows the high-yield areas to examine for upper extremity trauma. Probably the most three most common acute shoulder injuries are

fracture, shoulder separation (acromioclavicular separation), and dislocation of the humeral head.

Fractures

Most clavicular fractures occur either in the midportion or the distal third of the clavicle. Usually, the fractures are clinically obvious (Fig. 8–45). Rarely, there is dislocation of the proximal head of the clavicle from the sternoclavicular joint; however, this is also clinically obvious. Fractures of the scapula are reasonably rare, although they can occur as the result of a direct blow. Often this is apparent on a routine shoulder film and from the clinical history (Fig. 8–46). In many cases the fracture cannot be seen in its entirety as it traverses the blade of the scapula, and if there is any additional question, a Y view x-ray or a CT scan may be useful.

Fractures of the mid- or proximal humerus

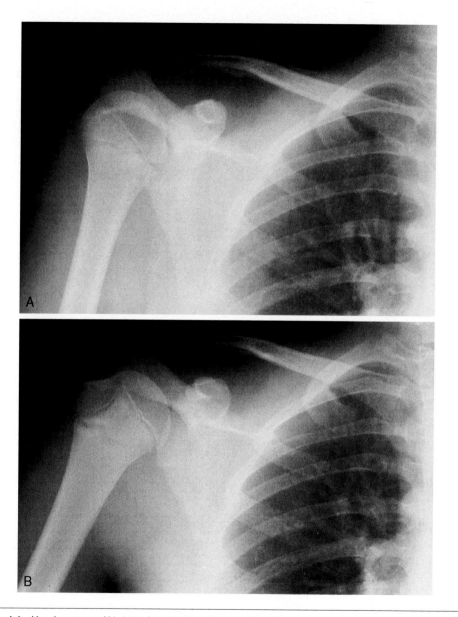

**FIGURE 8–39. Normal shoulder of an 11-year-old in internal rotation *(A)* and in external rotation *(B).* The epiphyseal plate of the proximal humerus should not be mistaken for a fracture.

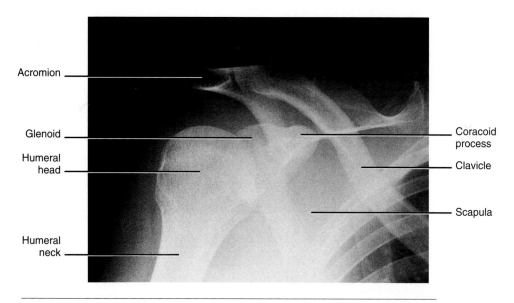

Acromion

Glenoid

Humeral
head

Humeral
neck

Coracoid
process

Clavicle

Scapula

FIGURE 8–40. Normal anatomy of the adult shoulder in the PA projection with the humerus in internal rotation.

FIGURE 8–41. Normal apophysis in the shoulder of a teenager. An apophysis with a lucent line can be seen in the distal acromion as well as the coracoid process. This should not be mistaken for an avulsion fracture.

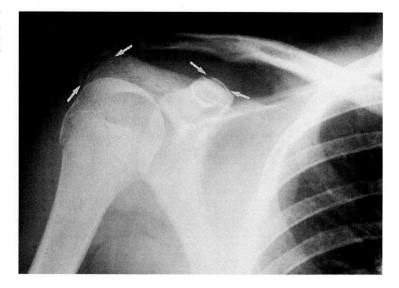

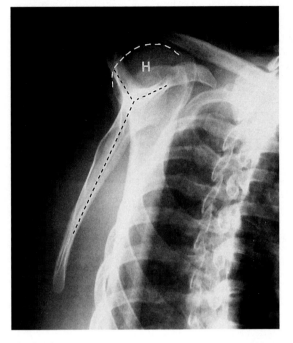

FIGURE 8–42. Normal oblique or Y, view of the shoulder. On this view, the elements of the scapula form a Y and the humeral head should overlap the intersecting arms of the Y.

FIGURE 8–43. Normal axillary view of the shoulder.

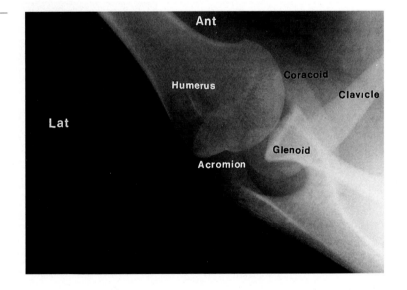

TABLE 8–3. Examination of an X-ray of the Upper Extremity Done For Trauma

Shoulder
AP View
　Anterior dislocation—humeral head inferior and medial
　Posterior dislocation—humeral head not round and slightly lateral
　AC separation
　Clavicular fracture
　Scapular fracture
　Rib fracture
Y View
　Dislocation
　Scapular fracture

Elbow
AP View
　Radial head fracture
　Supracondylar fracture
Lateral View
　Posterior fat pad (always abnormal)
　Bulging anterior fat pad
　Olecranon fracture
　Coronoid fracture
　Radial head alignment

Wrist
PA View
　Distal radius
　Ulnar styloid
　Navicular
　Widening between navicular and lunate
　Two distinct rows of carpals present
　Base of thumb
Lateral View
　Alignment of radius, ulna, lunate, and distal carpals
　Dorsum (for triquetral fracture)

Hand
AP View
　Fifth metacarpal (boxer's fracture)
　Base of first metacarpal (Bennett's or Rolando fracture if intra-articular)
　Base of first proximal phalanx (gamekeeper's thumb)
　Proximal interphalangeal joints—dislocations
　Distal phalanx—tuft fracture
Lateral View
　Base of phalanges (volar plate fracture)

present few problems in radiographic interpretation and thus will not be considered further.

Acromioclavicular (AC) Separation

In this injury, there is superior dislocation of the distal clavicle relative to the acromion (Fig. 8–47). Since the clavicle is slightly anterior relative to the acromion, if the patient is leaning back when the film is taken, it sometimes looks as though there is a separation when there is not. If you have any question, a single view that includes both shoulders often is useful. Sometimes, AP x-rays of the shoulders with the patient holding weights in both hands are ordered to see if this will accentuate a separation, but in practice this is rarely necessary.

Dislocations

Over 95 per cent of shoulder dislocations occur with anterior dislocation of the humeral head relative to the glenoid. This is in contrast to the hip, in which the vast majority of femoral head

dislocations are posterior. In an anterior shoulder dislocation, the humeral head usually is seen to be inferior to the glenoid on the AP projection, and there is medial displacement of the humeral head from its normal position relative to the glenoid (Fig. 8–48). As mentioned earlier, on the oblique view of the shoulder (the Y view), the humeral head should sit over the central portion of the Y. A Y view will clearly show the anterior and inferior dislocation of the humeral head (Fig. 8–49).

There are two specific abnormalities that you should be looking for in addition to the dislocation. As a dislocation occurs there sometimes is a fracture of a portion of the humeral head or of the glenoid. Some physicians relocate a dislocated shoulder without obtaining a prereduction film. If you do this, and the postreduction film demonstrates a fracture, the patient may accuse you of having been responsible for the fracture during the reduction. The second major abnormality that you should be looking for occurs in patients who have had repeated dislocations.

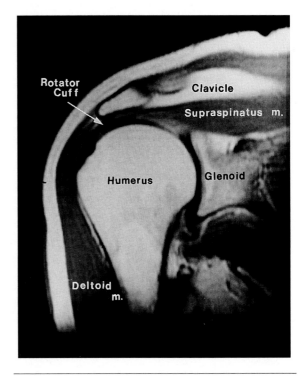

FIGURE 8–44. Normal coronal view of the shoulder with a T1 weighted MR scan. The osseous structures, including the humeral head, glenoid, acromion, and clavicle, are well seen. The muscular structures of the deltoid and supraspinatus are also seen, and the rotator cuff can be identified.

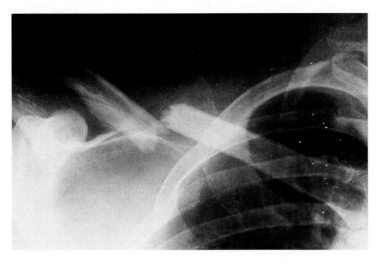

FIGURE 8–45. Midclavicular fracture.

FIGURE 8–46. Scapular fracture. A Y view of the shoulder clearly shows a fracture through the blade of the scapula *(arrows)*.

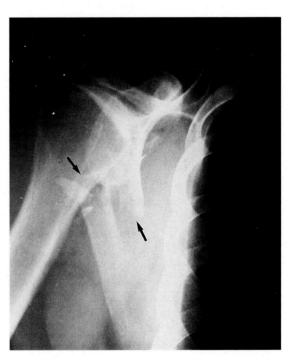

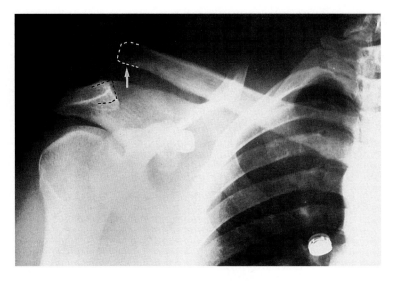

FIGURE 8–47. Acromioclavicular separation. The distal end of the clavicle is superiorly dislocated relative to the acromion.

Chronic trauma caused by interaction of the inferior edge of the glenoid with the humeral head produces a deformity or groove in the superolateral portion of the humeral head. This is known as a Hill-Sachs deformity (Fig. 8–50).

Posterior shoulder dislocations are rare, and they are quite tricky to identify on a standard AP shoulder radiograph. Remember that with internal rotation the humeral head on the AP projection is typically like the top half of a sphere. In a posterior shoulder dislocation, the humeral head simply does not appear to be rounded (Fig. 8–51), and there is slightly increased space between the humeral head and the glenoid. The Y view will clearly show you the posterior dislocation.

Degenerative Changes

A degenerative change that can be seen on the plain radiograph is calcification of tendons. This

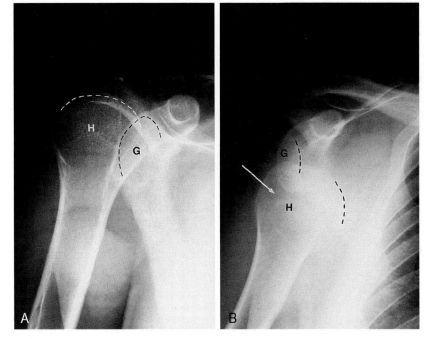

FIGURE 8–48. Anterior dislocation of the shoulder. A, In the normal AP view of the shoulder, the humeral head is located lateral to the glenoid, but there is a small amount of overlap. B, In the same patient with an anterior dislocation, the humeral head goes inferiorly and medially with respect to the glenoid.

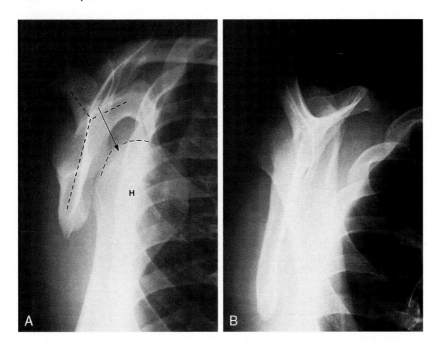

FIGURE 8–49. Anterior dislocation on the Y view. *A,* On the Y view, the humeral head is clearly anterior and inferior to the intersection of the Y of the scapula. *B,* After relocation, the humeral head overlaps the Y formed by the scapula.

usually appears as amorphous white densities over the superolateral aspect of the humeral head (Fig. 8–52). The major form of degenerative change is post-traumatic or degenerative arthritis. Since the glenohumeral joint is off axis relative to an AP x-ray beam, minimal joint space narrowing is not easily evaluated. However, if the changes are severe enough (Fig. 8–53), it is easy to see that the joint is narrowed. Typically, there is associated sclerosis and often spurring and deformity of the humeral head and the inferior aspect of the glenoid. Degenerative change also includes rotator cuff tears. These are best visualized utilizing MR scanning. With a rotator cuff tear there may be a narrowing of the acromiohumeral space to less than 6 mm, an eroded inferior aspect of the acromion, and abnormal communication of the joint space with the subdeltoid bursa.

Tumors

Of the number of lesions that can be found in the shoulder, one of the most common benign

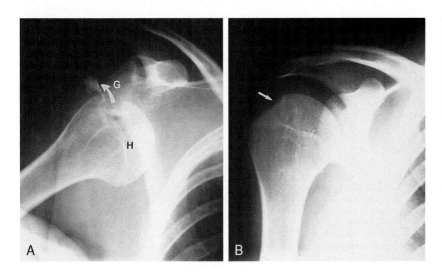

FIGURE 8–50. Complications of shoulder dislocation. *A,* In a patient with an anterior dislocation of the humeral head, a fracture fragment arising from the humerus *(arrow)* can be identified. *B,* In a different patient chronic anterior dislocations caused a Hill-Sach's deformity seen as a groove in the upper outer portion of the humeral head *(arrow).*

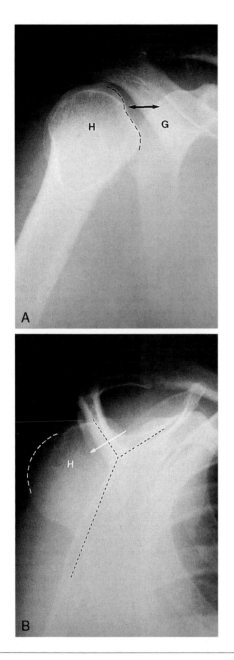

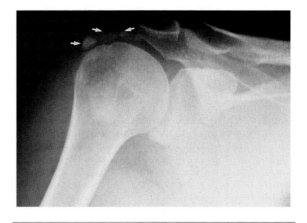

FIGURE 8–52. **Calcific tendinitis.** Small clumps of amorphous calcification can be identified over the superior and lateral portion of the humeral head *(arrows).*

quela of trauma or an intraosseous hematoma. It is usually discovered incidentally or when a fracture occurs through the weakened bone. As the child grows, the tumor usually becomes

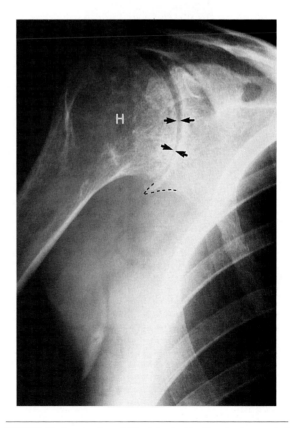

FIGURE 8–51. **Posterior dislocation of the humeral head.** *A,* An AP view of the shoulder initially looks fairly normal. However, there is an increased space *(double-ended arrow)* between the humeral head and the glenoid; the fact that the humeral head is not spherical *(dotted line)* is another clue. *B,* On the Y view of the shoulder, the humeral head can clearly be seen to be displaced posteriorly relative to the central portion of the Y formed by the scapula.

tumors is the unicameral bone cyst (Fig. 8–54). This expansile, lytic, well-demarcated lesion almost always occurs in the proximal portion of the humerus in children or young teenagers. It probably is not a true cyst but may be the se-

FIGURE 8–53. **Degenerative arthritis of the shoulder.** There has been marked narrowing of the normal joint space *(arrows).* There is flattening of the humeral head, and there is spurring deformity of the inferior portion of the glenoid.

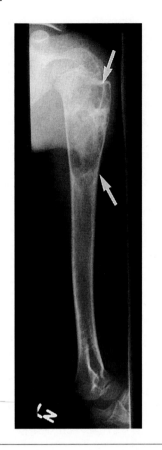

FIGURE 8–54. **Unicameral bone cyst.** The proximal portion of the humerus is a common location for this lesion *(arrows)*. The lesion is lucent, is quite well defined, and can be slightly expansile. A fracture can occur through this area owing to the weakened bone.

smaller and appears to progress down the shaft of the bone. Actually, it stays in the same place but appears to move with time because of the longitudinal bone growth that occurs at the epiphyseal plate.

Malignant lesions also develop in the shoulder. Since the scapula is a flat bone, Ewing's sarcoma can occur here. You should remember that the proximal humerus is the third most frequent site of osteogenic sarcoma in children. This particular lesion will be discussed further in the section on the knee, because the knee is a more common location.

Infection

Septic arthritis of the shoulder presents initially as swelling of the shoulder joint with an effu-sion, followed by cartilage destruction and then bony destruction of both the glenoid and the humeral head.

ELBOW

Normal Anatomy and Imaging

Most x-rays of the elbow relate to trauma. The normal images obtained include an AP and oblique view with the elbow extended and a lateral view with the elbow flexed at 90 degrees (Fig. 8–55). The lateral view is the most promising view to look for pathology in the elbow. There is a small dark area seen just anterior to the distal humerus. This is the anterior fat pad, and while it is normal to see this, it should be right up against the bone. A posterior fat pad is never seen normally. In a teenager, lack of fusion of the normal epiphyses and presence of apophyses can cause confusion. The last areas of fusion include the radial head and the coronoid apophysis, which is located on the medial aspect of the elbow. In addition, there is an olecranon apophysis that can be seen on the lateral view (Fig. 8–56). Normally, these apophyses are not mistaken for fractures if you realize that they have well-defined margins without sharp edges and that the anterior fat pad is in normal position and a posterior fat pad is not seen.

Trauma

As mentioned earlier, the place to begin looking for traumatic injuries in an adult is on the lateral view. You should immediately look for the anterior fat pad, which should lie against the anterior portion of the distal humerus. Anterior displacement of the fat pad is often referred to as the sail sign. This is because when it is pushed forward by an effusion or hemorrhage it resembles the spinnaker on a sailboat. When you see either anterior displacement of the anterior fat pad or any visualization whatever of the posterior fat pad, you should indicate that a fracture is likely to be present, even if you do not see it on any of the views. Sometimes, repeating the x-ray 7 to 10 days later will allow decalcification

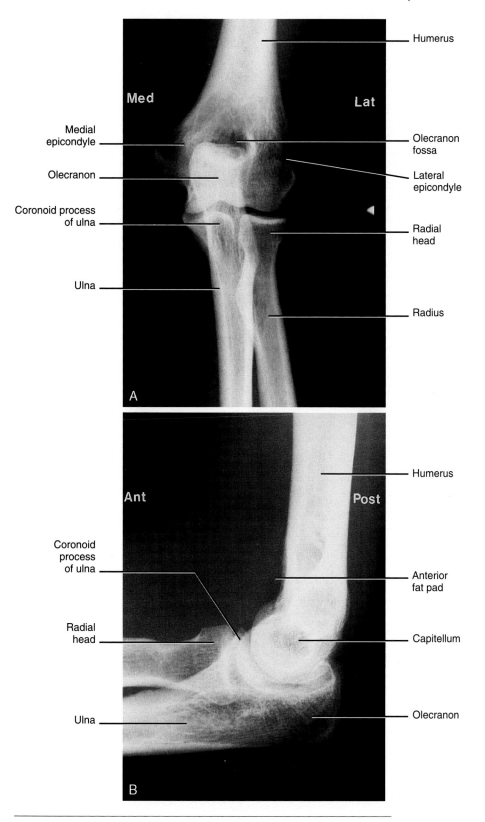

Humerus

Med

Lat

Medial
epicondyle

Olecranon
fossa

Olecranon

Lateral
epicondyle

Coronoid process
of ulna

Radial
head

Ulna

Radius

A

Humerus

Ant

Post

Coronoid
process
of ulna

Anterior
fat pad

Radial
head

Capitellum

Ulna

Olecranon

B

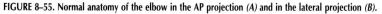

FIGURE 8–55. Normal anatomy of the elbow in the AP projection *(A)* and in the lateral projection *(B)*.

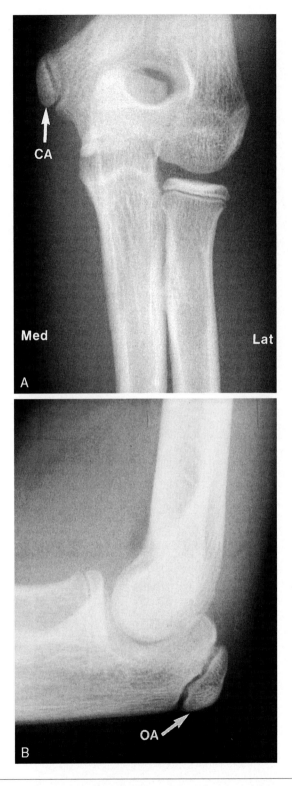

FIGURE 8–56. Normal apophyses. On the AP projection *(A)*, a coronoid apophysis can be seen along the medial aspect of the distal humerus. On the lateral view *(B)*, an olecranon apophysis is often visualized in older children. The epiphysis has not yet fused.

FIGURE 8–57. Radial head fracture. The lateral view of the elbow *(A)* shows anterior displacement of the dark stripe of the anterior fat pad *(arrows)*; a posterior fat pad is also seen *(posterior arrows)*. On the AP view *(B)*, a lucent fracture line is seen going obliquely across the humeral head.

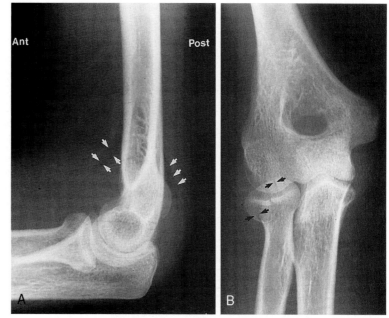

of the fracture to occur so that it will be more easily seen.

The most common fracture of the elbow seen in the adult is a radial head fracture (Fig. 8–57). Less common are fractures of the coronoid process of the ulna (Fig. 8–58) and fractures of the olecranon. Olecranon fractures are typically caused by falling directly on the elbow when it is flexed. Orthopedic hardware utilized to fix elbow injuries includes screws, wire, and fixation pins (Fig. 8–59). In evaluation of postreduction and postfixation x-rays, you should be looking at alignment and residual angulation to see that there is healing across the fracture, that the wires and screws have not migrated, and, finally, that there is no increasing lucency or dark areas around either the screws or the pins to suggest osteomyelitis or loosening.

FIGURE 8–58. Coronoid fracture. The AP view in this patient looked normal; however, on the lateral view, the coronoid process of the ulna has a lucent (dark) fracture line extending through it *(arrows)*.

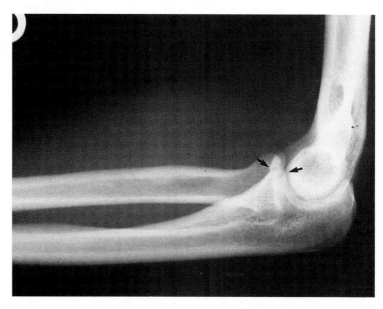

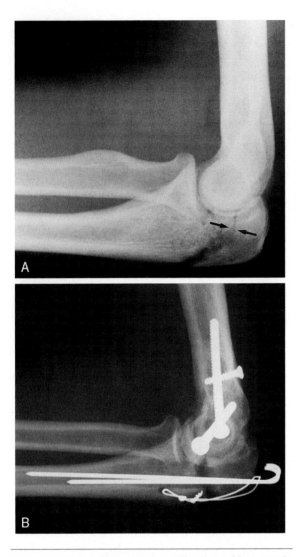

three classic fractures that you should be aware of. The first is the "nightstick" fracture. This is a single fracture through the midportion of the ulna (Fig. 8–60). It is called the nightstick fracture because it easily occurs when an individual raises his or her arm to protect against being hit with a stick. A direct blow to the upraised and slightly flexed forearm means that the impact of the stick will be directly on the midportion of the ulna, causing a fracture. Fractures of the forearm often heal by a simple reduction and casting, although occasionally a compression plate and fixation screws are utilized. In a compression plate the holes for the screws are somewhat elliptical, and this allows placement of the screws in such a manner that the ends of the fracture will be compressed together.

There are two other classic (although un-

FIGURE 8–59. Olecranon fracture. *A,* The initial lateral view of this patient who fell directly upon the elbow demonstrates a fracture line extending into the joint space *(arrows). B,* In a different patient, an olecranon fracture has been repaired by using two fixation pins and a tension wire. This particular patient also had a supracondylar fracture, accounting for the screws in the distal humerus.

FOREARM

Typical normal views of the forearm are obtained in AP and lateral projections. If you suspect trauma or abnormalities of either the elbow or the wrist, a forearm view alone is not satisfactory. You should order forearm views only when you think that the abnormality is in the midportion of either the radius or the ulna.

Trauma

Traumatic injuries are, by far, the most common reason for ordering forearm x-rays. There are

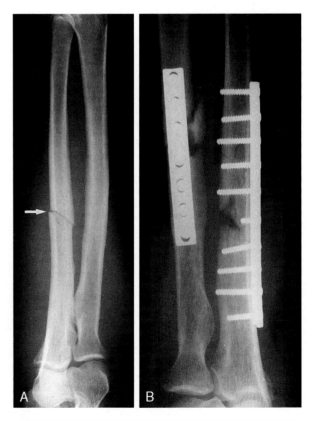

FIGURE 8–60. Nightstick fracture. *A,* An AP view of the forearm demonstrates a single fracture across the midportion of the ulna. This is called a nightstick fracture because it occurs when the person lifts the forearm to protect against being hit with a stick. *B,* In a different patient with a much more severe fracture of the radius and ulna, the fracture has been fixed utilizing a plate and screws. Notice the asymmetric holes in the plate, which allow for compression of the fracture fragments.

common) fractures of the forearm. The Monteggia fracture is a fracture of the proximal ulna with dislocation of the radial head (Fig. 8–61). The dislocation of the radial head can be missed unless you realize that the radius and radial head should point toward the capitellum. The usual mechanism of this fracture is falling forward while carrying weight in the hands, such as a load of books. During the fall, there is a direct blow to the ulna by a sharp object, such as the corner of a stair. The weight of the body is transmitted down the humerus to the elbow while the weight of the books is in the hands, and the corner of the stair is a fulcrum located at the proximal portion of the forearm between the two weights. The Galeazzi fracture is a fracture of the distal radius with dislocation of the ulnar head from the wrist joint (Fig. 8–62). The mechanism is somewhat similar to that of a Monteggia fracture but with the fulcrum located more distally.

HAND AND WRIST

Normal Anatomy and Imaging

The typical views obtained when either hand or wrist x-rays are ordered are AP, oblique, and lateral (Fig. 8–63). Usually x-rays of the hand are done for assessment of trauma or degenerative changes. The wrist has lots of little bones that have unusual shapes and that overlap. In the case of trauma, however, you should have examined the patient first and will have the advantage of knowing the location of interest. Examination of the wrist on the AP view begins with examination of the distal radius and ulna, particularly the styloid processes of each. Next, you should examine the two rows of carpals (with the proximal row being crescentic). The carpal joint spaces are usually quite uniform, and you should look across the carpal-metacarpal and interphalangeal joints in a sequential process.

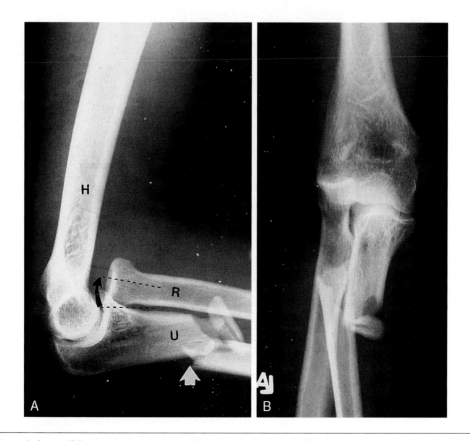

FIGURE 8–61. Monteggia fracture/dislocation. *A,* The lateral view of the elbow shows a fracture of the ulna that occurs at the direct point of impact *(large white arrow)* and dislocation of the radial head from its normal position *(curved black arrow). B,* On the AP projection, the ulnar fracture is clearly identified, but the radial head dislocation is impossible to see.

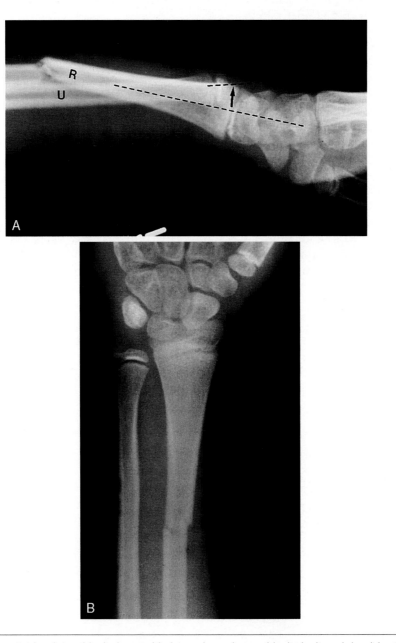

FIGURE 8–62. Galeazzi fracture. *A,* A lateral view of the distal aspect of the forearm shows a fracture of the distal radius and ulnar dislocation from the normal axis of the wrist. *B,* On the AP projection, only the radial fracture is seen.

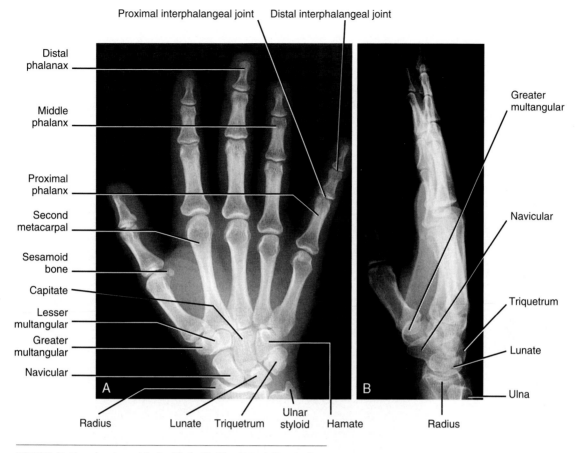

FIGURE 8-63. Normal anatomy of the hand in the PA *(A)* and lateral *(B)* projections.

Trauma

There are some general processes about fractures that you should understand. A fracture often becomes more apparent a week or so after the initial injury (Fig. 8–64). The reason is that in the early stages of a fracture, there is hyperemia, which is accompanied by resorption of calcium along the fracture line. This is why radiologists will sometimes indicate that although they do not see a fracture on a particular examination, if pain persists, a repeat view in 7 to 10 days may be useful. A second phenomenon is a more general loss of calcium and coarsening of the trabecular pattern in bones around a joint that has a fracture. This process may occur over several weeks and is the result of disuse osteoporosis (Fig. 8–65). Sometimes, even if there is minor trauma, there can be joint pain that persists for months with associated vasodilatation. This is termed reflex sympathetic dystrophy (RSD). The radiographic manifestations are focal osteoporosis and a coarse trabecular pattern, in an articular and periarticular distribution (Fig. 8–66).

Common fractures of the wrist include the Colles' fracture. This is a fracture of the distal radius with dorsal angulation of the distal fragment and an associated fracture of the ulnar styloid (Fig. 8–67). The mechanism of injury is typically falling on an outstretched hand with the palm facing down at the time of the fall. A Smith fracture is essentially a reverse Colles' fracture, with the distal radial fragment angulated toward the palmar surface (Fig. 8–68).

The most common fracture of the carpal bones is a fracture of the midportion of the carpal navicular. The navicular has an unusual blood supply. The arteries supply the more distal aspect of the bone and then circle back to

Text continued on page 314

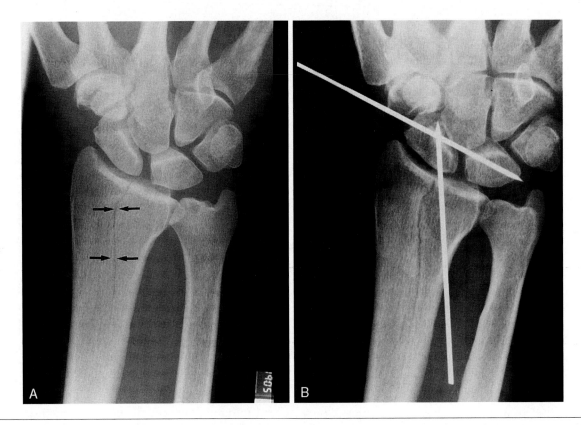

FIGURE 8–64. Increasing fracture visibility with time. *A,* Initial PA view of the wrist shows a longitudinal fracture with intra-articular extension *(arrows).* A film obtained 1 week later with fixation pins in place shows that the fracture line is much more evident owing to interval decalcification, which is a normal process. This may make fractures much more visible a week or so after the injury than on the initial films.

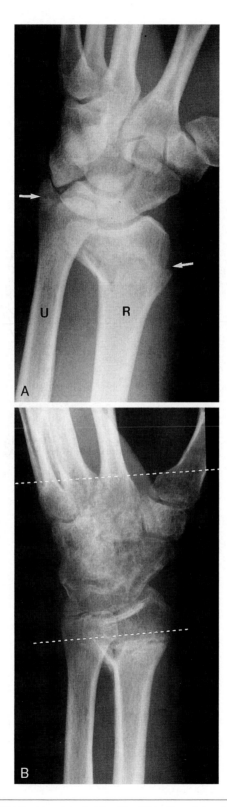

FIGURE 8–65. Interval disuse osteopenia. *A,* An initial film demonstrates fractures of the distal radius and ulnar styloid *(arrows).* The carpal bones are well mineralized and clearly delineated. *B,* A repeat film 3 weeks later shows that there has been marked resorption of calcium in a periarticular distribution *(between the dotted lines).* This is due to disuse and increased blood flow.

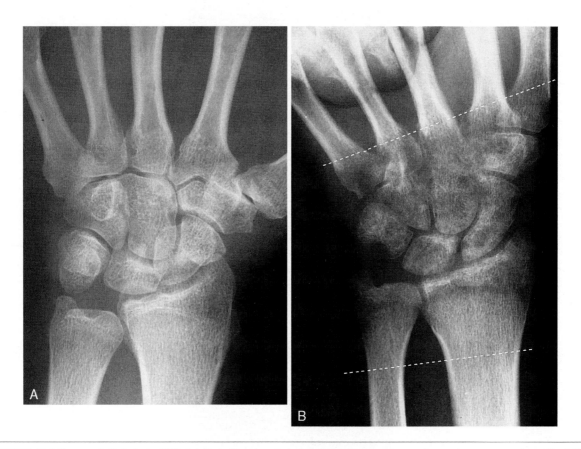

FIGURE 8–66. Reflex sympathetic dystrophy (RSD). *A,* A film in this patient who had relatively minor forearm trauma does not demonstrate any abnormality. *B,* The patient continued to complain of pain over the next 2 months, and another film of the wrist shows periarticular and carpal decalcification due to increased blood flow. The exact cause of RSD is debatable.

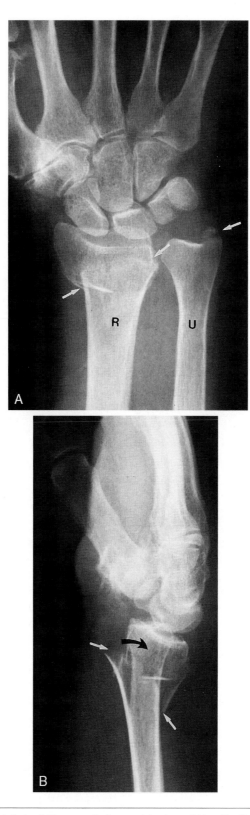

FIGURE 8–67. Colles' fracture. *A,* An impacted distal radial fracture and a fracture of the ulnar styloid are identified on the PA view in this patient who fell on the outstretched hand. *B,* The lateral view of the wrist shows that there is dorsal displacement and angulation as well as some impaction of the distal radius. If the fracture of the distal radius extends into the joint, this would be termed a Barton's fracture.

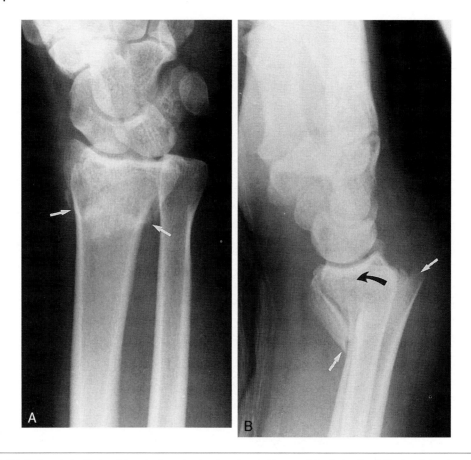

FIGURE 8–68. Smith's fracture. *A,* An AP view of the wrist shows that there is an impacted fracture of the distal radius. *B,* The lateral view shows that there is volar displacement of the distal fragment. If the fracture had extended into the articular surface, this would have been called a reverse Barton's fracture.

the more proximal portion. A fracture through the midportion of the navicular can disrupt the blood supply to the proximal portion and cause aseptic necrosis. When this occurs, the proximal portion of the navicular becomes dense or white relative to the rest of the carpal bones (Fig. 8–69).

An injury that can result from impaction of the distal radius and the carpal bones is disruption of the ligaments between the navicular and the lunate. Sometimes this can be a subtle finding, but you simply need to remember that the space between the distal radius and the carpal bones should be about the same as the distance between the lunate and the navicular. If you have a question as to whether this space is widened, an AP radiograph of the other wrist can be used for comparison (Fig. 8–70).

Tenderness over the dorsal aspect of the wrist should raise the possibility of a triquetral

fracture. This fracture is usually seen only on the lateral view and may be just a small avulsion fragment (Fig. 8–71).

Major falls can cause either lunate or perilunate dislocations of the carpal bones. The key to initial recognition of these dislocations on the AP view is the fact that you no longer see a distinct proximal crescentic row of carpal bones and then a distal row. The lateral view usually makes the type of dislocation reasonably clear. In perilunate dislocation, the lunate is in normal position at the end of the radius, but the remainder of the carpals are dislocated posteriorly and are usually overriding with some shortening of the wrist (Fig. 8–72). In a lunate dislocation, the rest of the carpals remain in a line along the axis of the radius; however, the lunate is usually rotated and dislocated toward the palmar surface (Fig. 8–73). Trauma of the lunate can also result in aseptic necrosis. This is typically re-

Text continued on page 319

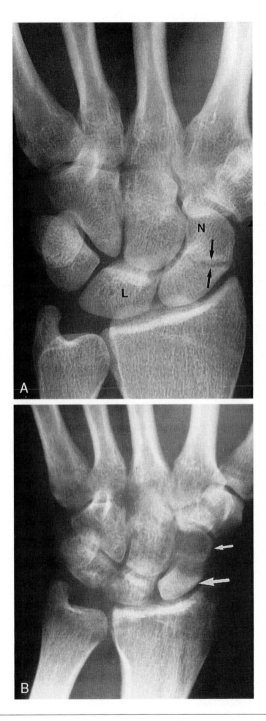

FIGURE 8–69. Scaphoid or navicular fracture. *A,* A PA view of the wrist in a patient who fell on his outstretched hand shows a lucent line extending through the midportion of the navicular. *B,* A later complication in this patient is aseptic necrosis of the proximal fragment *(large arrow)*. Note that this fragment has maintained normal mineralization because the blood supply has been interrupted. In contrast, the remainder of the carpal bones are demonstrating loss of calcium due to hyperemia and disuse after the fracture.

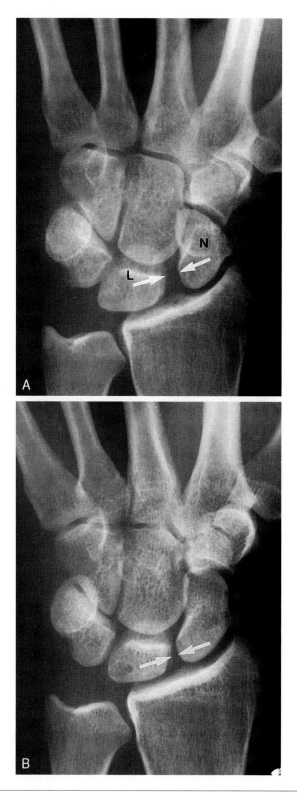

FIGURE 8–70. Scapholunate disassociation. *A,* A PA view of the wrist demonstrates a widened space between the navicular and the lunate *(arrows).* This is due to ligamentous disruption from an impaction injury. *B,* A normal wrist shows that the normal distance between the navicular and lunate *(arrows)* should be about the same as that between the navicular and the radius.

FIGURE 8–71. Triquetral fracture. This is an avulsion fracture of the dorsum of the wrist that is typically seen only on the lateral view. You should look very carefully in this location, since this is a fracture that is easily missed.

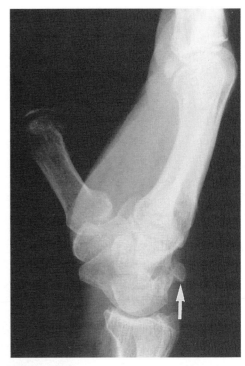

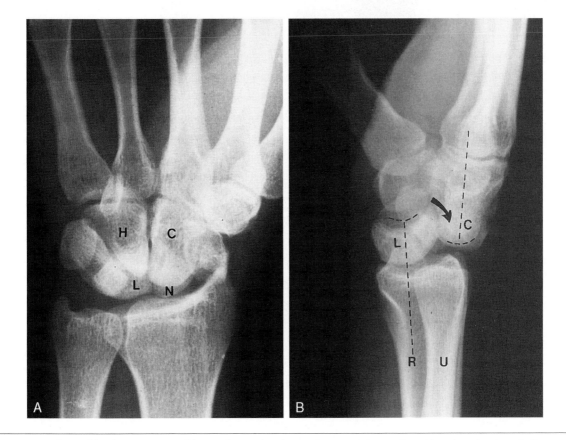

FIGURE 8–72. Perilunate dislocation. *A,* A PA view of the wrist does not show the normal two crescentic rows of carpal bones but rather shows significant overlap of the hamate and the lunate as well as the capitate with the navicular. *B,* A lateral view shows that the lunate remains in alignment with the end of the radius, but the remainder of the carpal bones have been dislocated dorsally.

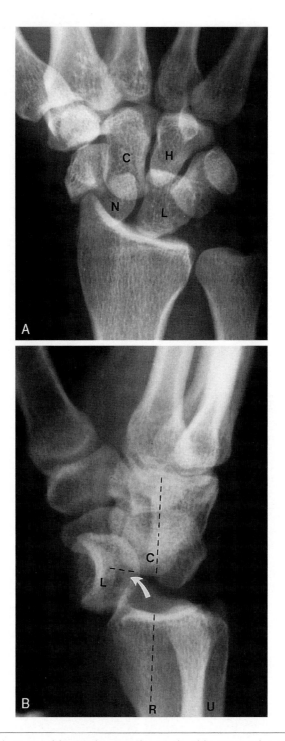

FIGURE 8–73. Lunate dislocation. *A,* On the PA view of the wrist, there is significant overlap of the capitate and navicular as well as the hamate and the lunate. Furthermore, there is clear overlap between the navicular and the radial styloid. All these findings suggest dislocation. *B,* On the lateral view, the carpal bones remain in alignment with the distal radius, but the lunate has rotated and dislocated in the palmar direction *(arrow).*

ferred to as Kienböck's malacia. This may occur as a result of repeated minor traumas or one single episode of trauma. The entity is recognized by irregularity and increased density of the lunate relative to the other carpal bones (Fig. 8–74).

HAND

Normal Anatomy and Imaging

X-rays of the hand and fingers taken for trauma should include AP, lateral (see Fig. 8–63), and oblique views. If the clinical issue is related to arthritis, an AP view of both hands is all that is needed. There is a relatively common finding in the hand that involves shortening of a metacarpal, typically the fourth (Fig. 8–75). This is

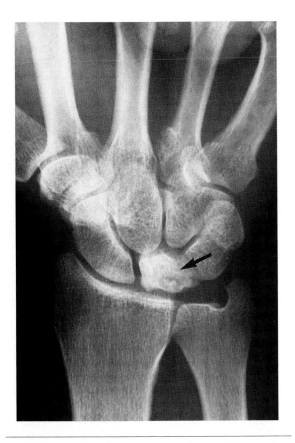

FIGURE 8–74. Aseptic necrosis of the lunate. A PA view of the wrist shows irregularity and increased density or sclerosis of the lunate *(arrow)*. This is also referred to as Kienböck's disease.

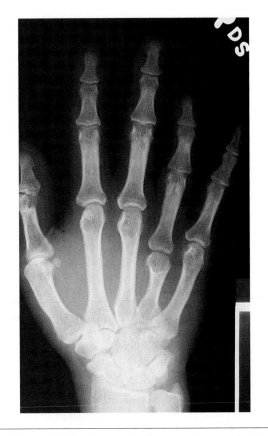

FIGURE 8–75. Short fourth metacarpal. While this can be a normal variant, it has also been associated with Turner's syndrome, sickle cell disease, infections, and some metabolic bone diseases, such as pseudohypoparathyroidism.

usually a normal variant, but the differential diagnosis includes Turner's syndrome, pseudohypoparathyroidism, and a few other much less common entities.

Trauma

X-rays of the hands may be taken for evaluation of foreign bodies. The most common are glass, pencil lead, metallic slivers, and pieces of wood. Glass is usually somewhat radiopaque and can be recognized by its very sharp corners or a geometric shape (Fig. 8–76). Metallic fragments are, of course, easy to spot, since they are so dense. Wood and pencil lead are typically not visible on an x-ray. The reason that pencil lead is not visible is because it is actually graphite and not lead.

There are two relatively frequent fracture

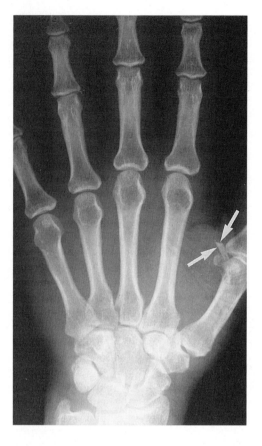

FIGURE 8–76. Glass within the soft tissue of the hand. Most glass has enough density that it is radiopaque and can be recognized by the sharp corners *(arrows)* and the patient history. Remember that objects made of either wood or graphite usually are not visible on an x-ray.

FIGURE 8–77. Boxer's fracture. This hand film was obtained on a teenager who had hand pain after punching a wall. The fracture usually occurs at the neck of the fifth metacarpal, with volar angulation of the distal fragment. Contrary to its name, it is not often seen in professional boxers.

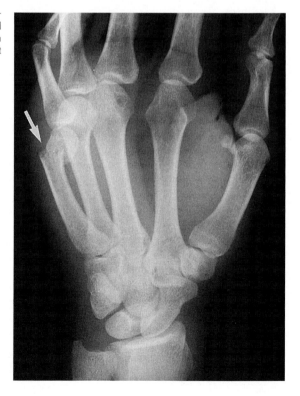

sites of the metacarpals. The most common of these is a fracture of the distal fifth metacarpal (the so-called boxer's fracture). The head of the fifth metacarpal is angled toward the palmar surface and may be somewhat impacted (Fig. 8–77).

The second common location for hand fractures is the base of the thumb. Bennett and Rolando fractures are triangular fractures of the base of the first metacarpal, with extension into the articular surface. There can be oblique fractures of the first metacarpal base that do not extend into the joint (Fig. 8–78). There is another rather classic fracture of the thumb. This is an avulsion fracture of the base of the proximal phalanx. Although this is called a gamekeeper's thumb, the most common mechanism of injury is getting a ski pole caught in the snow with the thumb being pulled backward.

Fingers can not only be fractured but also dislocated. Often, on AP projection, dislocation cannot be appreciated except as slight joint space narrowing and soft tissue swelling; how-

ever, on the lateral view, the dislocation is usually obvious (Fig. 8–79). All dislocations are clinically obvious but if there is unusual associated deformity or angulation, it may be useful to get a prereduction x-ray to see if there is an associated fracture.

In children, fractures about articular surfaces can occur in a variety of ways. They may involve only the epiphyseal plates or various combinations of the epiphyseal plate and the metaphysis. The Salter-Harris classification, shown schematically in Figure 8–80, is used for describing childhood fractures about most joints. A Salter-Harris type II fracture of the fifth digit is shown in Figure 8–81. Another relatively common fracture of the fingers involves the base of the middle phalanx on the palmar surface. This is a small avulsion fracture referred to as a volar plate fracture (Fig. 8–82). It is easily missed unless you look carefully at the lateral view. Of course, fractures of the terminal tuft of the distal phalanges occur very frequently from people slamming their fingers in doors and other

FIGURE 8–78. **Extra-articular fracture of the first metacarpal base.** There has been an oblique fracture at the metacarpal base *(arrows)* but without extension into the joint space. If there had been extension into the joint space with a single linear fracture, this would be termed a Bennett's fracture; if it were a comminuted fracture extending into the joint space, it would be termed a Rolando's fracture.

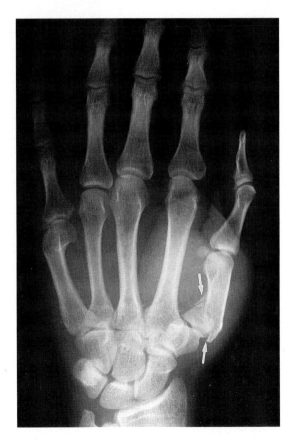

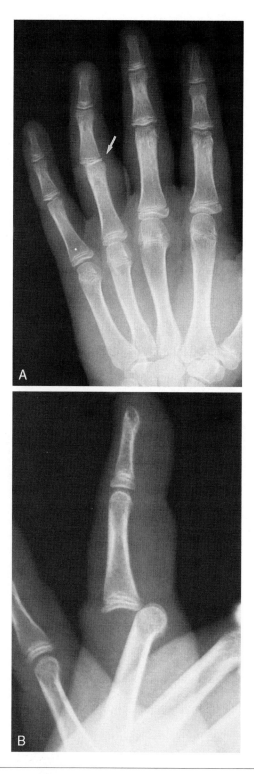

FIGURE 8–79. Complete dislocation of a proximal interphalangeal joint. *A,* A PA view of the hand shows some soft tissue swelling in what looks like only narrowing of a joint space. *B,* A lateral view clearly shows the dislocation, although this, of course, would be clinically obvious. This case should serve as a lesson in why two views are needed before you come to a conclusion about the position of various structures on an x-ray.

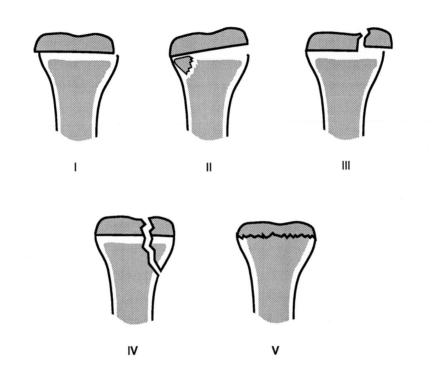

I

II

III

IV

V

FIGURE 8–80. Salter-Harris classification of epiphyseal fractures in children. A type I fracture is straight across the epiphyseal plate and may have some lateral displacement of the epiphysis. This occurs 5 per cent of the time. A type II fracture involves a portion of the epiphyseal plate and a corner fracture through the metaphysis. This occurs 75 per cent of the time. A type III fracture involving part of the epiphysis occurs only about 10 per cent of the time. A type IV fracture involving part of the epiphysis and part of the metaphysis occurs about 10 per cent of the time. A type V fracture is direct impaction and has the most serious consequences for further growth.

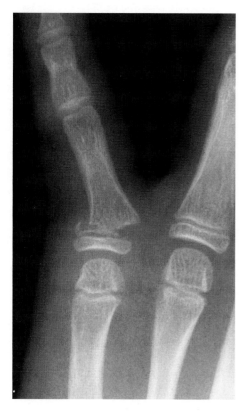

FIGURE 8–81. A Salter-Harris type II fracture of the fifth proximal phalanx.

FIGURE 8–82. **Volar plate fracture.** This fracture is seen only on the lateral view and is a small avulsion fracture, most commonly occurring at the base of the middle phalanx.

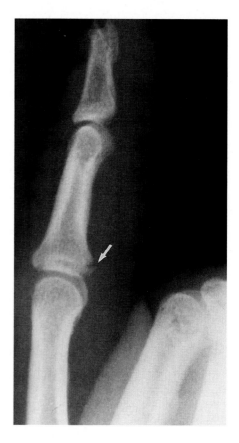

objects. These are quite obvious on the radiograph.

Infection

Infections are quite frequent in the hands as well as the feet. Often, the clinical problem is differentiating between cellulitis, osteomyelitis, and septic arthritis. When the x-ray shows destruction of a single joint space with involvement of the bone on both sides of the joint, septic arthritis should be considered (Fig. 8–83). Osteomyelitis usually is radiographically identified by soft tissue swelling, lucent or destructive areas within the bone itself, or focal periosteal reaction. An illustration of osteomyelitis of the foot appears later. With cellulitis there is only soft tissue swelling without bone or joint changes.

Arthritis

Evaluation of the hands for arthritis can provide some general ideas about the type of arthritis, although commonly there are a number of patients whose laboratory findings of rheumatoid arthritis conflict with an x-ray appearance that looks like degenerative arthritis. The reverse is also true. Thus, the radiographic diagnosis should not be leaned on too heavily.

Rheumatoid arthritis (RA) occurs most frequently in females, and they clinically present with morning stiffness, swelling of one or more joints, and subcutaneous nodules. General radiographic findings of rheumatoid arthritis include narrowing of the carpal joints, subchondral cysts, and erosion of the bones at the lateral edges of the joints. Patients with clinically obvious rheumatoid arthritis can often present with normal-looking x-rays of the hand and then un-

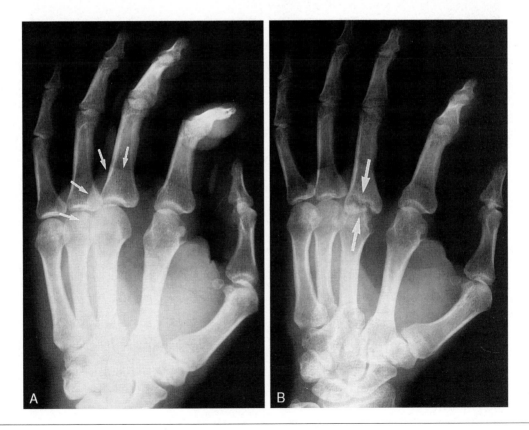

FIGURE 8–83. Septic arthritis. *A,* A film obtained 1 day after a human bite over the third metacarpal phalangeal joint shows only some soft tissue swelling *(arrows).* *B,* A repeat x-ray 4 weeks later shows that there has been destruction of both the distal metacarpal and the proximal phalanx because of an infection within the joint space.

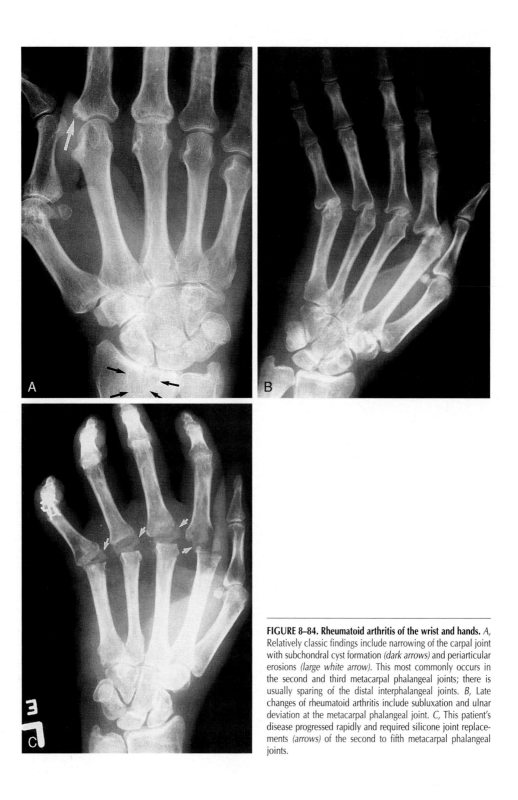

FIGURE 8–84. Rheumatoid arthritis of the wrist and hands. *A,* Relatively classic findings include narrowing of the carpal joint with subchondral cyst formation *(dark arrows)* and periarticular erosions *(large white arrow).* This most commonly occurs in the second and third metacarpal phalangeal joints; there is usually sparing of the distal interphalangeal joints. *B,* Late changes of rheumatoid arthritis include subluxation and ulnar deviation at the metacarpal phalangeal joint. *C,* This patient's disease progressed rapidly and required silicone joint replacements *(arrows)* of the second to fifth metacarpal phalangeal joints.

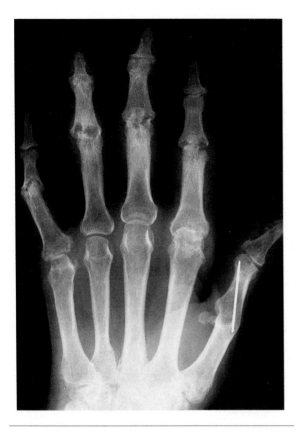

FIGURE 8–85. Psoriatic arthritis. Involvement of the distal and proximal inter-phalangeal joints is most common. Asymmetric changes are also common. Erosions can be aggressive and usually involve the intra-articular joint spaces.

dergo rapid progression. In addition to the findings already described, ulnar deviation at the metacarpo-phalangeal joints is relatively characteristic (Fig. 8–84), but it can occasionally occur with systemic lupus erythematosus (SLE). Any arthritis but RA can present with normal mineralization of bones. Diffuse osteoporosis is mostly seen with RA but periarticular demineralization is also quite common.

In advanced RA the patient's hands may develop the so-called boutonnière deformity, which is hyperextension of the DIP joint and flexion in the PIP joint. Another deformity is almost the reverse of this. The "swan-neck" deformity can also result from hyperextension of the PIP joint and flexion of the DIP joint. If the metacarpophalangeal joints have been completely destroyed, it is possible to replace these with silicone prostheses.

Findings of rheumatoid arthritis in other bones include penciling or erosion of the distal

clavicle and narrowing and erosions of the shoulder, hip, and knee joints as well as atlantoaxial subluxation. Finally, there can be a widened space between the carpal lunate and navicular bone (the Terry Thomas sign). Remember that these patients also can have interstitial lung changes, pulmonary nodules, and various forms of carditis.

When an arthritis involves distal interphalangeal joints with relative sparing of the proximal ones, erosive osteoarthritis and psoriatic arthritis become the more likely diagnoses (Fig. 8–85). Pseudogout can cause calcification within cartilage (chondrocalcinosis). This is not a finding specific to pseudogout, because it also occurs in hypercalcemic states. In the wrist and hand, the calcification is most often seen in the ulnar carpal region (Fig. 8–86). The other common site is the knee joint.

Tumors

Tumors of the hand and wrist are quite rare. The most common tumor is a benign enchondroma. This typically occurs in either the metacarpals or the proximal phalanges. It causes a lucent area in the central portion of the shaft with some expansion and inner table thinning of the cortex. There can be pathologic fractures through these areas as a result of the bone thinning (Fig. 8–87).

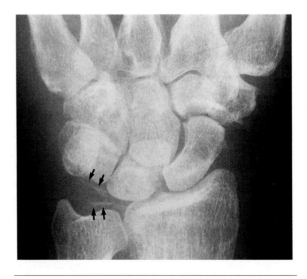

FIGURE 8–86. Calcium pyrophosphate deposition disease. In this disease there may be acute synovitis, sometimes called pseudogout. Here, calcification is seen in the cartilage of the wrist.

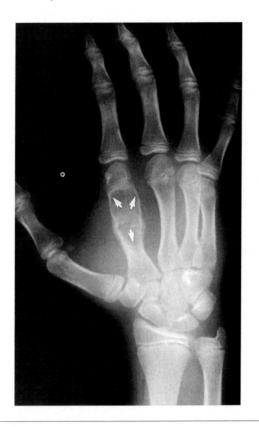

FIGURE 8–87. Enchondroma. A lucent lesion in a metacarpal or phalanx is most likely to be an enchondroma. It may be somewhat expansile *(arrows)*, and there may be fracture through the area of weakened bone. A healing fracture with some periosteal reaction is seen in the midportion of this lesion.

PELVIS

Normal Anatomy and Imaging

When you order a radiograph of the pelvis, only an AP view normally is obtained. On the AP view, there is clear demonstration of the iliac wings, ischium, pubis, and both hips as well as the lower lumbar spine. You should be able to look at the pelvic x-ray and determine not only whether the person is male or female but also the general age of the patient. The inlet of the male pelvis is generally somewhat triangular (Fig. 8–88), whereas the female pelvis has a much more ovoid shape (Fig. 8–89). Occasionally the genitalia are included on the film.

The general age of the patient is ascertained by the presence or absence of degenerative changes in the lower lumbar spine and hip joints. In children, there is incomplete fusion of the acetabulum; in slightly older children, you will be able to see clearly the apophysis of the greater trochanter and the epiphyseal plate of the hip. In the mid- to late teens, an apophysis appears on the iliac crest as well as on the inferior ischium (Fig. 8–90). Although these apophyses can sometimes be mistaken for avulsion fractures, the symmetry from one side of the pelvis to another and their location are usually enough to clearly identify them. There are several normal variants or results of very common conditions that you should be aware of. These are symmetric sclerotic areas (white) about the pubis or the sacroiliac (SI) joint. These are essentially normal findings and occur much more commonly in women, probably as the result of pelvic widening during childbirth (Fig. 8–91).

Trauma

A number of traumatic lesions can occur in the pelvis. A relatively common, and probably inappropriate, x-ray to order is a view of the coccyx. Demonstration of a coccyx fracture does not change treatment.

When a pelvic fracture is suspected, an AP radiograph is the initial view to order. You should examine the symphysis pubis. A widening of the symphysis of more than 1 cm is definitely abnormal. If the symphysis is widened, you should also look for widening of one of the SI joints (Fig. 8–92). The reason is that the pelvis is essentially a bony ring, and it is difficult to widen it or break it in one place without causing a traumatic injury elsewhere.

Many pelvic fractures are accompanied by internal pelvic hematomas. When a fracture in the pubic region is identified, you should exclude urethral and bladder injury. A cystogram is often performed to rule out bladder rupture. Sometimes the resultant hematoma is large enough to displace the bladder superiorly and laterally (Fig. 8–93).

Most pelvic fractures can, and should, be visualized on the plain radiograph of the pelvis, although occasionally it is necessary to get a CT scan (Fig. 8–94). This is done when a fracture is suspected but is not identified on the plain x-ray or when there are multiple fragments around the hip or SI joint. Pelvic fractures may heal

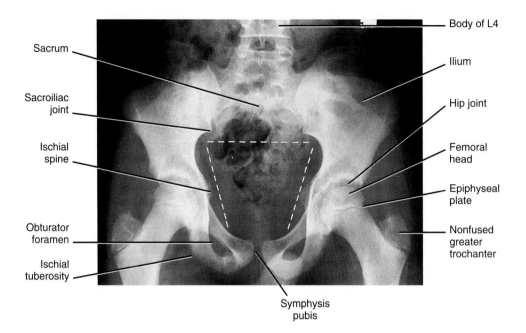

Sacrum

Sacroiliac
joint

Ischial
spine

Obturator
foramen

Ischial
tuberosity

Body of L4

Ilium

Hip joint

Femoral
head

Epiphyseal
plate

Nonfused
greater
trochanter

Symphysis
pubis

FIGURE 8–88. Normal anatomy of the teenage male pelvis. Note the generally triangular (android) shape of the pelvic inlet.

FIGURE 8–89. Normal anatomy of the adult female pelvis. Note the general ovoid (gynecoid) shape of the pelvic inlet.

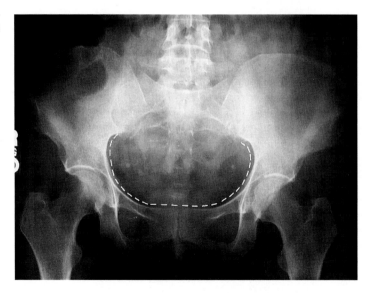

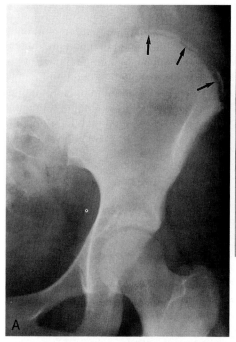

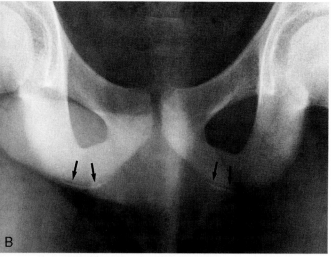

FIGURE 8–90. Normal apophyses. During the mid- and late teen years, an apophysis can be seen over the iliac crest *(A)* and along the inferior aspect of the ischium *(B)*. These should not be mistaken for avulsion fractures.

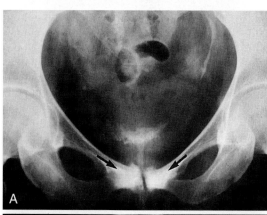

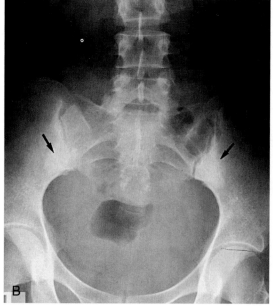

FIGURE 8–91. Benign sclerotic pelvic lesions. *A,* Osteitis condensans pubis. There is sclerosis along both sides of the pubis *(arrows)*. This condition commonly occurs in women and is believed to be the result of childbirth trauma. This film is from a postvoid view of an intravenous pyelogram, accounting for the contrast in the bladder and left ureter. *B,* Osteitis condensans ilii is seen in a different patient as sclerosis lateral to both sacroiliac joints *(arrows)*.

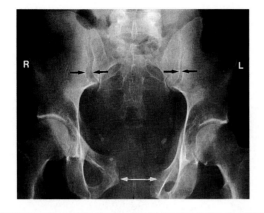

FIGURE 8–92. Pelvic fracture. There is marked diastasis of the pubis *(white arrow)* and widening of both sacroiliac joints, but the right is greater than the left *(black arrows)*. Whenever the pelvic ring is interrupted (as in this case), the fracture is unstable.

without fixation devices, or they may have external pins or plates and screws placed for stabilization.

Benign Lesions

Paget's disease is a common benign lesion of the pelvis. Usually there is involvement of only the right or left half of the pelvis. The iliopectineal line becomes thickened; there is coarsening of trabecular pattern; and the cortex becomes thickened (see Fig. 8–94). If a nuclear medicine bone scan is done, markedly increased blood flow to the bone will result in increased radioactivity in the affected areas. A generalized coarse trabecular pattern and patchy sclerosis of the whole pelvis and other bones can be due to renal failure. A diffuse increase in bone density can occur as a result of myelofibrosis, fluoride poisoning, osteopetrosis ("marble bone" disease) (Fig. 8–95), or diffuse sclerotic metastases.

Malignant Lesions

Focal lesions of the flat bones of the pelvis are often malignant. The differential diagnosis depends to a large extent upon the age of the patient. In a young patient, you may suspect Ewing's sarcoma (Fig. 8–96). Chondrosarcomas tend to arise in the pelvis of adults. On x-ray these tumors often have cauliflower or popcorn calcifications extending from the bone (Fig. 8–97). In older patients, favorite choices for multiple lytic or destructive lesions are metastases from lung, breast, or renal cell carcinoma and multiple myeloma (plasmacytoma). Dense or sclerotic lesions of the pelvis include metastases from prostate carcinoma (Fig. 8–98) and occasionally breast cancer.

HIP

Radiographs of the hip are done in the AP and "frog leg" (abducted) projections. Lateral views

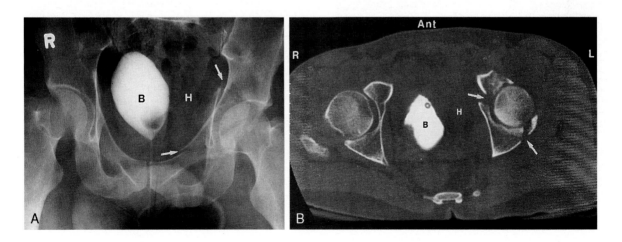

FIGURE 8–93. Fracture of the acetabulum. An AP view of the pelvis *(A)* clearly shows the corners of the fracture *(arrows)* as well as a hematoma displacing the bladder to the right. In order to see the exact nature of the acetabular injury, often a CT scan *(B)* is required; in this case it shows a complex fracture involving both the anterior and the posterior portions of the acetabulum.

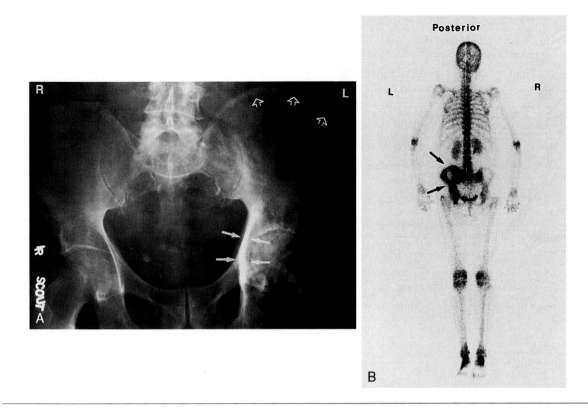

FIGURE 8–94. Paget's disease. *A,* On an AP view of the pelvis, enlargement of the left iliac crest with cortical thickening *(arrowheads)* and sclerosis and thickening of the left iliopectineal line *(arrows)* can be seen. These findings typically affect only one side of the pelvis. A posterior view from a nuclear medicine bone scan *(B)* shows markedly increased activity in the left hemipelvis as a result of the increased blood flow that occurs in this disease.

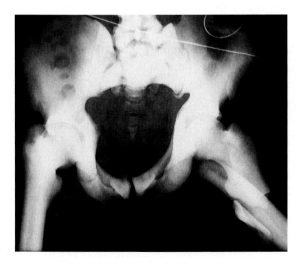

FIGURE 8–95. **Osteopetrosis.** In this disease, which is also called marble bone disease, there is an abnormality in osteoclast function. As a result, the bones become very dense or white, but they are almost chalklike and fracture easily. The patient broke his femur by just falling out of bed. Differential diagnosis of uniformly increased bony density would include fluorosis and myelofibrosis.

FIGURE 8–96. Ewing's tumor. An AP view of the pelvis in this 17-year-old female shows a destructive lesion above the left acetabulum with some surrounding sclerosis *(arrows)*. In a young individual, Ewing's tumor should be considered when there is a tumor in any flat bone, such as pelvis, ribs, scapula, or skull.

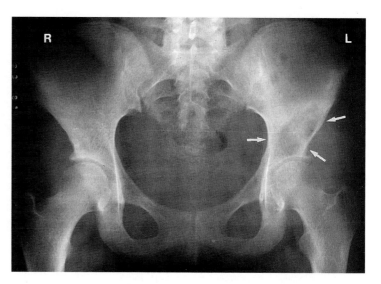

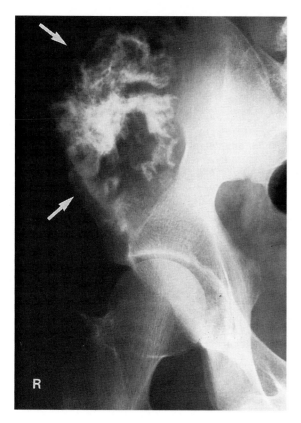

FIGURE 8–97. Chondrosarcoma of the pelvis. Chondrosarcomas may occur within the medullary cavity of the bone or may arise extending out of the bone. In this middle-aged male who noted a painful bulge, there is an extraosseous mass with irregular calcification or chondroid matrix *(arrows)* arising from the right ilium.

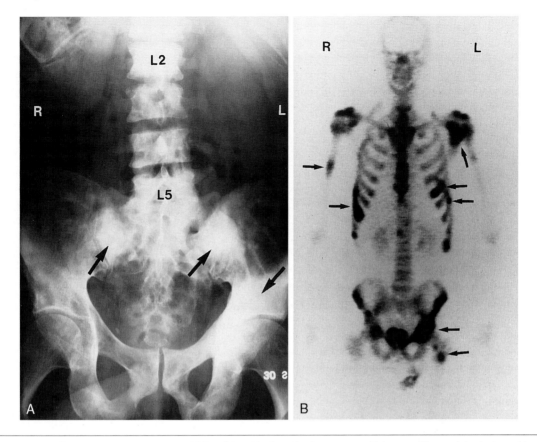

FIGURE 8–98. Metastatic prostate cancer. *A,* An AP view of the pelvis and lumbar spine demonstrates multiple areas of increased density *(arrows)* in a patchy distribution. Vertebrae L2 and L5 are also abnormally white or increased in density. *B,* A nuclear medicine whole-body bone scan most commonly shows the metastatic deposits as areas of increased activity *(arrows).*

usually are difficult to obtain and even more difficult to interpret. You should examine the relationship of the femoral head to the acetabulum, look for cortical discontinuities to suggest fractures, and examine the trabecular pattern to look for potential osseous lesions. In young teenagers, you should notice the apophysis of both the greater and the lesser trochanter. Children under the age of 10 or 12 years will not have fusion of the midportion of the acetabulum (Fig. 8–99).

Trauma

Table 8–4 shows the high-yield areas to examine for lower extremity trauma. Dislocations of the hip are usually the result of motor vehicle accidents. By far the most common dislocation is posteriorly, and on the AP x-ray the head of the femur appears to be superiorly and laterally displaced. When the hip is anteriorly dislocated, the femoral head appears inferior and medial to the acetabulum (Fig. 8–100). With any dislocation, there may be associated fracture fragments from the rim of the acetabulum. As the hip is relocated these small fragments may be caught in the joint space. Sometimes they are difficult to see on a plain x-ray, but if the fragment is in the joint, the distance from the head of the femur to the acetabulum will be widened. CT scanning can be of value in such cases (Fig. 8–101).

Fractures of the hip are most common in the region of the femoral neck and in the intertrochanteric region. Stress fractures of the femoral neck may appear only as an ill-defined sclerotic (white) band extending across the femoral neck. In older persons, a hip fracture may be difficult to see because there is so little calcium in the bone (Fig. 8–102).

A number of orthopedic devices are used to

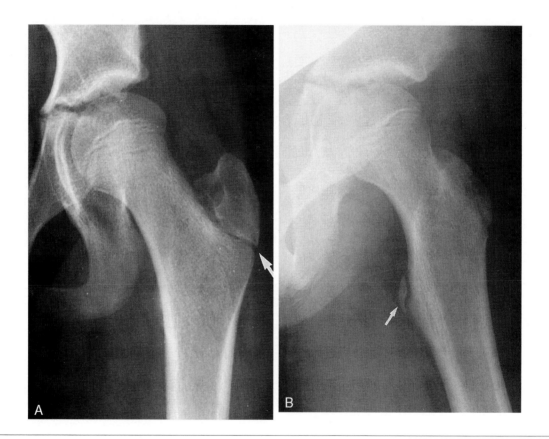

FIGURE 8–99. Normal apophyseal structures in a 10-year-old child. *A,* An AP view of the hip clearly shows the apophysis of the greater trochanter. *B,* An oblique view shows another apophysis of the lesser trochanter. Also notice that at this age, the acetabulum is not completely fused.

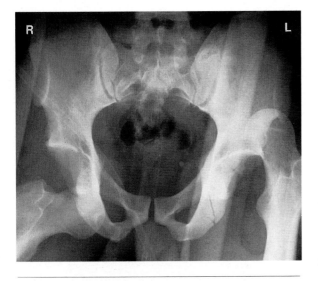

FIGURE 8–100. Hip dislocation. In this patient who was in a motor vehicle accident, there is both an anterior and a posterior dislocation of the hips. Posterior dislocation occurs 90 per cent of the time and is seen here on the left, with the femoral head displaced superior and lateral to the acetabulum. On the right, there is an anterior dislocation, with the femoral head displaced inferiorly and medially.

fix hip fractures. These include plate and screws or multiple pins through the femoral neck. Prosthetic replacement of the femoral head and neck (Fig. 8–103) is often necessary for degenerative changes. The prosthetic devices may or may not utilize cement in the femoral shaft. Depending on the degree of degenerative change in the acetabulum, orthopedic surgeons may also use an

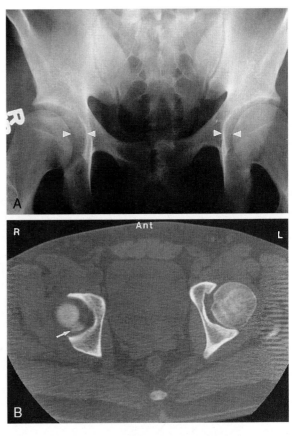

FIGURE 8–101. Fracture fragment after hip dislocation. A, In this patient there had been a posterior right hip dislocation, but after relocation there was pain and limitation of motion. There is asymmetric widening on the right between the femoral head and the acetabulum. No fracture fragment could be seen; however, with a transverse CT scan (B), a bony fracture fragment could be seen in the joint space (arrows).

acetabular component or an articulating (bipolar) section in the prosthetic femoral neck.

Common problems associated with prosthetic hips are loosening, infection, and dislocation. Dislocations are easily visualized on a plain radiograph. Pain may occur with loosening of the prosthesis or infection. If the prosthesis is loose and wiggling, the distal tip will move more than the rest of the shaft. A plain x-ray may show thinning of the bone cortex near the tip of the prosthesis. With loosening, a nuclear medicine bone scan will show increased activity near the distal tip of the prothesis. A nuclear medicine abscess scan can be ordered to exclude infection.

Aseptic necrosis of the hip is most commonly manifested by flattening, irregularity, and sclerosis of the superior aspect of the femoral

---

TABLE 8–4. Examination of an X-ray of the Lower Extremity Done For Trauma

Hip
AP and Frog-leg View
Widening of joint space
Posterior dislocation (femoral head up and out)
Anterior dislocation (femoral head in and down)
Fractures—femoral neck or intertrochanteric
Pelvic or acetabular fracture

Knee
AP View
Tibial plateau fracture
Tibial spine fracture
Patellar fracture
Lateral View
Joint effusion
Fat-fluid level
Patellar fracture

Ankle
AP View
Medial and lateral malleolus for fracture
Ankle mortise and joint space for asymmetric widening
Lateral View
Posterior malleolar fracture
Distal fibular fracture
Bulging of fat planes about joint (effusion)
Talar neck for fracture
Calcaneus
Base of fifth metatarsal fracture

FIGURE 8–102. Intertrochanteric fracture of the hip. With extracapsular hip fractures, an intertrochanteric fracture *(arrows)* occurs 70 per cent of the time, whereas a subtrochanteric fracture occurs 30 per cent of the time. Intracapsular fractures most commonly affect the femoral neck.

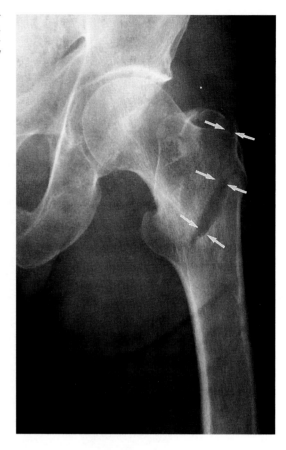

head. It can have a number of causes, and a mnemonic is ASEPTIC. This refers to *a*nemia (sickle cell), *s*teroids, *e*thanol, *p*ancreatitis, *t*rauma, *i*diopathic, and *C*aisson's disease (Fig. 8–104). The most sensitive imaging study for early aseptic necrosis is MRI. If this is not available, a nuclear medicine bone scan can be used. Late changes of aseptic necrosis with femoral head deformity can easily be seen on plain x-rays.

FEMUR

Normal Anatomy

The normal osseous anatomy of the femur is quite obvious and does not need to be discussed here. The normal x-ray projections are AP and lateral. Fractures of the femur also are very obvious. As expected, they may be transverse, spiral, or comminuted, with various degrees of angulation and overriding of the fragments.

Benign Lesions

It is important to be able to assess bone lesions and the likelihood of their being benign or malignant. Signs that a bone lesion may be benign are as follows: (1) It is small; (2) it does not have associated reaction of the periosteum; (3) it has a narrow zone of transition between the normal bone and the lesion; and (4) it has a thin, well-defined sclerotic (white) margin.

The bones of the leg are favored places for a benign fibrous cortical defect. These are usually located near but not at the ends of the bones and are usually well marginated. As the name suggests, they are present predominantly in the cortex of the bone rather than having their epicenter in the marrow space (Fig. 8–105). There is another lesion, called a nonossifying fibroma,

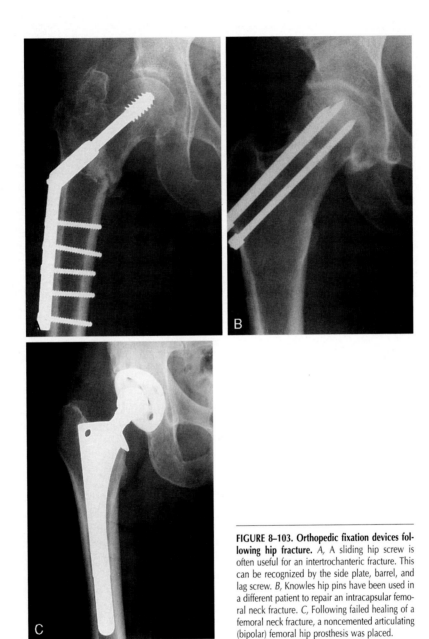

FIGURE 8–103. Orthopedic fixation devices following hip fracture. *A,* A sliding hip screw is often useful for an intertrochanteric fracture. This can be recognized by the side plate, barrel, and lag screw. *B,* Knowles hip pins have been used in a different patient to repair an intracapsular femoral neck fracture. *C,* Following failed healing of a femoral neck fracture, a noncemented articulating (bipolar) femoral hip prosthesis was placed.

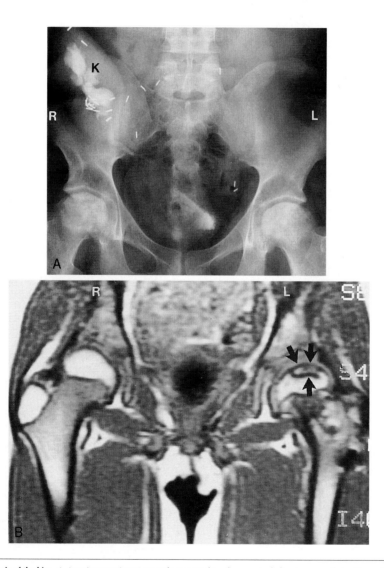

FIGURE 8–104. Aseptic necrosis of the hips. *A,* Aseptic necrosis can occur from a number of causes, including trauma and steroid use. In this patient, an AP view of the pelvis shows a transplanted kidney (K) in the right iliac fossa. Use of steroids has caused this patient to have bilateral aseptic necrosis. The femoral heads are somewhat flattened, irregular, and increased in density. *B,* Aseptic necrosis in a different patient is demonstrated on an MRI scan as an area of decreased signal in the left femoral head. This is the most sensitive method for detection of early aseptic necrosis.

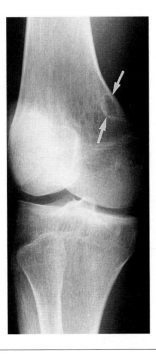

FIGURE 8–105. Fibrous cortical defect. This is probably the same lesion as a nonossifying fibroma. These are most commonly seen in the lower extremity of teenagers, particularly the femur and tibia. Here, the lesion is lucent and seen to have a sclerotic or dense margin. These lesions will fill in and become dense with time and they are clinically insignificant.

with the same characteristics, but it is bigger. Whether these lesions are truly different or simply a spectrum of the same lesion is unknown.

Fibrous dysplasia usually is a lytic lesion that looks like a hole in the bone. Fibrous dysplasia may present as a single lesion (monostotic) (Fig. 8–106), or it may be in multiple areas throughout the skeleton (polyostotic). It is centered in the marrow cavity and can be single or lobular. Lytic fibrous dysplasia thins the cortex on the inner margins. Most fibrous dysplasia lesions are found in children or young adults. In addition to the lucent, sort of cystic, variety, there can be a form in which the bone is diffusely involved and softened. When this happens in the femur, there is deformity with lateral bowing. This is referred to as a shepherd's crook deformity.

Amorphous or scattered calcifications projecting within the marrow space are usually the result of benign lesions, such as enchondroma (Fig. 8–107) or bone infarcts (Fig. 8–108). Bone infarcts are relatively common in patients with

sickle cell disease and also can be a result of decompression sickness from diving.

Malignant Lesions

A lytic (destructive) lesion that does not have a sclerotic margin in an adult should be regarded as a malignancy until proven otherwise. Breast cancer, lung cancer, and a host of other neoplasms commonly produce lytic lesions of bone. There are also a number of primary bone lesions that can produce this appearance, including plasmacytoma and eosinophilic granuloma.

Chondrosarcomas tend to occur in the femur, pelvis, and ribs. In the femur they are most common in the metaphysis. They can be very

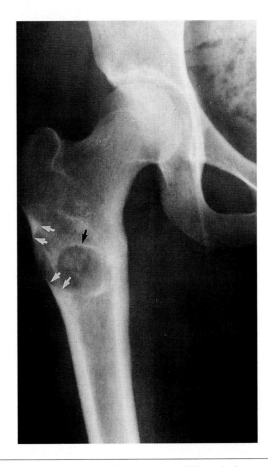

FIGURE 8–106. Fibrous dysplasia. Bone lesions of fibrous dysplasia can be single (monostotic) or multifocal (polyostotic) and represent a benign developmental anomaly with fibrous tissue in the medullary space. Typically, the lesions have a very narrow zone of transition between the lesion and normal bone (*black arrow*), and the lesion may scallop or thin the normal cortex from the inner side (*white arrows*). The bone also may be slightly expanded.

FIGURE 8–107. Enchondroma. This lateral view of the knee shows a dense lesion that is somewhat amorphous and projects within the medullary space of the bone. A well-defined lesion such as this is most likely an enchondroma, although a low-grade intramedullary chondrosarcoma also must be considered.

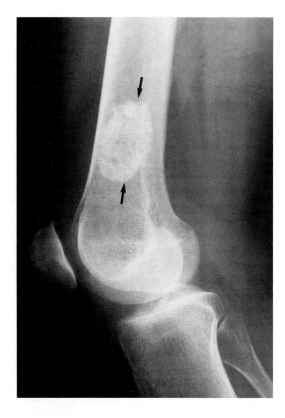

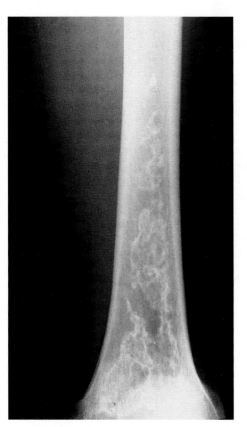

FIGURE 8–108. Bone infarcts. Diffuse and amorphous calcification within the medullary space is seen here in the distal femur. Bone infarcts such as this can occur in patients with sickle cell disease or as a result of decompression sickness following underwater diving accidents.

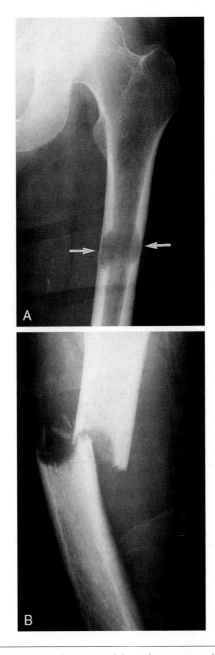

FIGURE 8–109. Lytic bone metastases. *A,* A view of the femur in this patient with known lung carcinoma shows a destructive lesion expanding from the marrow space and thinning the cortex *(arrows).* This lesion has no clear margin or white rim to distinguish it from normal bone. Lesions such as this in weight-bearing bones are important to find so that therapy can be undertaken to prevent pathologic fracture. *B,* A view of the femur in the same patient who returned 2 weeks later with a pathologic fracture.

variable in appearance from purely destructive, destructive with a chondroid (irregular calcification) matrix, to exostotic, or projecting from the cortex of a bone. The mean age for occurrence is 40 to 45 years.

Even if a patient has known metastatic disease elsewhere, it is important to identify metastatic sites in the pelvis and lower extremities. This is because these sites are weight bearing and are susceptible to pathologic fractures that can disable the patient (Fig. 8–109). Early detection can allow placement of a medullary rod or radiation therapy, which will allow a terminal patient to ambulate rather than being bedridden for the remaining months of life.

Periosteal Reaction

Periosteal reaction can be due to either benign or malignant lesions. Obviously, local periosteal reaction will be seen about a healing fracture. However, this is normally quite obvious and does not cause any confusion in interpretation.

Generalized periosteal reaction can occur along the long bones of the extremities in patients with lung cancer. This condition is known as hypertrophic pulmonary osteoarthropathy (HPO). The reason for the periosteal reaction is unclear.

Infections can also cause periosteal reaction. Osteomyelitis that has been present for several weeks can cause minimal periosteal reaction, and chronic osteomyelitis that has been present for months and years can cause a florid calcified periosteal reaction (Fig. 8–110).

In young patients (age 5 to 20 years), periosteal reaction in the midportion (diaphysis) of a long bone should raise the suspicion of a Ewing tumor; if located around the joint such as the knee, it should raise the suspicion of an osteogenic sarcoma (Fig. 8–111). Sunburst (radiating) type periosteal reaction is particularly worrisome for malignancy.

Myositis Ossificans

Calcification can occur in soft tissues. The muscles of the thigh are particularly prone to

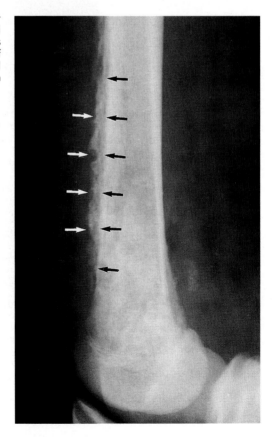

FIGURE 8–110. Chronic osteomyelitis. A lateral view of the knee shows florid periosteal reaction (arrows). The periosteal reaction that is dense and extends over a long area suggests chronic osteomyelitis. The bone of the distal femur has a mottled appearance as a result of the infection. Note also that the distal femoral epiphysis is not fused; given the periosteal reaction, the location in the distal femur, and the patient's age, you must also consider an osteogenic sarcoma.

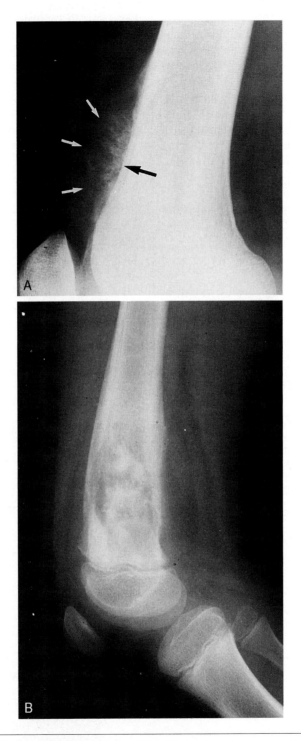

FIGURE 8–111. Osteogenic sarcoma of the knee. A lateral view of the knee *(A)* in a 19-year-old male shows a sunburst type periosteal reaction *(arrows)*. Knowing that the distal femur is the most common site of osteogenic sarcoma, that periosteal reaction is a feature, and that this patient is a teenager should make osteogenic sarcoma very high on your differential diagnostic list. Another common presentation *(B)* is a predominantly destructive central lesion seen here in the distal femur of an 8-year-old girl.

trauma, and bleeding within the soft tissue can subsequently calcify. This condition is referred to as myositis ossificans (Fig. 8–112) and may require surgery after the calcification has matured.

KNEE

Normal Anatomy

The normal x-ray projections that are obtained of the knee are AP and lateral views (Fig. 8–113). The lateral view is taken with the knee partially flexed. The AP view is important for assessing whether there is joint space narrowing. This is also the view that will show whether there is calcification of the cartilage in the joint space. Sometimes the tibial plateaus are at slightly different angulations so that the x-ray beam does not go horizontally through both medial and lateral compartments.

The lateral view is utilized to evaluate the patella and to determine whether a joint effusion is present. Both views are used to assess degenerative changes, fractures, and the general matrix of the bone of the distal femur, proximal tibia, and proximal fibula. Both views are also

needed to see whether there is a bony fragment within the joint space. This is necessary because in order to be sure that the fragment or loose body is within the joint space, it needs to be triangulated utilizing both projections.

There are two special views of the knee that are commonly requested. The first of these is the "sunrise" view. This is a tangential view of the anterior portion of the flexed knee, looking from the top down. The advantage of this view is that the relationship of the patella to the anterior femur is clearly shown. Another view that is available is the "tunnel" view. In this, the knee is flexed more than on the routine lateral view, and the x-ray beam is directed horizontally across the tibial plateau through the "tunnel" created by the femoral condyles. This affords a very good look at the anterior and posterior tibial spines as well as the femoral condyles.

In children, the epiphyseal plate of the distal femoral epiphysis and the proximal tibial epiphysis is well seen until at least 10 years of age. Complete fusion typically occurs in girls at about the age of 15 and in boys, several years later (Fig. 8–114). In teenagers, it is important to note on the lateral view that the anterior portion of the proximal tibial epiphysis folds down to form the attachment for the inferior

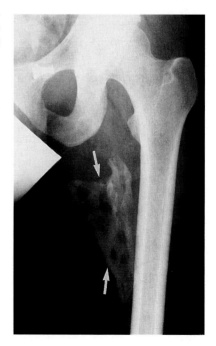

FIGURE 8–112. Myositis ossificans. The soft tissues of the thigh are a common location for blunt traumatic injury. In this case, dystrophic calcification has developed within the soft tissue *(arrows)*, significantly limiting the range of motion of this young soccer player.

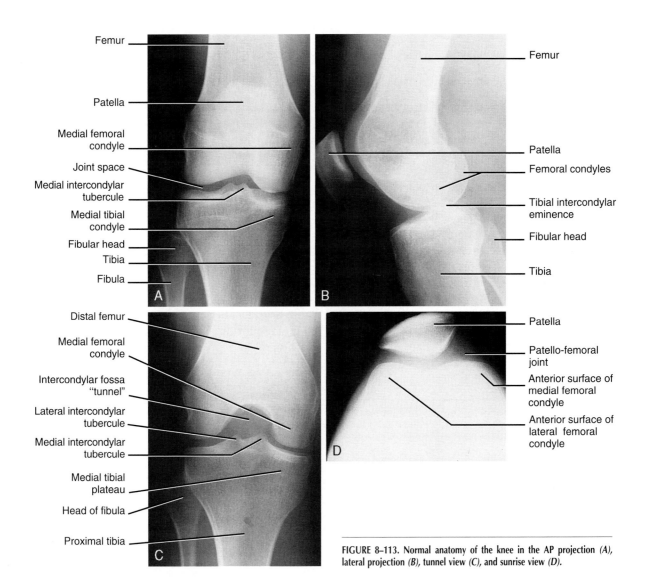

Femur

Patella

Medial femoral condyle

Joint space

Medial intercondylar tubercule

Medial tibial condyle

Fibular head

Tibia

Fibula

A

Femur

Patella

Femoral condyles

Tibial intercondylar eminence

Fibular head

Tibia

B

Distal femur

Medial femoral condyle

Intercondylar fossa "tunnel"

Lateral intercondylar tubercule

Medial intercondylar tubercule

Medial tibial plateau

Head of fibula

Proximal tibia

C

Patella

Patello-femoral joint

Anterior surface of medial femoral condyle

Anterior surface of lateral femoral condyle

D

FIGURE 8–113. Normal anatomy of the knee in the AP projection *(A)*, lateral projection *(B)*, tunnel view *(C)*, and sunrise view *(D)*.

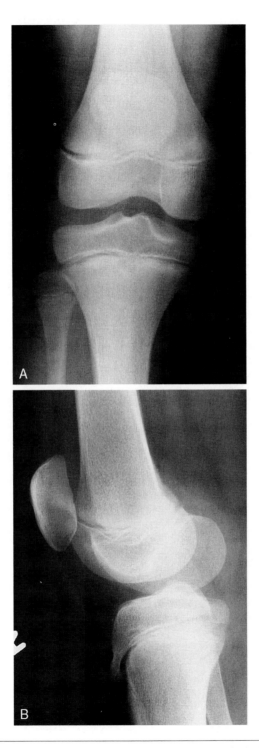

FIGURE 8–114. Normal knee in an 11-year-old child. *A,* An AP view clearly demonstrates the epiphyses of the distal femur, proximal tibia, and fibula. *B,* A lateral view shows the normal downward projection of the proximal tibial epiphysis along the anterior portion of the tibia to form the tibial tubercle.

aspect of the patellar tendon. It almost looks like a horn projecting downward from the anterior portion of the proximal tibia, and this is normal. A fairly common normal variant is the fabella. This is a small sesamoid bone in the tendons posterior to the knee joint. It is easily seen on the lateral view (Fig. 8–115).

With MRI, the soft tissues, including the tendons, ligaments, and cartilage of the knee, can be exquisitely visualized (Fig. 8–116). Structures of particular interest on these images are those that are commonly involved in trauma, such as the cruciate ligaments and the medial and lateral meniscus.

Trauma

The most common reasons for ordering knee x-rays involve trauma or degenerative change. In children, there may be questions about tumor and infection, which is dealt with later in the pediatric bone section of this chapter.

A knee joint effusion is easiest to identify superior to the patella and anterior to the distal femur. You should look for this on the lateral view (Fig. 8–117). The effusion is basically water or blood, which has the same density as muscle, and it is visualized only because there is anterior displacement of the normal fat line. It is not appropriate to order a knee x-ray to exclude or identify an effusion, since this is much better done by clinical examination. Knee effusions are usually identified as an incidental finding in patients who have had trauma and for whom the x-ray was ordered because a fracture was suspected.

The two most common soft tissue injuries of the knee involve the cruciate ligaments and the menisci. As mentioned earlier, the imaging study of choice for these is MRI, with which the cruciate ligaments can be well seen, and tears or partial tears of these ligaments can be easily identified (Fig. 8–118). Repair of cruciate ligaments often involves transplantation of a tendon and insertion of a bone plug. The x-rays that are obtained in follow-up of these patients demonstrate several screws in the femoral intracondylar notch and proximal tibia.

Normal cartilage looks quite black on MRI, and it typically is triangular. When there are tears within the cartilage, an area of increased signal (white) can be seen (Fig. 8–119). Not all areas of increased signal represent a tear, and there are a number of subtle criteria that are utilized by radiologists to differentiate between degenerative change and a tear.

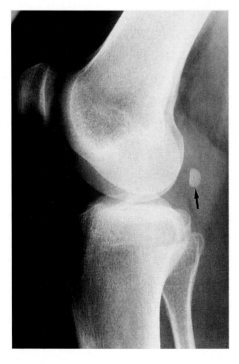

FIGURE 8–115. Fabella. On the lateral view of the knee, a small oval bone can be seen posterior to the knee joint *(arrow)*. This essentially is a sesamoid bone and is a normal variant of no clinical significance.

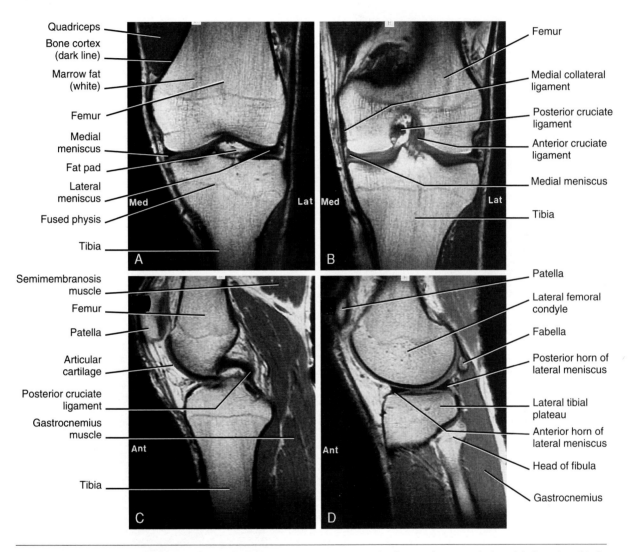

FIGURE 8–116. Normal anatomy of the knee on a magnetic resonance scan. Images are presented in the coronal view near the front of the knee *(A)*, and in the midportion of the knee *(B)*. Additional sagittal or lateral MR views are identified through the middle of the knee *(C)* and in the lateral compartment *(D)*.

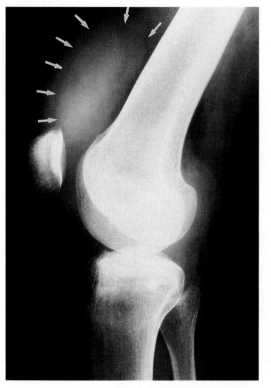

FIGURE 8–117. Large knee effusion. Knee effusions are best detected on the lateral view by looking above the patella and seeing anterior displacement of the dark fat line by soft tissue or water density *(arrows)*. Knee effusions are even more easily and accurately detected by clinical examination.

FIGURE 8–118. Posterior cruciate ligament tear. A lateral or sagittal view of the knee on MRI scan demonstrates disruption *(arrow)* of the normal dark posterior cruciate ligament.

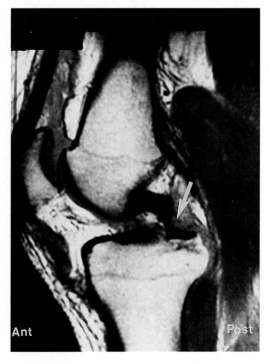

FIGURE 8–119. Tear in the posterior horn of the lateral meniscus. A sagittal view of the lateral knee on an MR scan shows increased signal *(arrows)* extending to the edges of the normally black or dark meniscus.

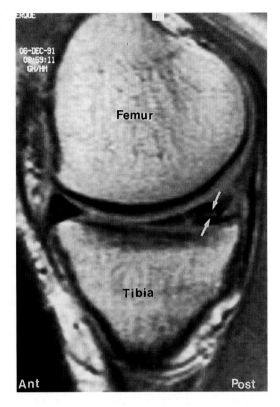

Patellar fractures are usually caused by a direct blow to the patella during a fall. The fractures are seen as dark lines across the bone, with sharp corners and edges. Repair of these fractures is done by utilizing fixation pins and wire (Fig. 8–120). A normal variant that is often confused with a patellar fracture is the bipartite patella. It is an abnormality in growth and results in a rounded or oval bony fragment in the upper and outer portion of the patella (Fig. 8–121). It usually is not a problem to differentiate from a fracture because of its location (upper outer portion) and its rounded and well-marginated edges.

Tibial plateau fractures are best visualized on the anterior view. They are reasonably common, and you should look for a vertical lucent line located slightly lateral to the center of the tibial spines. Sometimes, if the fracture is oblique to the x-ray beam, it can be difficult to see, but you may notice depression of one of the tibial plateaus, and you may see a step-off as you trace the tibial cortex along the joint surface. With tibial plateau fractures, there is often a collection of fluid above the patella. Remem-

ber that because lateral knee x-rays for trauma are done with the patient lying down, you can often see a horizontal "fat-fluid" level above the patella (Fig. 8–122). This probably does not represent fat from the marrow space coming from the site of the fracture, but rather represents layering of the various components of blood into cells and serum in a hemorrhagic effusion. Since tibial plateau fractures can sometimes be difficult to see, if you see a "fat-fluid" level on the lateral knee x-ray, you should look very hard to find a tibial plateau fracture.

Degenerative Changes

Degenerative changes of the knee are manifested by joint space narrowing and sclerosis of the nearby cortex. It is actually quite common to have only the medial or lateral compartment involved while the other compartment appears quite normal (Fig. 8–123). Other signs of degenerative change are small overhanging spurs at the edges of the joints. Occasionally, degenerative changes of the joint can involve disruption

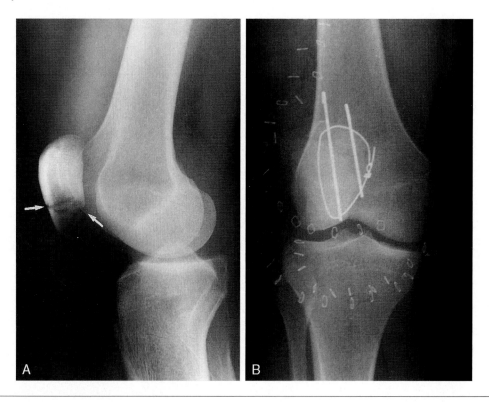

FIGURE 8–120. Patellar fracture. A lateral view *(A)* of the knee shows lucent or dark lines with sharp corners along the inferior portion of the patella *(arrows)*. An AP view *(B)* post surgery shows fixation pins and a tension wire in the patella. Multiple skin staples are also seen overlying the soft tissues.

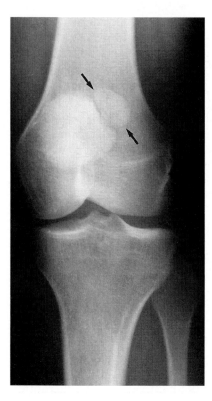

FIGURE 8–121. Bipartite patella. On this AP view of the knee, a fragment can be seen in the upper outer portion of the patella *(arrows)*. Note that this is rounded and that the location in the upper outer portion of the patella indicates that this is a normal variant of no clinical significance; it should not be mistaken for a patellar fracture.

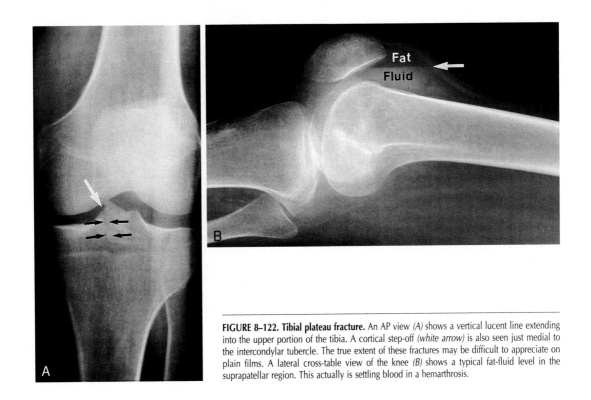

FIGURE 8–122. Tibial plateau fracture. An AP view *(A)* shows a vertical lucent line extending into the upper portion of the tibia. A cortical step-off *(white arrow)* is also seen just medial to the intercondylar tubercle. The true extent of these fractures may be difficult to appreciate on plain films. A lateral cross-table view of the knee *(B)* shows a typical fat-fluid level in the suprapatellar region. This actually is settling blood in a hemarthrosis.

FIGURE 8–123. Degenerative osteoarthritis. In this standing view of both knees, there is significant narrowing and sclerosis of the medial compartment of the left knee and of the lateral compartment of the right knee.

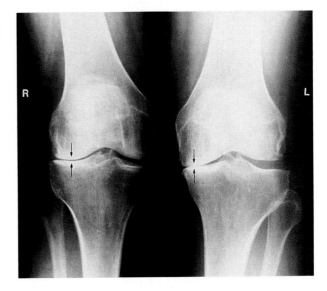

of pieces of cartilage that come loose and are a nidus of calcification. These calcifications are often within the joint space and can be single or multiple (Fig. 8–124). If they are single, they are called a "loose body." If they are multiple and extensive, the condition is termed synovial chondromatosis.

Arthritis

A number of arthritides can affect the major joints. Rheumatoid arthritis is a major player and can cause synovial destruction with joint space narrowing. One of the tip-offs to rheumatoid arthritis is the presence of subchondral cysts just under the bony cortex on both sides of the joint space (Fig. 8–125).

Sometimes, calcification can be seen within the articular cartilage of the knee. This finding is called chondrocalcinosis (Fig. 8–126); it is usually easy to distinguish from loose bodies

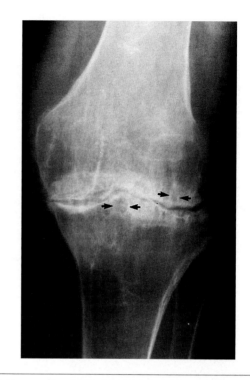

FIGURE 8–125. Rheumatoid arthritis of the knee. There is diffuse joint space narrowing with subchondral cyst formation *(arrows)*. A distinguishing feature between this and degenerative arthritis is that in rheumatoid arthritis, degenerative osteophytes or spurs are not usually seen.

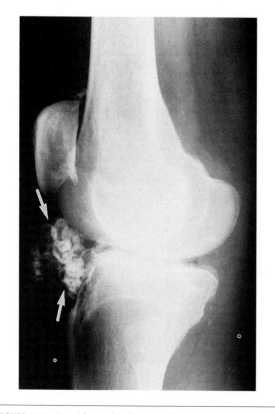

FIGURE 8–124. Synovial osteochondromatosis. These are small calcified loose bodies within the joint space *(arrows)*. This is sometimes referred to as "housemaid's knee" or "nun's knee."

within the joint space, since it is calcification that is in a horizontal linear fashion. Chondrocalcinosis may be due to degenerative change, hypercalcemic states, and pseudogout as well as some other less common entities.

When degenerative changes of the knee are extensive enough, a prosthetic knee replacement may be required (Fig. 8–127). A number of prostheses are available, but, in general, they have a femoral condylar component as well as a proximal tibial and patellar component. Sometimes the patellar component is not installed. On the AP view, these prostheses may look like they are not touching each other when, in fact, they are in contact. This is because of a plastic surface that is not visible on the x-ray. Abnormalities to look for with a prosthesis involve infection and loosening. Both are seen as a lucent line or rarefaction of bone around the screws or the base of the implant.

Tumors

There is a benign tumor, called a giant cell tumor, that commonly occurs around the knee,

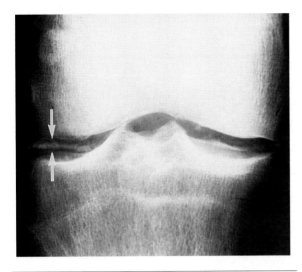

FIGURE 8–126. Chondrocalcinosis. Calcification of the cartilage in this knee is seen particularly well in the lateral compartment *(arrows)*. This is due to calcium pyrophosphate deposition disease (CPPD). Calcification is not seen in all patients with CPPD, and not all patients with chondrocalcinosis have CPPD.

particularly in the proximal tibia. It is a lytic lesion that is often quite large and characteristically occurs between the ages of 20 and 35 years. The tumor appears to arise from the old epiphyseal plate and to extend in both directions. It is not seen before epiphyseal closure, and when it is present, it typically crosses the fused epiphyseal plate (Fig. 8–128). Usually it is not confused with a malignant lesion, since it typically occurs during the late teens or in young adults. This is beyond the age for most osteogenic sarcomas and before the age for most metastatic lesions. In addition, its single focus and location peripherally in an extremity would be very unusual features of a metastatic lesion.

Osteogenic sarcoma is discussed later in the pediatric section of this chapter. A few unusual forms of osteogenic sarcoma do occur at older ages. Parosteal osteosarcomas, which constitute about 4 per cent of all osteosarcomas, are broadly based, typically in the posterior aspect of the femoral shaft. They occur in persons of about 40 years of age. Periosteal osteosarcomas are about half as common, have a saucer-shaped depression of the cortex, and occur at 10 to 20 years of age. You should remember that osteosarcomas in older adults can be produced by malignant degeneration of Paget's disease and may occur at any age as a consequence of radiation therapy.

TIBIA AND FIBULA

Normal Anatomy

Typical plain x-ray views include AP and lateral projections. You should be sure that the x-ray includes the entire length from the tibial plateau to the ankle joint. The anatomy is fairly obvious.

Trauma

There are a few points about tibial fractures that need to be discussed. Spiral fractures usually involve the distal tibia and often occur as the result of boot-top ski injuries. When a spiral tibial fracture is present, you should look very carefully to see if there is overriding of the fragments (Fig. 8–129). Many times, only an ankle x-ray has been ordered, and the tibial fracture is clearly identified. What you should notice is that it is not possible to shorten the tibia without associated trauma of the fibula, since the two bones are essentially hooked together at both ends. If you see only a tibial fracture, you should order a complete view of the tibia and fibula, and often you will find an associated fracture of the proximal portion of the fibula. Typical orthopedic hardware used in the fixation of fractures of the mid- or distal tibia includes intramedullary rods (Fig. 8–130). These rods also can be utilized for fractures in the midportion of the femur. Occasionally, fractures of long bones do not heal because fibrous tissue grows in between the ends of the bone. This is called a nonunion. Radiographically, this can be identified by the presence of a lucent line that is persistent and extends across the fracture site several months after the fracture occurred (Fig. 8–131).

Tumors

There are some benign bone tumors that occur in long bones, particularly in the lower extremity. The first of these is simply an outgrowth of bone and is called an osteochondroma. The cortex of the bone typically sticks out on a stalk and has a bulbous or mushroom-shaped cap on it. The cap is covered with cartilage. This growth almost invariably arises near a joint,

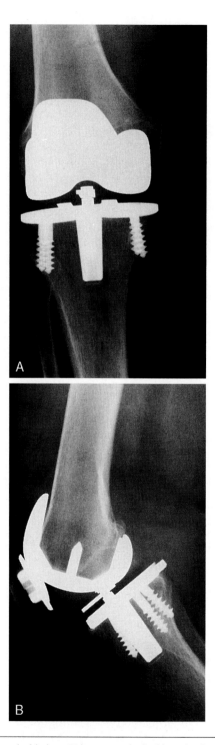

FIGURE 8–127. Total knee replacement. An AP radiograph of the knee *(A)* demonstrates the distal femoral and proximal tibial portions of a semiconstrained prosthesis. The two pieces do not appear to sit directly upon each other, because there is a plastic or Teflon spacer in between that is not seen on x-ray. The lateral view *(B)* demonstrates that this is a tricompartment replacement with a prosthetic posterior patellar portion as well.

FIGURE 8–128. Giant cell tumor. An AP view of the knee in this 25-year-old male demonstrates a destructive lesion that is centered at the fused epiphyseal plate and has extended into the metaphysis and the epiphysis. These lesions most commonly occur in the tibia or femur. The lesion is often expansile and can be locally aggressive. About one third of these patients will have a pathologic fracture.

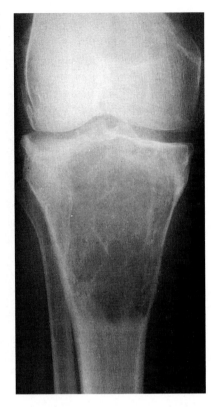

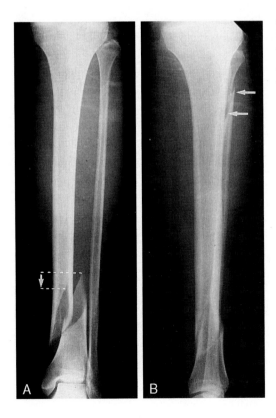

FIGURE 8–129. Spiral fracture of the distal tibia. An AP view of the tibia *(A)* in a skier shows a spiral fracture, but note that there has been override of the fragments, causing shortening *(arrow)*. This cannot possibly happen if the fibula is entirely intact. A lateral view *(B)* shows that there is an accompanying fracture of the proximal fibula with override as well. This fibular fracture would have been missed if only ankle views had been ordered and the significance of the override had not been appreciated.

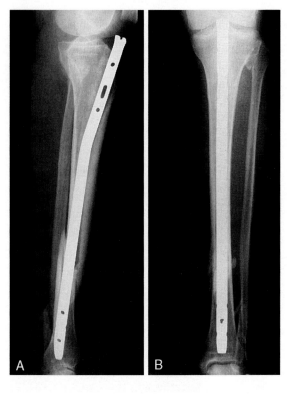

FIGURE 8–130. Intramedullary fixation of a tibial fracture. *A,* A lateral view of the tibia demonstrates an intramedullary rod that has been placed down through the anterior and proximal portion of the tibia. The holes at the top and bottom of the rod provide a place for cross-linking screws. A rod (as opposed to a plate and screws) is necessary because this is a weight-bearing bone with a lot of stress on it.

FIGURE 8–131. Nonunion of a tibial fracture. This AP view of the distal tibia and fibula obtained 3 months after the fracture occurred shows that there is no significant periosteal reaction bridging the fractures. In fact, there remains a dark lucent line across the original fracture site as a result of fibrous tissue having grown in and preventing healing.

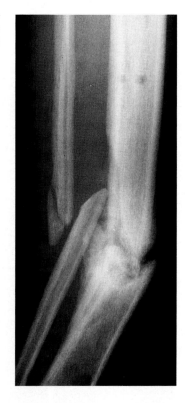

with the stalk always pointing away from the joint (Fig. 8–132). These lesions are usually asymptomatic unless they stick out far enough to be traumatized easily. If there is enlargement of such a lesion or associated pain without previous trauma, malignant transformation should be suspected. There is a form of hereditary multiple exostoses. The number of exostoses in a person with this condition may vary from a few to hundreds, but they are usually bilaterally symmetric.

An osteoid osteoma usually occurs along the cortex of a bone. It has a central area of lucency with a little sclerotic (white) nidus within it (Fig. 8–133). About 75 per cent of cases occur in persons between the ages of 11 and 26 years. This lesion incites a large amount of reaction, causing dense surrounding bone and sometimes local periosteal reaction. It is typically painful, and the pain is relieved by aspirin. On a nuclear medicine bone scan, these lesions are intensely hot. If all you see is an area of dense sclerosis near the cortex of a bone and you are unable to visualize a nidus or central lucent area, sometimes a CT scan can demonstrate the nidus.

With the exception of metastatic disease, most bone tumors are quite obvious and quite rare. Since the differential diagnosis depends upon the age, location, radiographic characteristics, and clinical history, you should always seek consultation with a radiologist before assuming that the lesion you are looking at is benign.

ANKLE

Normal Anatomy

Normal x-ray projections of the ankle are AP, lateral, and oblique. Although oblique views of most bones and joints are not normally obtained, this is important in the traumatized ankle since a number of oblique fractures that occur in the ankle are not easily seen on the AP or lateral view. The oblique view also allows a better look at the ankle mortise (Figs. 8–134 and 8–135).

There is an interesting phenomenon that occurs often on ankle x-rays, but also can occur on any x-ray where the dense cortex of bones

FIGURE 8–132. **Osteochondroma.** On this lateral view of the ankle, a benign osteochondroma is seen projecting posteriorly on a stalk. The end *(arrows)* is often covered with a cartilaginous cap. These lesions always occur near a joint but point away from it.

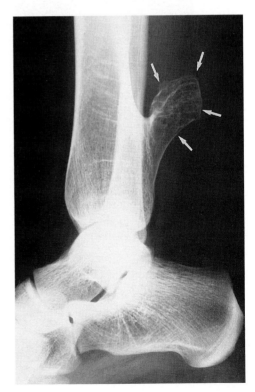

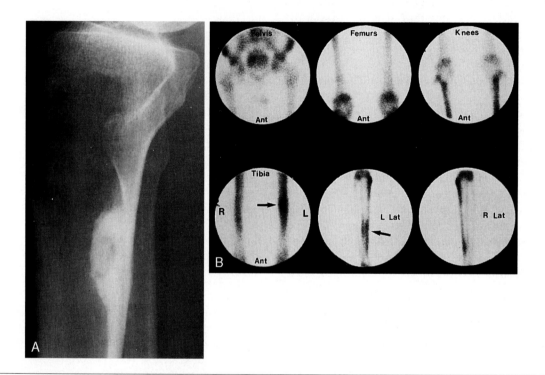

FIGURE 8–133. Osteoid osteoma. A lateral view *(A)* of the proximal tibia shows a very dense lesion in the posterior cortex. There is a darker central area that contains a white nidus. This lesion in a 20-year-old male caused pain in this area that was relieved by aspirin. Fifty-five per cent of these lesions occur in the femur and tibia. *B,* A nuclear medicine bone scan in a different patient with an osteoid osteoma in the left lower tibia shows increased activity *(arrows)* at the site of the lesion.

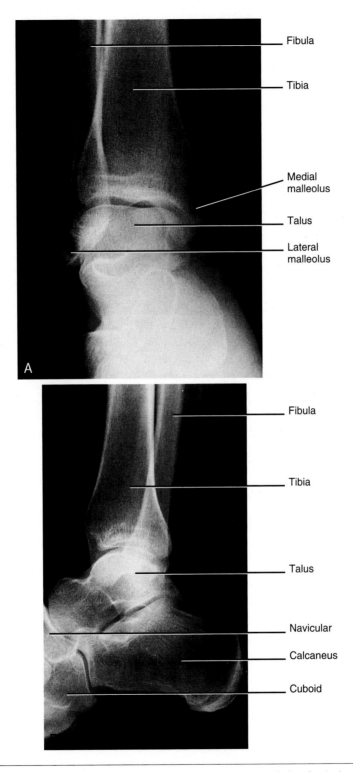

FIGURE 8–134. Normal anatomy of the ankle in the AP projection *(A)* and in the lateral projection *(B)*.

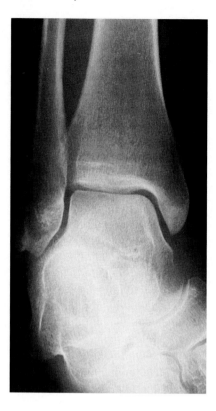

FIGURE 8–135. Oblique view of the ankle. This projection is the best one to show the ankle mortise and the relationship of the talus to the medial and lateral malleolus.

overlap. Where the cortices of two bones cross, occasionally there will be a dark or lucent line along the anterior edge of one cortex, and this dark line looks as though it is actually extending through the cortex of the other bone. This is an artifact called the "Mach effect." The point is that if you see a lucent line through the cortex of a bone, you should make sure that there is not another overlapping bone at this exact point causing a pseudofracture artifact (Fig. 8–136A). Sometimes a lucent line can be seen extending through the cortex of a bone as a result of a blood vessel passing through a nutrient canal (Fig. 8–136B) and these should not be mistaken for a fracture.

The ankle of a child demonstrates an epiphysis in the distal tibia and fibula. In children between the ages of 7 and 12 years, you will also see a calcaneal apophysis on the lateral view. This is seen as a crescentic density over the posterior aspect of the heel, and it should not be mistaken for a fracture (Fig. 8–137).

Trauma

The vast majority of ankle x-rays are obtained to evaluate the effects of trauma. On the lateral view of the ankle, you should look for an anterior thin dark fat line right in front of the joint space. If it is displaced or bowed forward, there is an effusion, hemorrhage, or infection in the ankle joint (Fig. 8–138).

The most common fractures of the ankle involve either the medial or the lateral malleolus. Less commonly, there are fractures of the medial and lateral malleolus (bimalleolar fracture; Fig. 8–139A). With very severe trauma, there will be fractures not only of both medial and lateral malleoli but also of the posterior aspect of the tibia (trimalleolar fracture). Whenever the posterior malleolus is fractured, there almost always is an associated medial or lateral malleolar fracture. The extreme force and disruption necessary to cause a trimalleolar fracture disrupts ligaments as well, often causing subluxation of the distal tibia relative to the talus (Fig. 8–139B).

Malleolar fractures can be treated in a number of ways, including screws and pins (particularly in the medial malleolus) and sometimes plates and screws. Occasionally, in the case of a compound fracture, antibiotic beads will be placed in the wound. These can be visualized

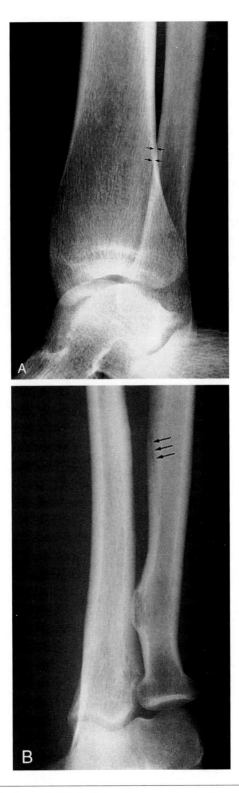

FIGURE 8–136. Pseudofractures. *A,* A Mach effect is an optical illusion that can be seen anywhere two bones cross each other. On this lateral view of the ankle where the cortex of the fibula and tibia project crossing each other, there is a dark line formed *(arrows)* that is an artifact and can be mistaken for a fracture of the posterior tibial cortex. *B,* A nutrient canal is seen in the radius as a dark oblique line *(arrows)* extending through one side of the bony cortex.

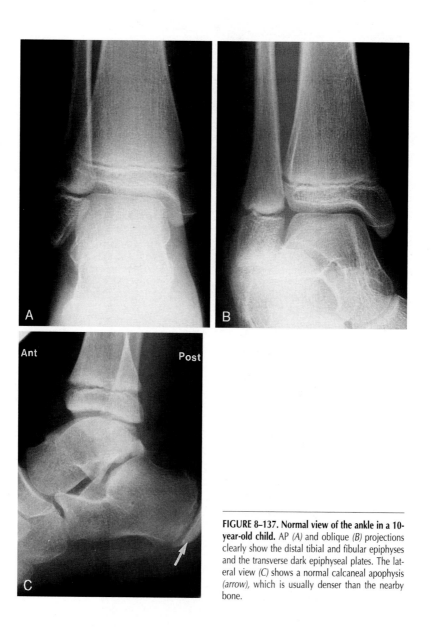

FIGURE 8–137. Normal view of the ankle in a 10-year-old child. AP *(A)* and oblique *(B)* projections clearly show the distal tibial and fibular epiphyses and the transverse dark epiphyseal plates. The lateral view *(C)* shows a normal calcaneal apophysis *(arrow)*, which is usually denser than the nearby bone.

FIGURE 8–138. Ankle effusion. An ankle effusion is best seen on the lateral view. The dark fat stripe *(arrows)* is displaced and bowed anteriorly by fluid within the joint.

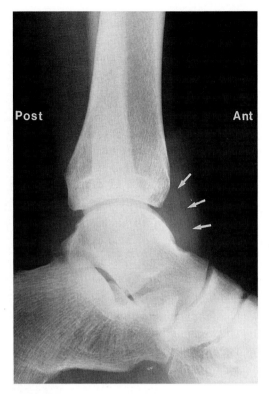

on the x-ray (Fig. 8–140). As with other joints, when orthopedic hardware is present and follow-up x-rays are performed, you should look for destructive areas along the shaft of the screws as well as sclerosis that is not associated with the fracture itself. These are findings that suggest infection and osteomyelitis (Fig. 8–141).

Just because the bony structures of the ankle look normal on the x-ray does not mean that there is no soft tissue pathology. There may be significant ligamentous disruption that is not appreciated. If clinical suspicion persists about ligamentous disruption and laxity of the ankle, stress views can be performed. These are x-rays taken while the ankle is being twisted, and they can show widening of the ankle joint (Fig. 8–142). MRI is rarely indicated for most ankle trauma.

Benign Nontraumatic Abnormalities

There are three fairly common dense bone abnormalities that are seen typically in the distal tibia. These lesions do occur in other bones, but

the ankle is so frequently x-rayed that questions about these come up more often relative to the ankle. The first of these are horizontal dense lines in the metaphysis of the tibia (Fig. 8–143). These are called "growth arrest" lines, and they represent a time when there was some interference with the normal longitudinal growth process of the bone, perhaps periods of sickness during the individual's life. Occasionally, dense lines such as these reflect heavy metal ingestion (lead poisoning or ingestion of bismuth or phosphorus). Growth arrest lines are of no clinical significance whatever at the time they are seen, since they are a representation of a historical event.

Small oval sclerotic or dense lesions can occur in most bones. These are called bone islands, and their origin is uncertain. They are completely benign lesions and should be regarded as a normal variant. They rarely measure more than 5 or 6 mm in width and 1 cm in length. The long axis of the oval is always in the long axis of the bone or aligned with the trabecular pattern (Fig. 8–144).

Benign fibrous cortical defects and nonossi-

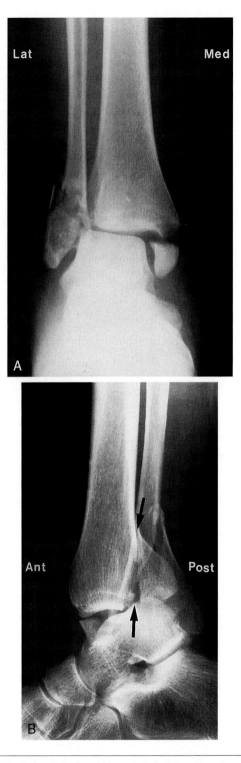

FIGURE 8–139. Ankle fractures. *A,* In this bimalleolar fracture the horizontal fracture medially and an oblique fracture laterally mean that this was an eversion injury. With an inversion injury, there would have been a horizontal fibular fracture and oblique fracture of the medial malleolus. *B,* Trimalleolar fracture in a different patient. The lateral view is necessary to show a fracture of the posterior malleolus *(arrows).* Also note that there has been anterior subluxation of the distal tibial on the talus.

FIGURE 8–140. Antibiotic beads. This AP view of the ankle demonstrates fixation screws and pin through the medial malleolus. The wire with beads *(arrows)* represents local antibiotic therapy, which is usually utilized for open fractures.

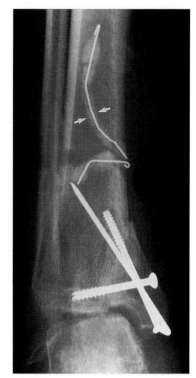

fying fibromas have been discussed in relationship to the femur (see Fig. 8–105). If the lesions are large they may fracture, but many heal spontaneously during young adult life, leaving behind an area of dense bone (Fig. 8–145).

FOOT

As with the ankle, typical x-ray projections of the foot following trauma include AP, lateral, and oblique. For purposes of an arthritis workup, AP and lateral views are sufficient (Fig. 8–146).

There is a special view of the foot called the calcaneal view. It is taken when a fracture of the calcaneus is suspected. The foot is flexed, and the x-ray beam is angled down through the posterior aspect of the heel. This provides a good view of at least the posterior half of the calcaneus (Fig. 8–147).

There are a few congenital and developmental abnormalities of the foot that you should be aware of. There can be fusion or a bony bridge across the proximal bones, for example,

between the talus and the calcaneus or between the calcaneus and the navicular. Many times these can be seen on plain films, although occasionally CT scanning is needed to identify the abnormality.

A wide variety of small accessory bones are seen about the ankle and tarsal bones (Fig. 8–148). These are variable but usually can easily be distinguished from fractures, since accessory bones are well corticated and typically round or oval. Another common developmental abnormality is a cystic-looking area that occurs in the anterior and midportion of the calcaneus. Although this sometimes is called a calcaneal cyst, MRI has shown that a large number of these, in fact, are intraosseous lipomas. Why they tend to occur in this location is unknown (Fig. 8–149). Generally they are not clinically significant, but if they are large, the weakened bone may result in a pathologic fracture.

Trauma

A number of foot x-rays are ordered to look for foreign bodies that the patient stepped on. If the

Text continued on page 372

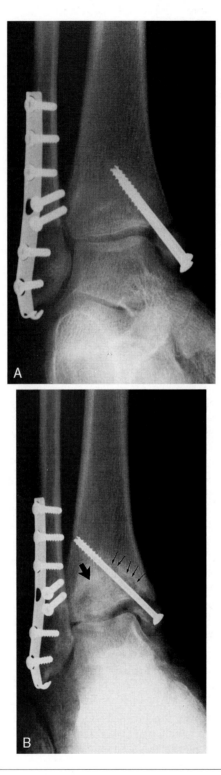

FIGURE 8–141. Developing osteomyelitis. *A,* An oblique view of the ankle immediately after repair of a bimalleolar fracture shows two screws through the medial malleolus and a plate and screws in the lateral malleolus. *B,* A repeat examination 6 weeks later, when the patient had developed a low-grade fever and pain, demonstrates destruction of bone around the edge of the screw *(small arrows)* and a larger destructive lesion *(large arrow)* of the distal tibial extending to the joint surface.

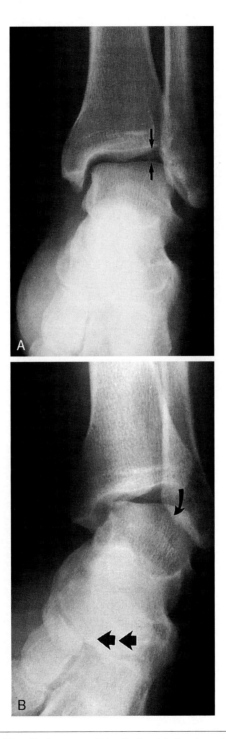

FIGURE 8-142. Ankle instability. *A,* An AP view of the ankle demonstrates slight widening of the lateral aspect of the ankle mortise *(arrows). B,* A stress view was obtained by inverting the foot (in the direction of the large arrows). This makes the ligamentous injury much more obvious by opening the ankle mortise even further *(curved arrow).*

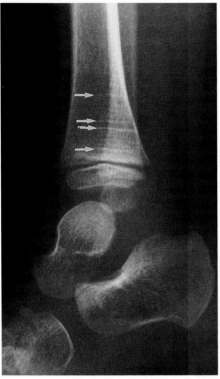

FIGURE 8–143. Growth arrest lines. These transverse dense lines in the metaphysis of a long bone are due to bouts of illness that this child had in the past. Similar horizontal lines can be due to episodic heavy metal ingestion, such as lead poisoning.

FIGURE 8–144. Bone island. This small oval dense area *(arrow)* of bone is essentially a normal variant. It is commonly seen around the ankle because the ankles are x-rayed so frequently for trauma. These benign lesions almost always are less than 1 cm in the longest axis, and the long axis of the elliptical lesion is parallel with the long axis of the bone.

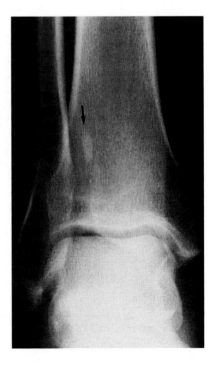

FIGURE 8–145. Healed nonossifying fibroma. These lesions are usually discovered incidentally in young adults. Ninety per cent are found near the metaphysis of the tibia or fibula. The dense nature and lack of periosteal reaction indicate that this is a benign lesion, and no further work-up is called for.

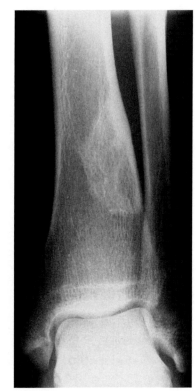

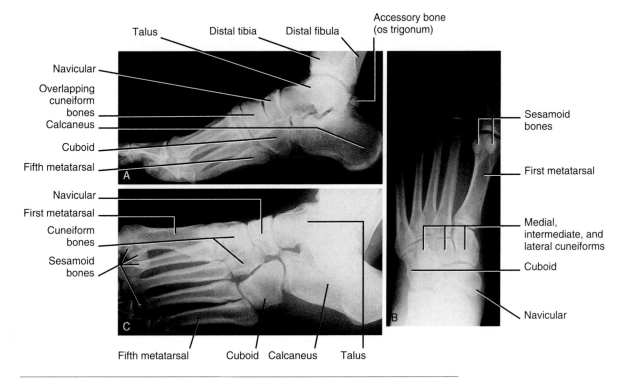

FIGURE 8–146. Normal anatomy of the foot in the lateral projection *(A)*, AP projection *(B)*, and oblique projection *(C)*.

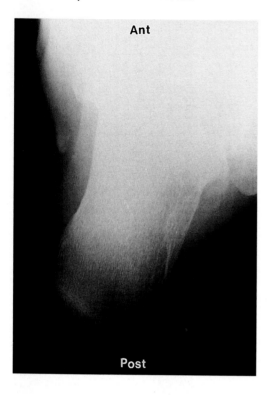

Ant

Post

FIGURE 8–147. Calcaneal view. This view is taken to look for subtle fractures of the posterior aspect of the calcaneus. It is taken by placing the foot on a film and shooting down along the backside of the ankle.

suspected object is metallic, it can normally be visualized (Fig. 8–150). As was discussed in the section on the hand, most glass can also be seen. If the object is not visible externally, a radiologist may operate a fluoroscope while another physician is locating the object. Digging around in the sole of the foot often causes residual painful scars, and the more easily an object can be located, the less scarring there should be. Remember that wooden objects or graphite from pencils will not be visualized by x-ray.

Fractures of the foot can involve any bone. Fractures of the talus are rare but almost always involve the neck of the talus (Fig. 8–151). This is the so-called aviator's fracture, since it occurred when early pilots crashed and slammed their feet into the front of the cockpit. Obviously, today the fracture is much more often due to motor vehicle accidents. Calcaneal fractures often can be difficult to appreciate on the lateral view and are almost impossible to see on an AP view. For this reason, the calcaneal view that we discussed earlier should also be ordered (Fig. 8–152). Sometimes there are patients with persistent foot pain who have normal plain x-rays. A nuclear medicine bone scan can sometimes localize a bone in which there is an occult fracture (Fig. 8–153).

A very common fracture of the foot involves the base of the fifth metatarsal. There is frequently an apophysis on the lateral aspect of the fifth metatarsal base, and this is often confused with a fracture. The way to tell the two apart is by noting that the long axis of the apophysis is parallel to the long axis of the metatarsal. Fractures, on the other hand, typically are transverse or perpendicular to the long axis of the bone (Fig. 8–154).

Most fractures of the metatarsals are fairly easy to recognize. Two unique fractures can occur in this region. The first is the so-called Lisfranc fracture. This is actually a fracture and lateral dislocation of the second, third, fourth, and fifth metatarsals relative to the tarsal bones. This usually happens as a result of falling out of a saddle while horseback riding and getting a foot caught in the stirrup (Fig. 8–155).

Another classic fracture of the metatarsals is the so-called march fracture. This is a stress fracture that typically occurs in army recruits who have to march long distances and are not used to it, but it is also seen in athletes and

Text continued on page 378

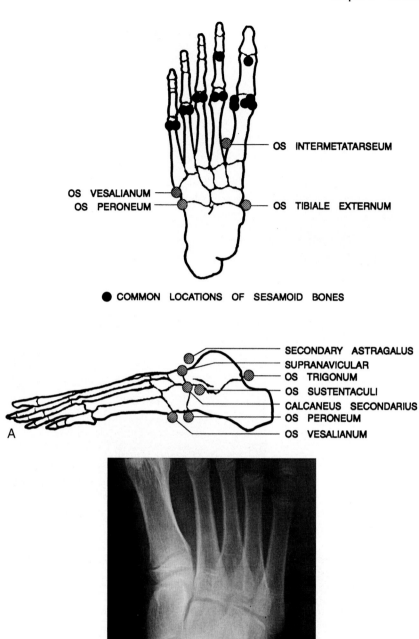

FIGURE 8–148. Accessory bones of the foot. *A*, Schematic representation of normal accessory and sesmoid bones. *B*, An x-ray of the foot of a child shows an accessory os naviculare *(arrow)*.

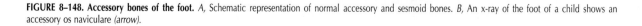

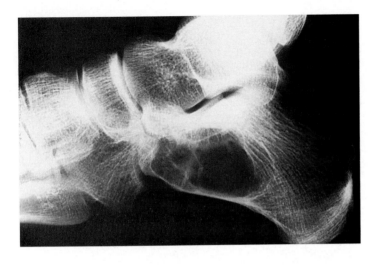

FIGURE 8–149. Calcaneal cyst. This lateral view of the foot shows a large well-defined lucent area in the anterior portion of the calcaneus. Although this has been referred to as a calcaneal cyst, often it has been shown to contain fat and to be an intraosseous lipoma. These lesions almost never occur at any other location.

FIGURE 8–150. Sewing needle in the foot. The lateral view of the foot shows two metallic needle fragments (arrow) in the sole of the foot.

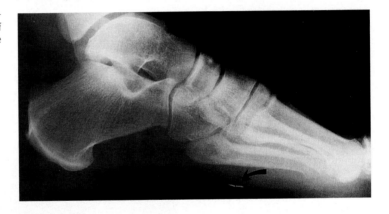

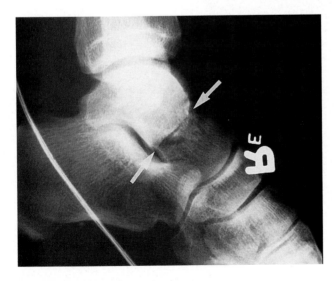

FIGURE 8–151. Talar neck fracture. A lucent line can be seen extending through the talus (arrows). This is the second most common fracture of the proximal foot, and historically it is referred to as an aviator's fracture.

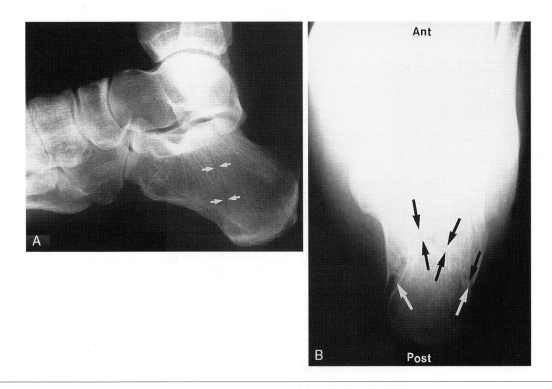

FIGURE 8–152. Calcaneal fracture. The lateral view of the calcaneus *(A)* shows a subtle lucent (dark) line through the calcaneus. This extends into the subtalar joint about 75 per cent of the time. This fracture has also been called a lover's fracture (probably from tales of disappointed lovers jumping off buildings or bridges). A calcaneal view *(B)* in the same patient makes the fracture much more obvious *(arrows)* particularly at the lateral margins.

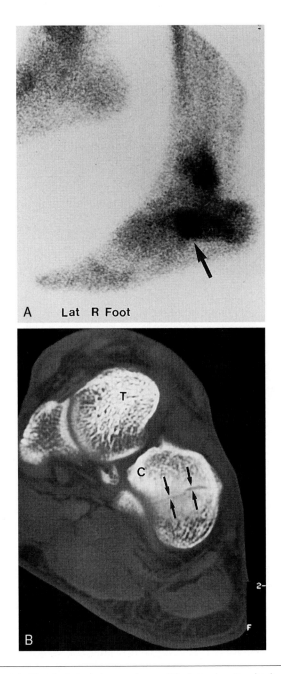

FIGURE 8–153. Occult calcaneal fracture. *A,* In this patient who had a normal x-ray of the foot and continued to have pain, a nuclear medicine bone scan was performed. A lateral image of the foot shows an area of markedly increased activity *(arrow)* along the anterior portion of the calcaneus. *B,* A CT scan was then performed with thin sections over the area of interest, and the calcaneal fracture was identified *(arrows).*

FIGURE 8–154. Fracture of the fifth metatarsal base. This fracture usually occurs from inversion of the foot and is transverse across the base of the metatarsal. This should not be confused with a normal fifth metatarsal apophysis, which this patient also has. The fracture is always transverse and is referred to as a Jones fracture. The apophysis is always parallel with the long axis of the metatarsal.

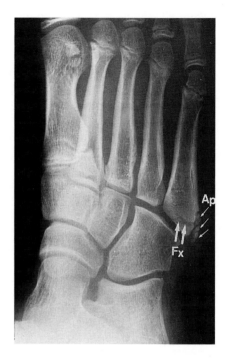

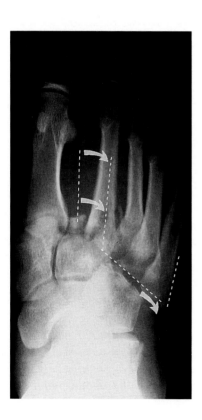

FIGURE 8–155. Lisfranc fracture/dislocation. This is a fracture/dislocation in which the second through fifth metatarsals are fractured and/or subluxed laterally (arrows).

dancers. The distal third of the second, third, or fourth metatarsal is the usual location. If you look very carefully in this region, sometimes you can see slightly increased sclerosis or periosteal reaction (Fig. 8–156). If the radiograph is normal, a stress fracture may still be present, and in this circumstance it is usually easily visualized as an area of intensely increased activity on a nuclear medicine bone scan.

There is a form of aseptic necrosis that most commonly involves the head of the second metatarsal. This is manifested as flattening of the articular surface with associated sclerosis (Fig. 8–157). This is called Köhler-Freiberg infarction. The lesion is seen less frequently in the head of the third or first metatarsal. This injury is believed to be a type of stress fracture, and it is often found during late adolescence. Degenerative joint disease is a late complication of this condition.

Degenerative and Arthritic Conditions

Views of the feet obtained for arthritis evaluation are often unrevealing or nonspecific, and if

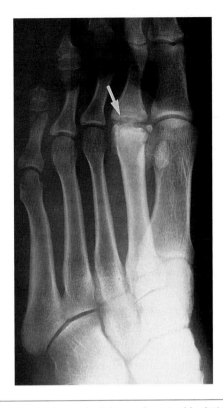

FIGURE 8–157. Aseptic necrosis of the second metatarsal head. This usually occurs in teenagers and is referred to as a Freiberg osteonecrosis. Subsequent degenerative arthritis in this region is common.

any x-ray is ordered for arthritis evaluation, the highest yield usually is obtained with an AP view of the hands. As pointed out earlier, the radiographic findings, while somewhat characteristic, are not as specific as laboratory findings. The major metabolic abnormality that occurs in the foot is gout (Fig. 8–158). This is typically manifested as swelling over the first metatarsophalangeal joint. On x-ray these are erosions in the periarticular region with overhanging edges. These are late findings, and again the diagnosis is best made by laboratory analysis.

Infection

Patients with diabetes may develop peripheral neuropathy as well as vascular insufficiency. The latter is particularly acute in the toes, and there often is concomitant infection. X-rays of the feet can demonstrate changes of osteomyelitis to help distinguish this from cellulitis. The characteristic signs of osteomyelitis include soft

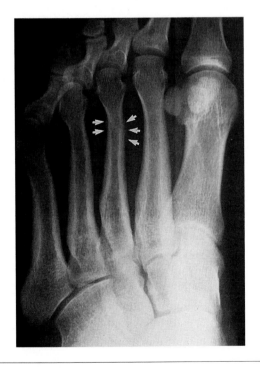

FIGURE 8–156. Stress fracture. This marine recruit complained of foot pain. A small amount of periosteal reaction is seen *(arrows)*, and there is slight sclerosis extending across the medullary cavity. Stress fractures commonly occur at the distal third of the second and third metatarsals. This is also referred to as a "march" fracture. They can be very difficult to appreciate even when you know where to look.

FIGURE 8–158. Gout. The first metatarsal phalangeal joint is the most commonly affected. Here, there is a large tophus that has caused erosion at the margins of the joints; in general, however, the joint space itself is reasonably well preserved.

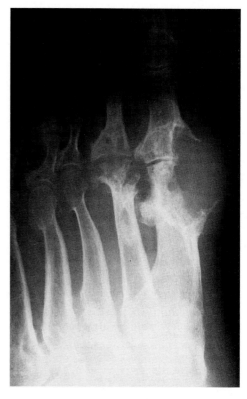

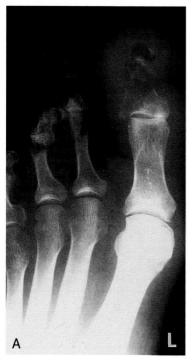

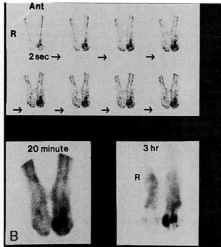

FIGURE 8–159. Osteomyelitis of the foot. *A,* In this diabetic patient, there is a significant soft tissue swelling and destruction of the bony structure of the distal phalanx of the great toe. *B,* When radiographs are normal, there still can be osteomyelitis. A nuclear medicine bone scan is more sensitive and will show increased blood flow in the first seconds after radionuclide injection, increased blood pooling at 20 minutes, and more focal and intense radioactivity on the 3-hour images.

tissue swelling, focal loss of trabecular pattern, periosteal reaction, and frank bone destruction (Fig. 8–159). The differentiation of osteomyelitis from cellulitis is important because the therapy for osteomyelitis involves weeks of intravenous therapy. If the bone changes that have been described are present, you can conclude that there is osteomyelitis. Osteomyelitis can be pres-

ent when there is a normal radiograph, and if clinical suspicion is high, evaluation with a three-phase nuclear medicine bone scan is often useful. Other plain x-ray changes that are characteristic of diabetic involvement of the foot include marked vascular calcification and occasionally air within the soft tissue due to infection and gangrene.

Pediatric Musculoskeletal Radiology

SKULL

Anatomy

Typical views of the skull in a child are the same as in adults—AP and lateral. The differences in normal anatomy consist of dark or lucent lines that represent the cranial sutures (Fig. 8–160) and a small face in comparison with the cranium. Cranial sutures usually remain partially open until at least midlife, and it is particularly important that they remain open in the early years of life to allow growth of the brain. The sutures of the skull can close prematurely (craniosynostosis). The sagittal suture is the most commonly involved, and the coronal suture less so. Premature closure of the sagittal suture results in growth of the skull in the areas where

the coronal and lambdoid sutures remain open, and the skull becomes much longer than normal (scaphocephaly) (Fig. 8–161). If the coronal suture closes prematurely, growth continues to occur along the sagittal suture, and the skull becomes much wider than normal. A skull film is often not necessary, since the shape of the skull and a ridge of bone over the closed suture are clinically apparent. On a skull film the prematurely closed suture may be dense (white) at the edges or may just be difficult to see.

Trauma

Fractures are seen as very sharply defined lucent lines that do not correspond to sutures. The

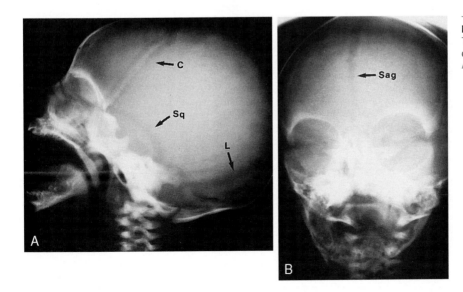

FIGURE 8–160. Normal newborn skull. *A,* The lateral view clearly shows the lambdoidal, squamous, and coronal sutures. *B,* An AP view clearly shows the sagittal suture.

FIGURE 8–161. Premature closure of the sagittal suture. Closure of the sagittal suture has allowed growth of the skull only in the AP direction; here the coronal and lambdoidal sutures can be seen to be widened.

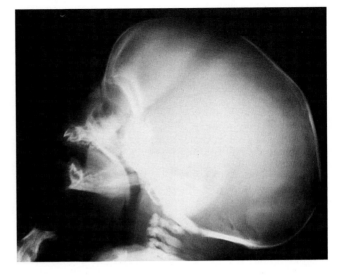

margins of the sutures are somewhat wiggly, especially as they near closure. Sometimes it can be difficult to differentiate between a fracture and a vascular groove. Most vascular grooves are seen on the lateral view of the skull and radiate superiorly and posteriorly from a position just above the ear. In addition, if you look carefully, the vascular groove is a lucent line that is bounded by a sclerotic (white) margin before you reach the normal bone of the skull. A skull fracture will be a lucent line (dark) and then normal skull.

Occasionally, a fracture line will widen progressively during the first weeks or months after injury. The widening is due to formation of an underlying leptomeningeal cyst, which causes pressure and subsequent atrophy of the bone at the edges of the fracture line. The dura is torn at the time of injury, allowing this process to occur. Sometimes, this lesion is referred to as a growing skull fracture of childhood, and it usually will not heal without surgery (Fig. 8–162).

Another common traumatic lesion of childhood is a cephalohematoma. These are caused by traumatic hemorrhage into the neonatal scalp during labor, although they can also occur following cephalic injury during infancy or childhood. With healing, there is usually a new shell of subperiosteal bone over the hematoma, which then thickens and calcifies. Clinically, cephalohematomas can disappear in weeks to months, although the x-ray finding may persist long afterward (Fig. 8–163).

Neoplastic lesions of the skull can occur during childhood. Almost all present as multiple lucent holes (Fig. 8–164). Typical malignant lesions in very young children are due to histiocytosis X, although with slightly older children, metastatic lesions occur from neuroblastoma.

Many clinicians order sinus views in order to look for sinusitis. This is often the result of parental concern rather than medical need. You should remember that the sinuses are not developed at birth and are progressively pneumatized over the first 10 years of life. The first sinuses to appear are the maxillary sinuses; the frontal sinuses come much later. For both children and adults, it is inappropriate to order sinus views for what clinically appears to be routine sinusitis (Fig. 8–165).

SPINE

There are two items that cause confusion in interpretation of cervical spine views in children. The first is that the odontoid process and the body of C2 form as separate ossification centers, and fusion occurs in the first year or so of life (Fig. 8–166*A*). Occasionally, nonfusion can persist into adulthood. The differentiation from an odontoid fracture can be made by the absence of sharp, angulated corners and the absence of soft tissue swelling. Another surprising but common finding in children is a pseudosubluxa-

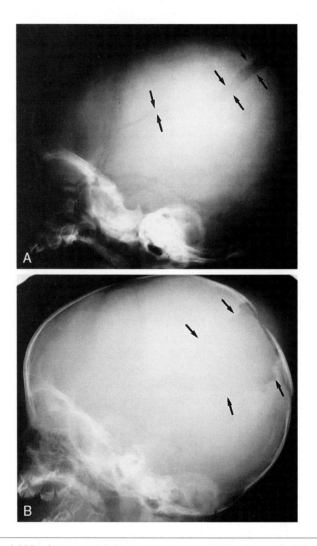

FIGURE 8–162. Growing skull fracture of childhood. *A,* A parietal skull fracture is easily seen on this lateral view of the skull *(arrows). B,* A repeat skull film 2 months later shows that the fracture line has become very wide *(arrows).* This is due to a leptomeningeal cyst and continued pressure erosion of the bone.

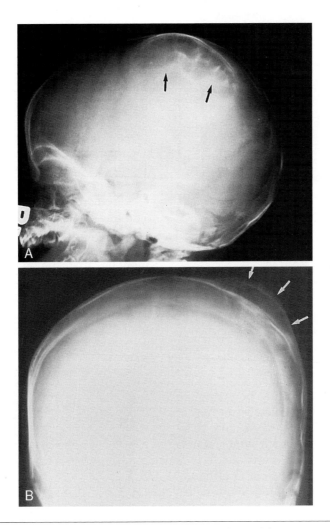

FIGURE 8–163. Cephalohematoma. *A,* A lateral view of the skull shows a lucent multilocular and expansile lesion *(arrows). B,* An AP tangential view of the skull shows that this lesion is primarily bulging out from the normal skull cortex because of calcification of the hematoma.

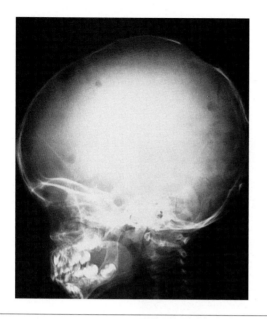

FIGURE 8–164. Histiocytosis X of the skull. Multiple lucent holes of varying sizes are seen in this lateral projection of the skull. A large scalloped lesion has destroyed the cortex over the posterior aspect of the skull and has beveled edges, which is characteristic of this disease.

tion at C2 and C3. This is simply a normal variant and occurs when the child has his or her neck slightly flexed (Fig. 8–166B). If this occurs in children over the age of approximately 5 years, you should suspect a traumatic cause rather than a normal variant.

There are a number of congenital spinal abnormalities that occur, including hemivertebra and butterfly vertebra, which often result in scoliosis. Severe abnormalities are usually diagnosed soon after birth, but more minor abnormalities may not be found until there is a scoliosis work-up in adolescence or adulthood.

There is a rather unusual spinal abnormality of childhood called diskitis. This usually occurs in the lumbar spine and appears radiographically as a decreased disk space (Fig. 8–167). On a nuclear medicine bone scan, there is increased activity of the vertebral body both above and below the affected level. The origin of this entity is uncertain, but it may represent a low-grade infection.

UPPER EXTREMITY

Humerus

Lesions in the proximal humerus that are lytic, somewhat expansive, and quite well demarcated

are usually unicameral bone cysts (see Fig. 8–54). Care should be taken, however, in the diagnosis, since the third most common site of osteogenic sarcoma is the proximal humerus.

Elbow

The pediatric elbow can cause difficulties in interpretation owing to the development of various ossification centers. The epiphysis of the radial head initially appears at approximately 3 to 5 years of age, and the olecranon appears between 8 and 11 years. The capitulum of the distal humerus appears at less than 1 year of age, the medial epicondyle at 3 to 6 years of age, the trochlea at 7 to 9 years of age, and the lateral epicondyle at 12 to 14 years of age. The development may even be asymmetric between right and left depending on which arm is dominant (Fig. 8–168). The asymmetric appearance of the lateral condylar ossification center can often be mistaken for a fracture, and clinical correlation is essential. Note should be made that avulsion fractures of the lateral condyle are quite rare, whereas avulsion fractures of the medial condyle are much more common. When

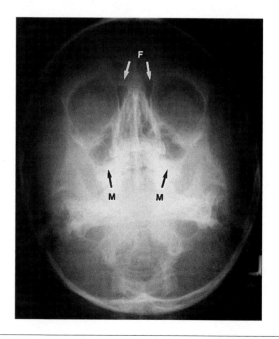

FIGURE 8–165. Normal sinuses in a 5-year-old child. The maxillary sinuses are poorly developed at this age and only partially pneumatized, and the frontal sinuses are only beginning to develop.

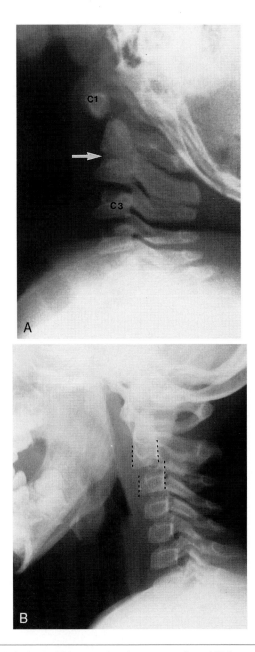

FIGURE 8–166. Normal variations of the cervical spine in children. *A,* A lateral view in a newborn child shows a cleft where the odontoid is not yet completely fused to the body of C2. This is normal. *B,* Pseudosubluxation of C2 on C3 is a very common normal variant in children; it occurs only at this level, particularly when the neck is straight or slightly flexed.

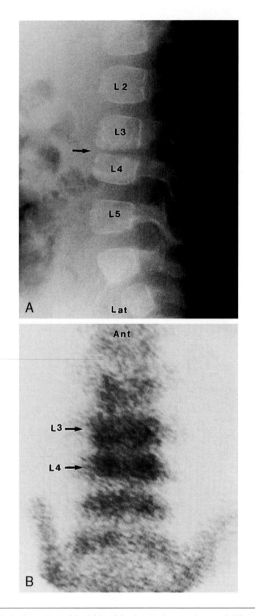

FIGURE 8–167. Diskitis. *A,* A lateral view of the lumbar spine in this child with back pain shows a decreased disk space at L3–L4 *(arrow).* Sometimes the disk space is not appreciably narrowed, and the diagnosis can sometimes be made with a nuclear medicine bone scan *(B).* Here, on an anterior view of the lumbar spine, increased radioactivity is seen at L3 and L4, compatible with the diagnosis of diskitis.

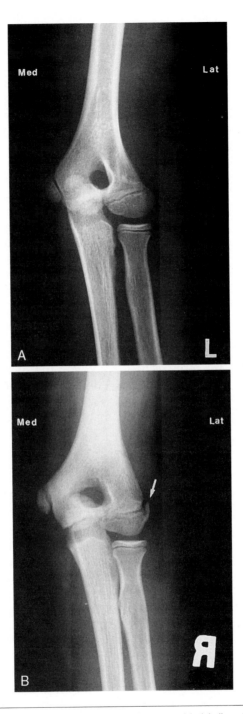

FIGURE 8–168. Normal variation and development of the elbow in children. *A,* On an AP view of the left elbow, the medial epicondyle is visualized, but the lateral is not. *B,* On the right side, the lateral epicondyle is seen. This asymmetric development from one side to the other can occur normally. Since lateral epicondyle fractures are rare, you should suspect that this is an apophysis.

this occurs, it is sometimes called "Little Leaguer's elbow" (Fig. 8–169).

In examining the elbow for fracture, remember that visualization of the anterior fat pad lying up against the anterior aspect of the distal humerus is a normal finding. A posterior fat pad should never be seen, and the anterior fat pad should not be displaced or bowed forward (Fig. 8–170A). In addition, the apophysis of the olecranon should not be mistaken for a fracture.

A relatively common fracture in children is a supracondylar fracture that extends across the distal aspect of the humerus. When this occurs, there almost always is bowing forward of the anterior fat pad and visualization of the posterior fat pad. You should evaluate the anterior humeral line. This line should extend down into the middle third of the capitellum (Fig. 8–170B).

Destructive lesions involving a joint space usually are produced by inflammatory lesions. They may be the result of infection in the joint space (septic arthritis) or of other chronic inflammatory processes, such as inflammation due to intermittent bleeding within the joint in patients with hemophilia (Fig. 8–171). Significant joint involvement also occurs in children who have juvenile rheumatoid arthritis.

Forearm, Wrist, and Hand

Fractures of the forearm and wrist are very common in children; a number of the types that occur in adults have already been discussed. Whenever there are multiple fractures, especially those that appear to be in different stages of healing, child abuse should be suspected. The fact that the fractures are of different ages can be ascertained by periosteal reaction or callus around some, but not around other, fracture sites. If child abuse is suspected, additional views of the skull, ribs, pelvis, and both upper and lower extremities should be obtained (Fig. 8–172).

Young children have bones that are relatively plastic, and two unique childhood fractures occur as a result of this plasticity. The first is a "buckle" or "torus" fracture. Sometimes, on a single view, all you will identify is a slight outward bulge of the cortex, whereas on other views, you may actually see a buckling of the

cortex (Fig. 8–173). The other fracture is the so-called greenstick fracture. In this, the bone is bent but typically fractured only on one side of the cortex, similar to breaking a green twig (Fig. 8–174).

At the end of any long bone there can be a number of the Salter-Harris type fractures described earlier (see Fig. 8–80). One of the most difficult fractures to see is a nondisplaced, or very minimally displaced, Salter-Harris type I fracture through the epiphyseal plate. Often the x-ray at the time of injury will be normal; however, a repeat examination 1 to 2 weeks later will reveal increasing sclerosis (white lines) across the epiphyseal plate, indicating a healing fracture (Fig. 8–175). Fortunately, nondisplaced Salter-Harris type I fractures are not important clinically.

Normal growth of the bones in the hand includes appearance and development of the carpal bones and of epiphyses at the end of the radius and ulna, the distal second through fourth metacarpals, the proximal first metacarpal, and the proximal aspects of the phalanges. At birth there are essentially no ossification centers of the carpal bones or epiphyses in the hand. As a general rule, one carpal bone appears each year from the age of 1 year to about the age of 7 years (Fig. 8–176). There can be variation in the appearance of the epiphyses and ossification centers between the two hands, and the growth pattern is usually somewhat more advanced in girls than in boys of the same age.

In a child under the age of 10 years, it is very rare to have fractures of the carpal bones. Typical hand fractures in children involve either Salter fractures of the fingers or fractures of the terminal phalanges (since children usually get their fingers caught in doors and other objects).

Osteomyelitis in very young children often involves both the distal metaphysis and the epiphysis of a bone. This is because the epiphysis receives its blood supply from the shaft of the bone. In older children, the epiphysis has its own separate blood supply, and osteomyelitis usually involves the metaphysis just proximal to the epiphyseal plate. With hematogenous spread of bacteria, multiple bones can be involved. The radiographic findings of osteomyelitis include soft tissue swelling, bone destruction, and periosteal reaction. As with adults, if

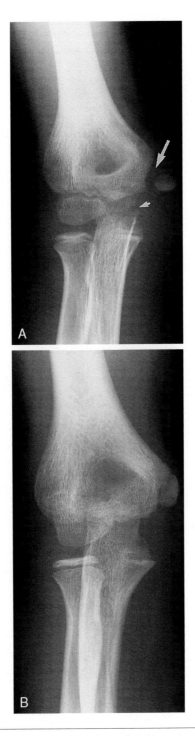

FIGURE 8–169. "Little Leaguer's elbow." *A,* An AP view of the elbow shows an abnormally wide space between the medial epicondyle and the distal humerus *(large arrow).* An olecranon fracture is also seen *(small arrow). B,* The opposite elbow is shown for comparison with the normal position of the medial epicondyle.

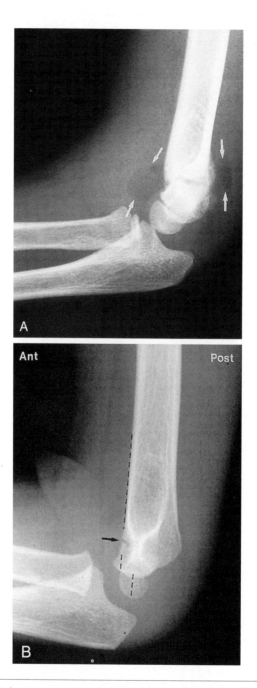

FIGURE 8–170. Supracondylar fractures. This is the most common elbow fracture in children. *A,* A lateral view of the elbow shows marked anterior displacement of the anterior fat and visualization of the posterior fat pad *(arrows),* a sign that a fracture is almost certainly present. *B,* In a younger child a fracture is seen because of the posterior displacement of the capitellum from the anterior humeral line. An incomplete cortical fracture is also seen *(arrow).*

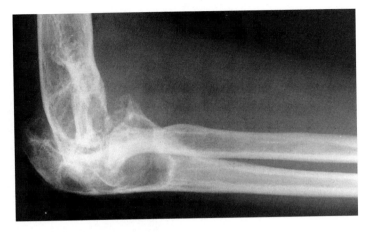

FIGURE 8–171. Hemophilia. A lateral view of the elbow shows marked destruction of the joint space. Chronic bleeding within the joint has destroyed the cartilage. Similar findings may be seen with juvenile rheumatoid arthritis.

a clinical question remains about the presence of osteomyelitis or even septic arthritis, a radionuclide bone scan is often helpful (Fig. 8–177).

PELVIS AND HIPS

Dislocation of the hip in children is usually congenital and occurs more often in girls than in boys. There are a number of ways to make the radiographic diagnosis. Radiographic diagnosis of a congenital hip dislocation is unreliable in the neonate because the ossification center for the femoral head is not developed. Perhaps the simplest radiographic method is evaluation of Shenton's line, which is formed by the medial aspect of the obturator foramen and the medial aspect of the femoral neck. Together, these should form a nice smooth curved arc (Fig. 8–178). A frog-leg view with the legs abducted is useless, because in this position the hip is reduced. Radiographic diagnosis of congenital hip dislocation should be done rarely, if ever, since the clinical finding of an audible click when the hips are abducted should be sufficient to make the diagnosis. If there is any doubt, ultrasound examination may be useful.

Occasionally, children can develop aseptic necrosis of the epiphysis of the femoral head (Legg-Perthes disease). Boys are more commonly affected than girls. Clinical signs are a limp and pain with limitation in motion of the hip. The radiographic findings are irregularity, sclerosis (increased density), and fragmentation of the epiphysis. There is often a resulting deformity that is followed by a disabling osteoarthritis decades later (Fig. 8–179).

Another pediatric hip abnormality is slipping of the epiphysis of the femoral head. The cause of this is unknown, and it usually does not happen in children under 9 years of age. The diagnosis is made radiographically by noting a thickened epiphyseal plate and medial displacement of the femoral head relative to the femoral neck (Fig. 8–180). The lateral or abducted frog-leg view of the hip offers the best view of these findings. When the epiphysis fuses, there is no more slippage, but the deformity that has occurred will be permanent, and later degenerative disease will be a complication.

LOWER EXTREMITIES

Although systemic bone diseases are quite rare in children, there are two entities that you should be aware of. The first is osteogenesis imperfecta. This is a hereditary disease, with abnormal collagen fibers and a disorder of the osteoblasts. There are fragile bones or teeth, thin skin, and sometimes blue sclera. There are two forms of the disease, one which is noted immediately at birth and one that appears later. The disease is radiographically characterized by multiple healing fractures and bowing deformities of the bone (Fig. 8–181).

Arthritic changes in children are very rare with the exception of juvenile rheumatoid arthritis and hemophilia. Both these diseases can

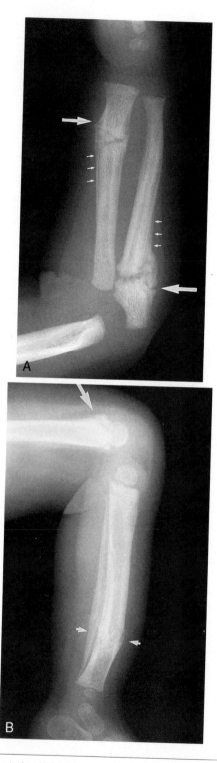

FIGURE 8–172. Child abuse. *A,* A view of the forearm in this child shows extensive periosteal reaction *(small arrows)* and transverse fracture lines *(large arrows).* Fractures of long bones in children, particularly with different stages of healing, are very suggestive of a battered child. *B,* A lateral view of the lower extremity in the same child also reveals fractures of the distal fibula and tibia *(small arrows)* as well as a metaphyseal corner fracture *(large arrow)* of the distal femur. This latter fracture is also typical of child abuse.

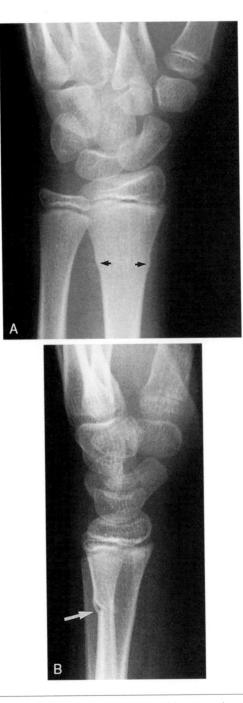

FIGURE 8–173. Torus or buckle fracture. *A,* An AP view of the wrist shows slight bulging of the cortex in the metaphyseal region *(arrows). B,* A lateral view of the wrist shows buckling of the dorsal cortex.

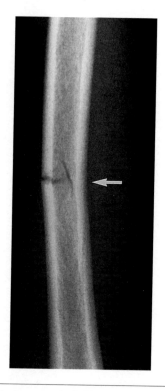

FIGURE 8–174. Greenstick fracture. In the humerus of this elementary school child, a direct blow from the direction of the arrow has caused an incomplete transverse fracture.

cause fluid collections within the joint and destruction of the cartilage, followed by degenerative change. There may also be hyperemia, which results in overgrowth of the epiphyseal region of the bone. The joint effusions, irregularity of the articular surface, and subsequent degenerative changes are easily visualized on radiographs (Fig. 8–182).

Ewing's tumor typically occurs in the shaft of the long bones or in flat bones, such as the pelvis, scapula, and ribs. In contrast, osteogenic sarcomas occur most commonly in the distal femur, less commonly in the proximal tibia and proximal humerus, and rarely elsewhere. An osteogenic sarcoma may present as a destructive lesion in the central portion of the bone or with periosteal reaction and soft tissue swelling (Fig. 8–183). Often, an MR scan is useful to show the soft tissue extent of the tumor.

A number of characteristic traumatic tibial lesions occur in children. As mentioned earlier, the proximal tibial epiphysis normally has an anterior projection that slopes down over the front of the tibia. Radiographically, this is best seen on the lateral view (see Fig. 8–114). This appearance can look a little bit irregular, however, if a small fragment is pulled off, and if the patient has pain, this is consistent with the diagnosis of Osgood-Schlatter's injury. This is relatively frequent in children 10 to 15 years of age, particularly in boys who participate in active sports. It probably represents a partial avulsion of the anterior tubercle by the inferior patellar tendon, and it heals with rest (Fig. 8–184).

In children between the ages of 3 and 5 years, a spiral or oblique fracture of the mid- or distal tibia may occur. This is usually referred to as a toddler's fracture. Sometimes there is a history of twisting the leg or jumping off a chair, but often these injuries are found in children who simply refuse to bear weight on the extremity. If this particular entity is suspected, AP, lateral, and oblique views of the tibia should be obtained (Fig. 8–185).

Salter-Harris type fractures are common in the ankle. As mentioned in the discussion of the wrist, the Salter-Harris type I fractures may not be displaced and may be seen only as increased

Text continued on page 403

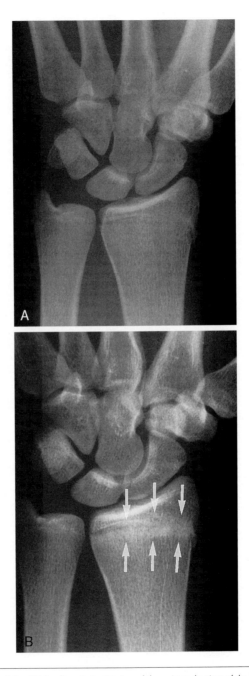

FIGURE 8–175. Occult Salter-Harris fracture of the distal radius. *A,* An AP view of the wrist at the time of the injury does not show any cortical disruption or displacement. *B,* A repeat examination 10 days later shows sclerosis across the epiphyseal plate, indicating healing of an occult Salter-Harris type I fracture.

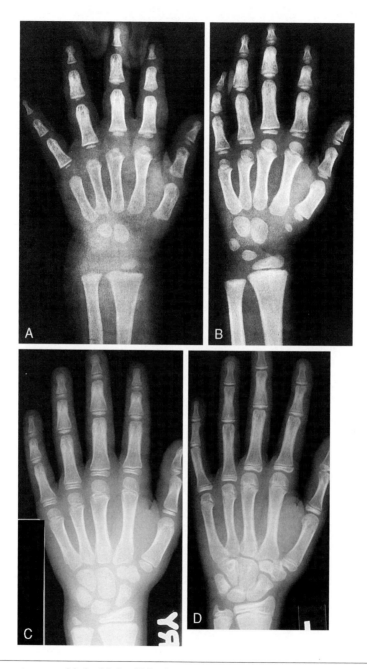

FIGURE 8–176. Normal development anatomy of the hand during childhood. A 2-year-old male *(A)*, 5-year-old male *(B)*, 7-year-old male *(C)*, and 15-year-old male *(D)*. In general, the approximate age can be guessed, since the number of carpal bones usually is close to the child's age in years up to about 7 years.

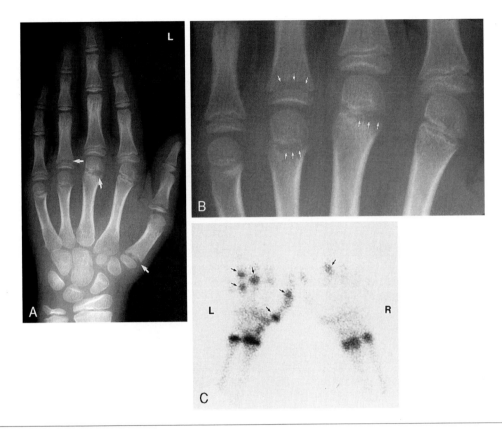

FIGURE 8–177. Multifocal osteomyelitis. *A,* An AP view of the hand demonstrates metaphyseal destruction of at least three sites. This hematogenously spread osteomyelitis usually will not cross the epiphyseal plate if the child is more than several years old. *B,* Detailed view of the hand showing the areas of metaphyseal destruction *(arrows). C,* A nuclear medicine bone scan of both hands in this child shows additional areas of abnormality *(arrows)* that were clinically unsuspected.

FIGURE 8–178. Congenital dislocation of the hip. An AP view demonstrates dislocation of the right hip. The dotted line, which should be continuous, is called Shenton's line. The right acetabulum is also at a steeper angle on the right than on the left. Diagnosis of congenital dislocation of the hip should be made on the basis of clinical examination.

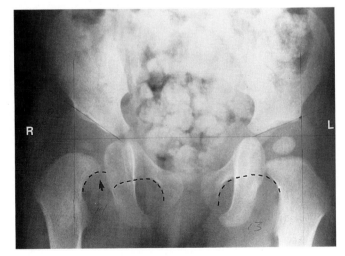

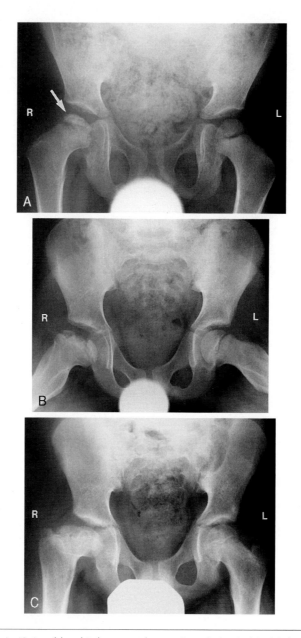

FIGURE 8–179. Legg-Perthes disease. *A,* An AP view of the pelvis demonstrates fragmentation and sclerosis of the right femoral epiphysis in this 6-year-old male. *B,* A follow-up film obtained 8 years later shows continuing deformity due to the osteonecrosis. The patient developed significant degenerative arthritis *(C)* by the age of 12 years.

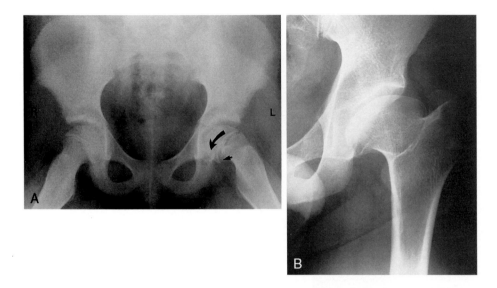

FIGURE 8–180. Slipped capital femoral epiphysis. *A,* An AP view of the pelvis in this overweight teenage male shows slipping of the left femoral epiphysis relative to the femoral neck *(arrows).* This essentially is a Salter-Harris type I fracture. *B,* Follow-up film of the left hip 10 years later shows significant deformity, which will result in degenerative arthritis.

FIGURE 8–181. Osteogenesis imperfecta. This lateral view of the lower extremities shows marked bowing of the bones due to softening. There are also multiple fractures that occur as a result of this congenital bone dysplasia.

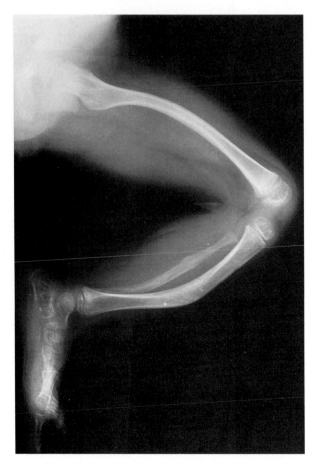

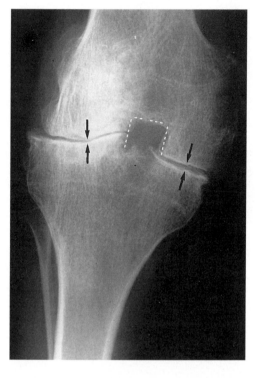

FIGURE 8–182. Hemophilia. An AP view of the knee shows marked joint space narrowing with destruction due to repeated bleeding into the joint space. There is also a very square intercondylar notch. Similar findings are seen in juvenile rheumatoid arthritis.

FIGURE 8–183. Central osteosarcoma. *A,* A destructive lesion is seen in the metaphysis on this AP view of the knee in a young teenager with pain. *B,* A magnetic resonance scan of both legs shows the soft tissue extent of the tumor *(arrows).*

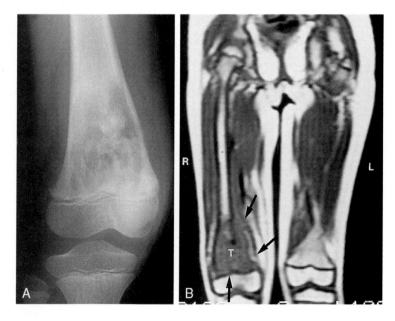

FIGURE 8–184. Osgood-Schlatter disease. A lateral view of the knee demonstrates a tiny avulsion fracture of the anterior tibial tuberosity in this young male athlete. This disease is quite common and usually is self-limited.

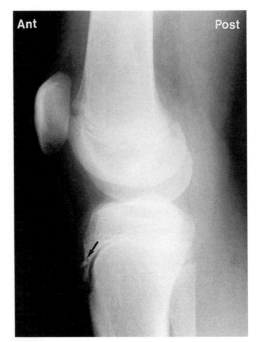

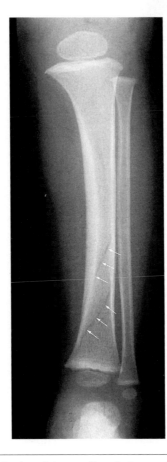

FIGURE 8–185. Toddler's fracture. This 3-year-old child refused to walk because of leg pain. An x-ray of the lower leg shows an oblique fracture *(arrows)* of the distal tibia. This fracture may be the result of weight bearing and should not be confused with the fractures of child abuse.

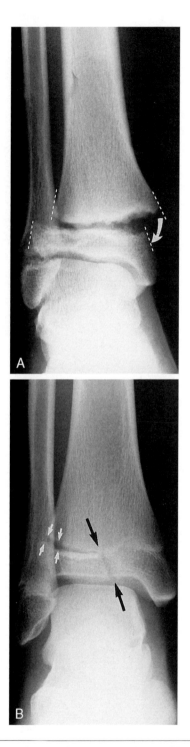

FIGURE 8–186. Salter-Harris fractures of the ankle. *A,* A Salter type I fracture is seen with marked lateral displacement of the epiphysis relative to the tibial metaphysis. *B,* A Salter type III fracture of the lateral tibial epiphysis. This is also called a Tillaux fracture and probably occurs because the growth plate fuses from medial to lateral, making the medial side stronger.

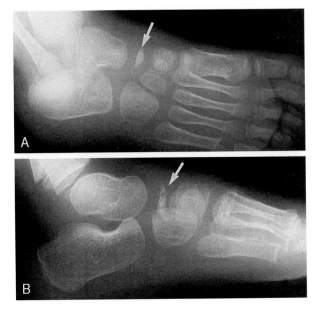

FIGURE 8–187. Aseptic necrosis of the tarsal navicular. This usually occurs between the ages of 4 and 8 years and most commonly is recognized incidentally. There may be increased density (A) or irregularity (B) of the tarsal navicular. This is also called Köhler's osteonecrosis. The abnormality is almost always self-limited and requires no therapy.

density about the epiphyseal plate 1 or 2 weeks post injury. If there is significant displacement and disruption of the epiphyseal plate, the radiographic diagnosis is usually not a problem. Sometimes even a Salter-Harris type III fracture can be subtle (Fig. 8–186). The fractures with the worst prognosis are the impacted Salter-Harris type V (see Fig. 8–80).

Occasionally, in a patient who has a history of foot trauma or pain, you may notice that there is irregularity and increased density or sclerosis of the tarsal navicular (Fig. 8–187). This is referred to as Köhler's disease. Whether this condition is a result of trauma or aseptic necrosis is uncertain; it is often seen incidentally in a child with a twisted ankle. The patient occasionally may have pain over the navicular. This condition essentially always heals without any inter-vention. For some reason, the other tarsal bones are rarely, if ever, involved in this process. You should almost regard this finding as a normal variant.

General Suggested Readings

Edeiken J, Dalinka M, Karasick D: Edeiken's Roentgen Diagnosis of Diseases of Bone, 4th ed. Baltimore, Williams & Wilkins, 1990.

Greenfield G: Radiology of Bone Diseases, 5th ed. Philadelphia, JB Lippincott, 1990.

Greenspan A: Orthopedic Radiology, A Practical Approach, 2nd ed. New York, Raven Press, 1992.

Ozonoff M: Pediatric Orthopedic Radiology, 2nd ed. Philadelphia, WB Saunders, 1992.

Resnick D: Diagnosis of Bone and Joint Disorders, 3rd ed. Philadelphia, WB Saunders, 1995.

Rogers LF: Radiology of Skeletal Trauma, 2nd ed. New York, Churchill Livingstone, 1992.

Chapter 9

Nonskeletal Pediatric Imaging

Most of the pediatric bone lesions have been covered in a special section at the end of Chapter 8. Congenital cardiac lesions have been covered in Chapter 5. This chapter discusses imaging techniques for other commonly encountered pediatric problems.

HEAD

Imaging of the fetal and infant brain can be done utilizing ultrasound as long as the fontanels remain open. Structures that can normally be visualized include the lateral ventricles, choroid plexus, thalamus, temporal lobes, and posterior fossa (Fig. 9–1). The two most common indications for ultrasound of baby heads are (1) evaluation of ventricular enlargement (hydrocephalus) and (2) hemorrhage either within the parenchyma of the brain or within the ventricles

(Fig. 9–2). The major advantages of ultrasound in this application are that the imaging can be done in the neonatal intensive care unit and that ionizing radiation is not used. This is important, since these studies are repeated multiple times for continuing evaluation.

Brain tumors in children are evaluated by CT or MRI. With MRI there is need for sedation, and pediatric monitoring of respiration and other functions in a very high magnetic field is difficult. CT scanning is easier to perform. About half of brain tumors in children are astrocytomas; medulloblastomas (20 per cent), ependymomas (10 per cent), and craniopharyngiomas (5 per cent) are less common.

NECK

Lateral soft tissue views of the neck are often done for evaluation of the pediatric airway. This

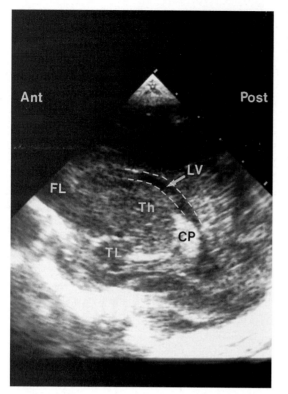

FIGURE 9–1. Ultrasound of normal neonatal head. A sagittal view obtained through an open fontanel clearly shows the frontal lobe, lateral ventricle, thalamus, temporal lobe, and choroid plexus.

is important in cases of suspected croup or epiglottitis. As you evaluate these lateral films, you should look to see that the child's neck has been extended. In a young child, when the neck is flexed, the trachea can buckle forward, causing the appearance of a retropharyngeal mass. Simply by extending the neck and lifting the chin, this artifact can be avoided (Fig. 9–3).

Acute epiglottitis usually occurs in older children (between 2 and 7 years of age) and most commonly is due to *Haemophilus influenzae*. This can be a life-threatening disease, and the clinical findings are severe sore throat, high fever, a muffled voice, and stridor. The patients often can breathe easier sitting up, and they drool. This is a true pediatric emergency. Since intubation can be necessary on very short notice, a physician should accompany the child to the x-ray department. The lateral soft tissue view of the neck shows a thickened epiglottis, often appearing bulbous (in the shape of a thumb) (Fig. 9–4). Remember that the normal epiglottis is a delicate, thin, curved structure. Other findings include ballooning of the hypopharynx and subglottic edema in about one fourth of cases.

Croup typically occurs in young children (between 6 months and 3 years of age), and it usually has a respiratory syncytial viral (RSV) origin. The children often have a brassy cough (like the barking of a seal) and inspiratory stridor. Occasionally the airway may have enough edema that placement of an artificial airway is necessary. The radiographic findings on the lateral view are marked ballooning of the pharynx and hypopharynx. On the AP view, the upper portion of the trachea is shaped like a steeple (Fig. 9–5). The "steeple sign," caused by subglottic edema, is not pathopneumonic, since it can also occur in some children who have epiglottitis.

CHEST

Normal Anatomy and Imaging

One of the major differences between the normal chest of an adult or child and a neonate is the presence of the thymus. The thymus is routinely

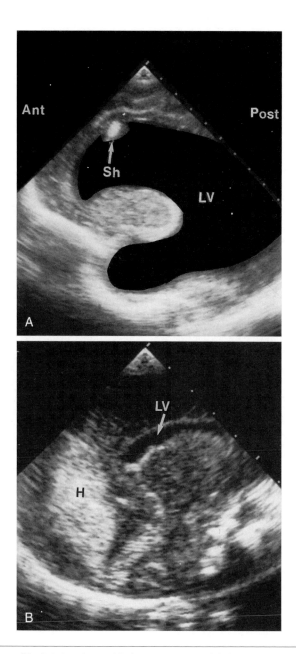

FIGURE 9–2. Ultrasound of abnormal neonatal head. *A,* Sagittal view of the brain in a neonate with hydrocephalus. A dilated lateral ventricle (LV) is seen as well as the shunt (Sh) catheter. *B,* Intraparenchymal hemorrhage. A sagittal view of the brain in a different infant shows a normal-sized lateral ventricle but an area of increased echoes representing hemorrhage (H) within the substance of the brain.

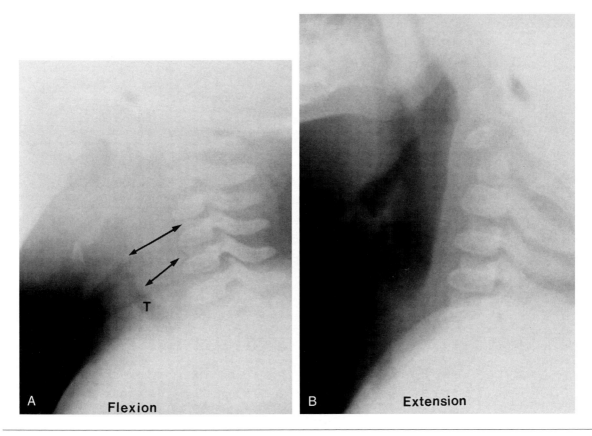

FIGURE 9–3. Pseudoretropharyngeal abscess. *A,* Lateral soft tissue view of the neck in a child with the neck slightly flexed shows the trachea (T) bowed forward, which suggests that there is a retropharyngeal soft tissue mass *(arrows). B,* A lateral view done a few minutes later of the same child with the neck extended shows a normal prevertebral soft tissue pattern.

FIGURE 9–4. Epiglottitis. A lateral soft tissue view of the neck shows a ballooned pharynx with a swollen epiglottis (E) in the shape of a large thumbprint *(arrows)*.

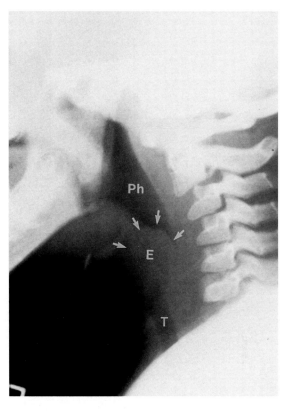

identified on chest films from birth to approximately 2 years of age. The thymus is usually seen as a widening of the soft tissues of the upper mediastinum, although occasionally it may appear to project out into the lung (the "sail sign") (Fig. 9–6). Some people think when they see the "sail sign" that it is an indication that a pneumothorax is present. This is not true.

Imaging of the chest in infants and children can be difficult owing to their uncooperative nature, especially when they are sick. In neonates, portable x-rays are usually obtained in the intensive care unit in a supine AP projection. Somewhat older children can be placed in a holder or restrained with Velcro straps while a film is obtained. In most of these instances, the film is taken randomly with respect to inspiration and expiration. Amazingly enough, hypoinflation of the chest on the x-ray is usually not a problem in interpretation of pediatric chest x-rays.

Most children with pneumonias, bronchiolitis, or reactive airway disease have hyperinflation. In most normal young children, the most superior portion of the hemidiaphragm is at the level of the posterior eighth rib. If the diaphragms are lower than this, hyperinflation should be considered, and pathology may well be present. Rotation of the patient can cause problems in interpretation. As the patient is rotated to the left, the right cardiac border projects over the spine, and the right lower lobe pulmonary vessels are indistinct and can mimic an infiltrate (Fig. 9–7).

A favorite x-ray examination is the "babygram." This is an AP view of both the chest and the abdomen. In very small babies the x-ray exposure can be adequate to visualize pulmonary vasculature, bowel gas, and skeletal structures. On the other hand, if you are interested only in the chest, that is what you should order to avoid unnecessary radiation exposure.

Foreign Bodies. Foreign bodies can be either aspirated or ingested. Most foreign bodies consist of vegetable material (such as peanuts) or plastic. You should remember that vegetable and plastic items are usually not visible on an x-ray. When a foreign body is aspirated into a

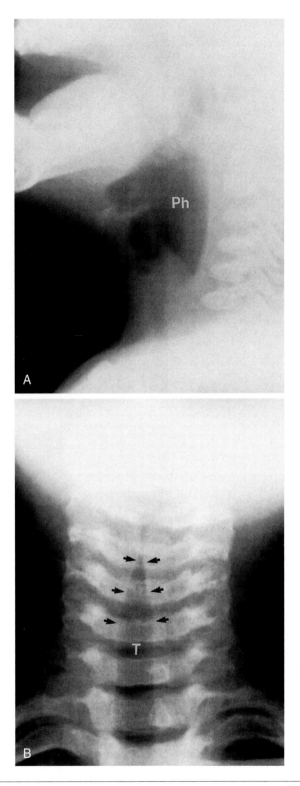

FIGURE 9–5. Croup. In a child with a "barking" cough, a lateral soft tissue view of the neck *(A)* demonstrates a markedly ballooned pharynx. *B,* An AP view of the neck shows a steeple-shaped trachea *(arrows)* caused by subglottic edema.

FIGURE 9–6. Normal thymic shadow. A PA view of the chest shows a very prominent thymic shadow *(arrows)*. Sometimes referred to as the sail sign, this is a normal finding.

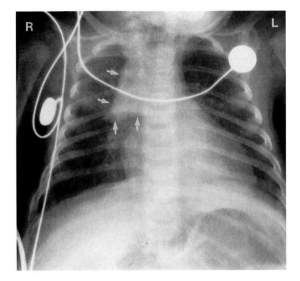

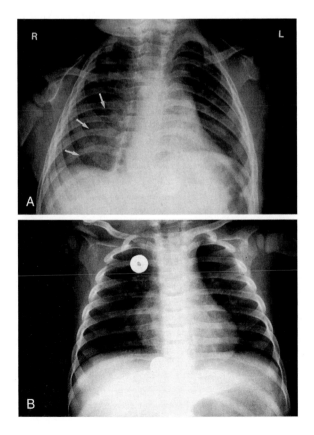

FIGURE 9–7. Pseudoinfiltrate due to poor positioning. *A,* An AP view of the chest was obtained but is slightly rotated. This throws the heart shadow to the left and makes the right pulmonary vascularity appear prominent, creating the impression of a right middle or lower lobe infiltrate *(arrows)*. *B,* A repeat view obtained on the same infant within 10 minutes shows that the chest is perfectly normal.

bronchus, there are two possibilities. The first is that the object will become completely impacted and will not allow air to pass during either inspiration or expiration. In this case, the air distally will become resorbed, and there will be postobstructive atelectasis or a focal infiltrate with associated volume loss.

The second possibility is that the object is only incompletely obstructing the bronchus. This occurs because, during inspiration, the bronchus gets larger in diameter, and air can pass around the object. During expiration, the bronchus gets narrower owing to pressure in the lung, and the air distal to the object cannot escape. The object acts as a ball-valve. Thus, if you are suspicious of an inhaled foreign body, be sure to order an inspiration and an expiration film. On the inspiration film, you may see postobstructive atelectasis, or the film may be normal. If the film is normal, there still may be a ball-valve phenomenon and on the expiration view, air will be trapped on the affected side, while the unaffected lung will decrease in vol-

ume. When this happens, there will be a resultant shift of the mediastinum toward the normal unaffected side (Fig. 9–8).

Swallowed objects may be caught within the esophagus. In children, the objects that are large enough to remain in the esophagus are typically coins. These may be lodged at the level of the thoracic inlet, or they may sit in the esophagus just above the level of the aortic arch (Fig. 9–9). Another common foreign object that may lodge in either the hypopharynx or the esophagus is a fish bone or chicken bone. Chicken bones may be visualized on x-rays, but most fish bones are composed of cartilage and are essentially invisible on x-ray.

Tubes and Lines. A discussion of central venous catheters, jugular catheters, and pleural tubes has been included in Chapter 3. The tubes and catheters that are of specific interest in children are endotracheal tubes and umbilical artery and vein catheters. The tip of an endotracheal tube should be at least as far down as the level of the

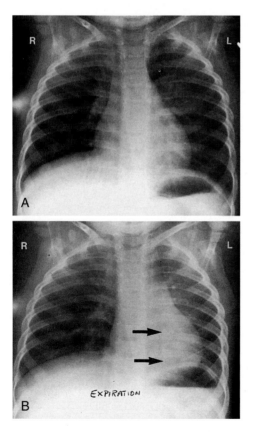

FIGURE 9–8. Foreign body in right mainstem bronchus. In this case the mother thought the child inhaled a peanut. A, An inspiration view of the chest looks essentially normal. B, An expiration view shows that the left lung has decreased in volume (as expected) but that there is a shift of the heart to the left. The right lung remains hyperinflated owing to the inability of the air to escape the ball-valve phenomenon caused by the foreign body.

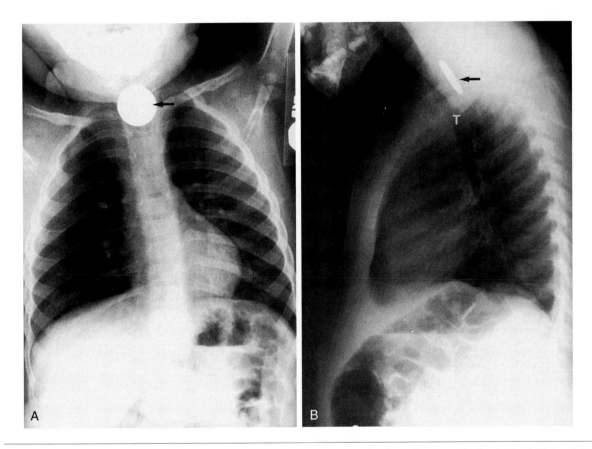

FIGURE 9–9. Coin in the esophagus. *A,* A PA view of the chest demonstrates a quarter that is lodged in the esophagus just at the thoracic inlet. *B,* The lateral view also shows the coin behind the trachea in the esophagus.

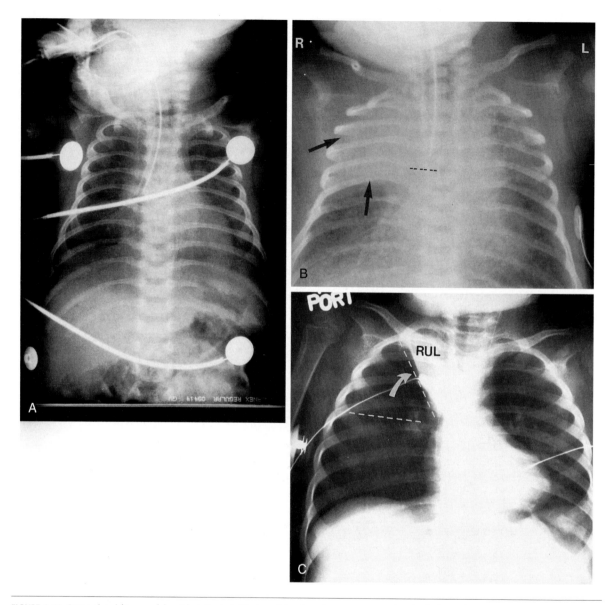

FIGURE 9–10. Progressive right upper lobe atelectasis. *A,* A PA view of the chest demonstrates an endotracheal tube with the tip down in the right mainstem bronchus. This will often obstruct the right upper lobe bronchus. *B,* Early atelectasis of the right upper lobe occurs with resorption of air, causing consolidation *(arrows)* and slight upward bowing of the minor fissure. *C,* As collapse of the right upper lobe becomes complete, the minor fissure rotates upward and medially, and the completely collapsed right upper lobe remains as a small density along the right paratracheal region.

medial clavicles or at the level of the vertebral body of T1 or T2. The endotracheal tube should also have its tip located 1 or 2 cm proximal to the carina. If the carina cannot be easily visualized, you should remember that on an AP or a PA chest x-ray, a tube with its tip projecting over the vertebral body of T5 is probably too low. Endotracheal tubes that are too low usually will go down the right mainstem bronchus, since this is more vertical in orientation than the left mainstem bronchus. Initially, an endotracheal tube positioned in the right mainstem bronchus may demonstrate a relatively normal-appearing lung. With time, however, selective obstruction of the right upper lobe bronchus will cause right upper lobe atelectasis with progressive collapse (Fig. 9–10) or generalized left lung collapse.

Umbilical artery and vein catheters are easily differentiated on the lateral view of the abdomen and chest. The umbilical artery catheter (UAC) proceeds inferiorly from the umbilicus down into the pelvis and then turns and comes up the aorta (Fig. 9–11). Usually, the tip of an umbilical artery catheter is positioned at approximately the level of the vertebral body of T8. If an umbilical artery catheter is advanced too far, either it can proceed up into the great vessels of the head and neck or it can go anteriorly in the aortic arch. An umbilical vein catheter (UVC) also is best identified on the lateral view. It can be seen progressing immediately superiorly from the umbilicus and then posteriorly along the liver and into the inferior vena cava and right atrium.

If both a UAC and a UVC are present on an AP view it is not often easy to tell them apart, especially since you will be seeing the portions of the catheters that are inside and outside the baby. What you should do is imagine where the umbilicus should be. A catheter that goes straight up and slightly to the right of the midline is a UVC, and one that goes down toward the pelvis and then toward the head is a UAC.

Another catheter that can sometimes be confusing is a ventriculoperitoneal shunt catheter. These shunts, which are placed for relief of hydrocephalus, extend from the lateral ventricle of

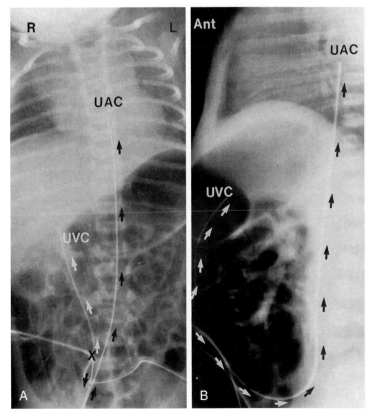

FIGURE 9–11. Differentiation of umbilical artery from umbilical vein catheters. *A,* On the AP view babygram, if you imagine the position of the umbilicus (at the position of the X), the catheter, which initially goes inferiorly and then turns and goes superiorly just to the left of midline, is the umbilical artery catheter *(black arrows).* A catheter that goes into the umbilical region and immediately progresses cephalad and slightly to the right of the midline *(white arrows)* is the umbilical vein catheter. *B,* A lateral view on the same infant demonstrates the inferior, then the posterior and superior, course of the umbilical artery catheter, and the immediate superior course of the umbilical vein catheter progressing toward the inferior portion of the liver.

the brain down along the soft tissues of the neck and anterior chest wall and then into the peritoneal cavity (Fig. 9–12). Less commonly, the distal shunt tip may be placed in the region of the right atrium.

Respiratory Diseases in the Newborn. A number of entities can cause neonatal respiratory difficulty (Table 9–1). You should be able to recognize a congenital diaphragmatic hernia, since it is a cause of respiratory distress in the neonatal period, and it carries a mortality rate well in excess of 50 per cent. Clinical manifestations are a scaphoid abdomen and bowel sounds in the chest. There can also be cyanosis due to pulmonary hypoplasia and pulmonary hypertension. These hernias occur more commonly on the left and will displace the heart and tracheal structures to the right. There will be an opacity within the chest, which often has visible bowel or at least air-filled spaces within it (Fig. 9–13).

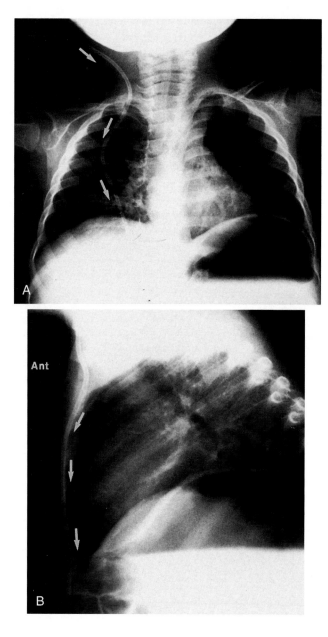

FIGURE 9–12. Ventricular peritoneal shunt for hydrocephalus. *A,* An AP view of the chest shows a catheter coming down from the cervical region and progressing across the chest, but not in a pathway that would represent vascular or other mediastinal structures. *B,* The lateral view of the chest shows the catheter progressing along the anterior soft tissues down into the abdomen.

TABLE 9–1. X-ray Findings of Respiratory Distress in the Newborn

Entity	Time	Lung Volume	Lung Findings
Diaphragmatic hernia	At birth	Compressed	Bowel in chest
Meconium aspiration	At birth	Increased	Coarse, patchy infiltrates
Transient tachypnea	0–2 days	Normal or increased	Homogeneous diffuse or linear infiltrates
Hyaline membrane disease	0–7 days	Decreased*	Granular infiltrates
Neonatal pneumonia	Variable	Variable	Granular or patchy infiltrates
Pneumothorax	Variable	Decreased	Lucent dark area at lung edge†

*Can be increased if the patient is on positive-pressure ventilation (PEEP).
†Pneumothorax almost always occurs in children who are on PEEP.
You should look carefully for a basilar, medial, or anterior pneumothorax, since the films are usually done supine.

At birth, there can be meconium aspiration. Meconium is the term used for the first stool evacuated after birth, and it is composed of mucus, epithelial cells, bile, and debris. In fetal distress there may be evacuation of meconium into the amniotic fluid. Only about 10 per cent of the time does this cause respiratory problems. At birth, as a result of this, there may be coarse patchy infiltrates as well as hyperinflation of the lungs, which clears in about 3 to 5 days. Pneumothorax or pneumomediastinum occurs in about 25 per cent of cases.

Another cause of respiratory distress within 48 hours of birth is transient tachypnea of the newborn (TTN). Lung volumes may be larger than normal, and there may be linear or streaky opacities that clear within 2 days. TTN is really a clinical and not a radiographic diagnosis; it is due to delayed resorption of intrauterine pulmonary liquid.

Hyaline membrane disease (HMD) is caused by surfactant deficiency and results in low lung volumes (unless the infant is intubated) and granular or ground-glass opacities of both lungs. Any opacity in the lungs of a premature infant should be considered to be HMD until another cause is established. Air bronchograms are often present, and, rarely, there is a pleural effusion. Hyaline membrane disease typically becomes radiographically apparent at 4 to 6 hours after birth.

With HMD or pneumonia, infants may need positive-pressure ventilation. The complications of this respiratory therapy include pulmonary interstitial emphysema and bronchopulmonary dysplasia. Pulmonary interstitial emphysema (PIE) refers to accumulation of air outside of alveoli and in interstitial or perivascular spaces. The imaging features include tortuous linear lucencies that radiate outward from the hilum and may extend all the way to the periphery of the lung. If you look carefully, these do not resemble the pattern of a typical bronchial tree but are more tortuous (Fig. 9–14). You should be able to recognize PIE, since it may rapidly result in life-threatening complications, such as pneumothorax, pneumomediastinum, or pneumopericardium (Fig. 9–15).

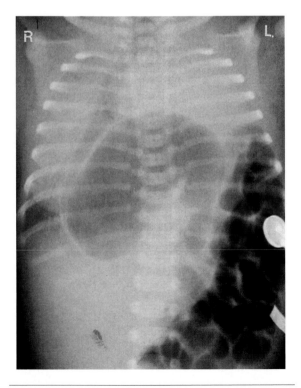

FIGURE 9–13. Diaphragmatic hernia. This newborn had significant respiratory difficulty. An AP view of the chest and abdomen demonstrates opacification of the left hemithorax, with bowel loops pushing up into the opacified left hemithorax. This condition carries a high fatality rate and should be recognized immediately.

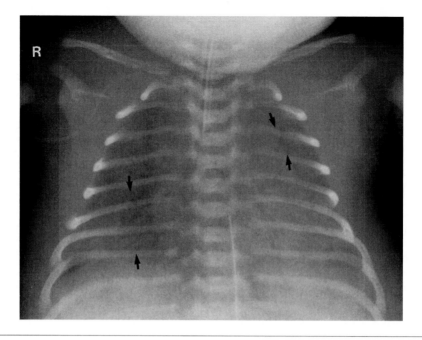

FIGURE 9–14. Pulmonary interstitial emphysema (PIE). This AP view of the chest shows generalized opacification of both lungs in a child with hyaline membrane disease. The arrows indicate linear air collections that do not follow the normal branching bronchial pattern and represent air in the interstitium. These patients often quickly progress to having a pneumothorax.

Since the AP chest x-rays of newborns or neonates are usually obtained with the infant in a supine position, a pneumothorax may be difficult to appreciate. This is because the air is usually located anteriorly (and not superiorly or laterally) in the pleural space. You may be able to see lucencies either at the base of the lung or along the medial aspect of the lung. Often, a lateral x-ray taken with the child lying on the back is necessary to show you the (anterior) pneumothorax (Fig. 9–16).

Bronchopulmonary dysplasia (BPD) is thought to be the result of oxygen toxicity or barotrauma associated with respiratory therapy. This usually progresses as either HMD or neonatal pneumonia is resolving. It is usually seen progressing from approximately 1 week to 1 month of life. The lungs typically become hyperinflated, in spite of the fact that they may have diffuse opacity with linear densities caused by fibrosis. There also may be areas of rounded lucency within the lung.

Pneumonia. Neonatal pneumonia may result in a lung that is low in volume, normal, or hyperinflated. The lung opacities are typically granular, and the time course is variable. Neonatal pneumonias are due to transplacental infection (from TORCH) or from perineal flora acquired as a result of premature rupture of the membranes or while passing through the birth canal.

Very young children (several weeks to 1 year of age) may have a viral pneumonia caused either by RSV or by *H. influenzae*. With these, the early stage is bronchiolitis. About 15 per cent of children under the age of 2 years will develop bronchiolitis and will present with rhinorrhea, sneezing, cough, and low-grade fever followed by the rapid onset of tachypnea and wheezing. Most cases occur during winter and early spring. These patients will not have infiltrates on the chest x-ray, and hyperinflation is the only radiographic clue. Bronchiolitis most commonly is due to RSV. As these viral pneumonias progress, children may also develop perihilar or peribronchial opacities. This can be seen as peribronchial cuffing or hilar adenopathy. Again, many of these patients show associated hyperinflation. The peribronchial cuffing can be seen by looking for an outline of a bronchus in the region of the hilum and noting that the bronchial wall is thicker than a line traced by a fine lead pencil.

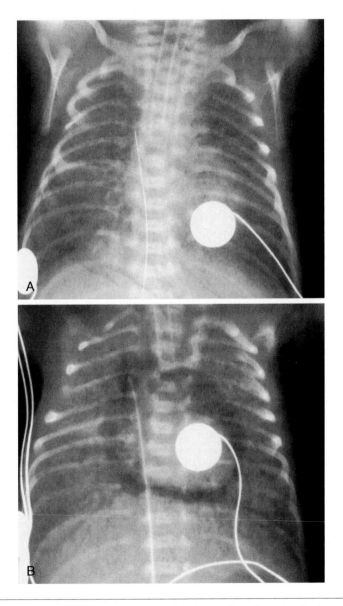

FIGURE 9–15. Complications of hyaline membrane disease. *A,* Most patients with hyaline membrane disease have low lung volume and bilateral infiltrates. This patient is hyperinflated, with the diaphragms down to the level of the posterior tenth ribs because of the need for positive pressure ventilation. *B,* A subsequent AP chest x-ray demonstrates development of a pneumopericardium, seen as a dark collection of air surrounding the heart.

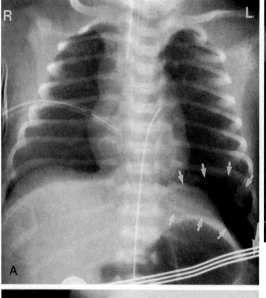

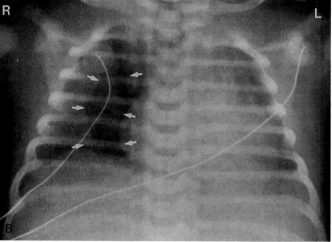

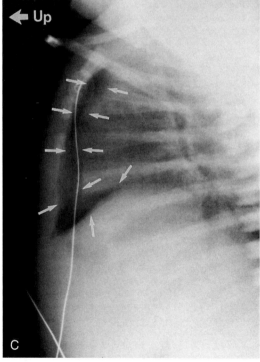

FIGURE 9–16. Pneumothorax on supine chest x-ray. *A,* In this infant, a right chest tube has already been placed because a pneumothorax is present. There is, however, a lucency at the left lung base *(small arrows)* representing a loculated pneumothorax. Note, in addition, a deep sulcus sign *(large arrow).* *B,* An AP view of the chest in another infant demonstrates a lucency or dark area overlying the medial aspect of the right lung and outlining the right cardiac border. This represents an anterior medial right pneumothorax. *C,* A lateral view of the chest with this patient supine is the best way to see an anterior pneumothorax. This will be seen as a dark collection of air in the retrosternal region and in the anterior costophrenic angle *(arrows).*

As children get somewhat older (aged 1 to 3 years), they develop bacterial pneumonias. Pneumococcus is a common pathogen at age 1 to 3 years, whereas *Staphylococcus aureus* and *H. influenzae* are usually seen during infancy. Bacterial pneumonias typically cause alveolar infiltrates with lobar or segmental consolidations, often with effusion. Staphylococcal pneumonias may cause pneumothorax and also may cavitate. Most of the bacterial pneumonias have appearances similar to those already described for adults. The two exceptions are the cavitating staphylococcal pneumonias and, occasionally, what is termed a round pneumonia. A round pneumonia is usually a bacterial pneumonia in an early stage, and later typical lobar consolidations may develop (Fig. 9–17).

Cystic Fibrosis. Cystic fibrosis is caused by a dysfunction of the exocrine glands producing thick mucus that accumulates in the lungs, causing bronchitis and recurrent pneumonias. It is an autosomal recessive disorder and is the most common lethal genetic disease affecting Caucasians. Pulmonary findings are present in essentially all cases by the time a child is 10 years of age or more. The most obvious finding is

hyperinflation. Essentially, the chest x-ray looks like that of an adult with COPD. There is an increased AP diameter and flattening of the hemidiaphragms. In addition, the lungs generally appear "dirty." There is peribronchial thickening and bronchiectasis with a lot of pulmonary markings at the lung bases (Fig. 9–18). These are not lobar or segmental infiltrates.

Children with cystic fibrosis also are prone to a wide variety of gastrointestinal problems, including meconium ileus, meconium peritonitis, rectal prolapse, volvulus, intussusception, pancreatitis, jaundice, and growth failure or vitamin deficiencies. You should suspect cystic fibrosis in any child with recurrent respiratory or gastrointestinal symptoms.

PEDIATRIC ABDOMINAL IMAGING

Congenital diaphragmatic hernia has already been mentioned, but you should be aware of a number of other congenital abnormalities of the bowel in neonates. Initial imaging studies of choice for various problems are listed in Table 9–2.

Esophageal Fistula. Tracheoesophageal fistula (TEF) may be suspected in an infant who has had polyhydramnios. This is usually clinically apparent, since there is excessive salivation and as soon as you attempt to feed the child there will be aspiration, coughing, and choking. Ninety-five per cent of patients with a TEF will have a blind-ending esophagus. The diagnosis is usually made by passing a small, soft feeding tube down the esophagus to the blind end and taking a lateral x-ray. If necessary, air can be injected to help visualization. Instillation of barium or other contrast material is rarely, if ever, indicated. In those few patients with an "H type" fistula and a patent esophagus it may take months to arrive at the diagnosis, but the disorder should be suspected in a child with recurrent pneumonias or chronic cough. You should remember that 40 per cent of patients with (tracheo-esophageal fistula) have associated cardiac and other gastrointestinal anomalies. The VATER syndrome describes the association between vertebral anomalies (hemivertebra), anal

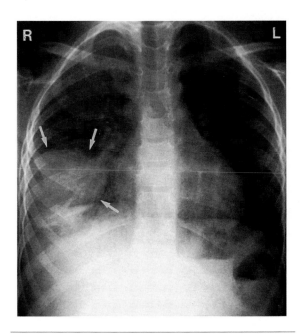

FIGURE 9–17. **Round pneumonia.** A PA view of the chest demonstrates a rounded density in the right lower lobe *(arrows)*. Usually this will progress to a standard lobar consolidation of a typical pneumonia.

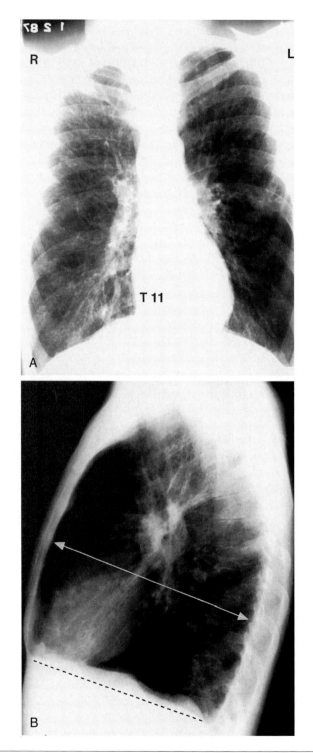

FIGURE 9–18. Cystic fibrosis. *A,* The PA view of the chest in this young teenager demonstrates marked hyperinflation, with the hemidiaphragms being flattened and pushed down to the level of the posterior eleventh ribs. There is also diffuse bronchial thickening throughout both lungs. *B,* The lateral view of the chest shows an increase in AP diameter and flattening of the hemidiaphragms. These findings in an adult would normally be associated with COPD, but in a teenager or child are almost certainly due to cystic fibrosis.

TABLE 9–2. Imaging of Pediatric Gastrointestinal Problems	
Suspected Problems	**Imaging Test of Choice**
Esophageal atresia or tracheoesophageal fistula	Lateral x-ray with soft feeding tube in place
Gastroesophageal reflux	Barium swallow or nuclear medicine reflux study
Pyloric stenosis	Ultrasound
Duodenal atresia, stenosis or midgut volvulus	Plain x-ray (use air as contrast)
Meconium ileus	Plain film and Gastrografin enema
Intussusception	Plain film followed by reduction utilizing air or Gastrografin
Necrotizing enterocolitis	Plain film of the abdomen and possible left lateral decubitus views (to look for free air)
Hirschsprung's disease	Barium or Gastrografin enema
Biliary atresia or neonatal hepatitis	Nuclear medicine hepatobiliary scan
Meckel's diverticulum	Nuclear medicine Meckel's scan

atresia, (*tracheo-e*sophageal fistula), and *r*adial limb dysplasia.

Bowel Obstruction. Air should normally be seen in the abdomen of the neonate in the following temporal progression: in the stomach 2 hours after birth, in the small bowel at 6 hours, and in the rectum by 24 hours.

Hypertrophic pyloric stenosis is the second most common gastrointestinal condition requiring surgery in the first 2 months of life. Pyloric stenosis is more common in male infants and should be suspected if there is a maternal or sibling history of the condition. The typical clinical symptom is nonbilious vomiting during the second to fourth week of life. There may be a palpable olive-shaped mass to the right of the umbilicus. A plain film of the abdomen will show a stomach that is dilated to greater than 7 cm, and peristaltic waves can sometimes be seen, giving the stomach a caterpillar appearance. The diagnosis is confirmed by using abdominal ultrasound to visualize the thickened pyloric muscle. The pyloric muscle should not be more than 4 mm in thickness (mucosa to outside wall) or greater than 18 mm in length (Fig. 9–19).

Duodenal atresias, midgut volvulus, and pyloric stenosis are apparent because they produce obstruction and vomiting. Under these circumstances, you should consult the radiologist as

to what imaging procedure would be best. The approximate level of obstruction in the bowel is typically determined on the plain film by seeing how far bowel gas has progressed through the gastrointestinal tract. If gas is seen only in the stomach or the stomach and duodenum (the "double-bubble" sign), a proximal obstruction is likely. Duodenal atresia or midgut volvulus should be suspected in a birth with polyhydramnios and an infant who has bile-stained vomiting. Duodenal atresia is the most common cause of the double-bubble sign, with annular pancreas being next most common. Duodenal bands, webs, and midgut volvulus are less frequent. Duodenal atresia has been associated with Down's syndrome. Midgut volvulus, although less common, is important to consider, because there is a high mortality rate without intervention. A midgut volvulus occurs when the small bowel and proximal colon rotate about the axis of the superior mesenteric artery; this can cause arterial compromise and gangrene.

If air is seen beyond the duodenum but not into the distal small bowel or colon, you should think of midlevel lesions. Atresias can occur in the jejunum and ileum. With any of these entities, even with x-ray contrast studies, it is not possible to tell with certainty either the site or the length of the atresia or even to differentiate an atresia from a midgut volvulus. As a result, most pediatric surgeons are content with the plain x-ray findings before proceeding to surgery. Occasionally some will request a barium enema to look for a microcolon prior to surgery.

If gas is seen throughout most of the abdomen of a neonate but not in the region of the rectum, a distal small bowel or colon obstruction should be suspected. This may be the result of either a meconium ileus or Hirschsprung's disease. A note of caution should be entered here relative to the appearance of bowel gas in a neonate or very young child. Gas in the small bowel and colon look exactly the same, and you should not allow yourself to think that you can tell the difference. Rather, differential diagnoses are made on the basis of whether you see gas in the proximal or distal "bowel."

Meconium ileus is seen in 50 per cent of patients with cystic fibrosis. On an enema performed with water-soluble contrast, the colon is seen to be very small (microcolon), since it was

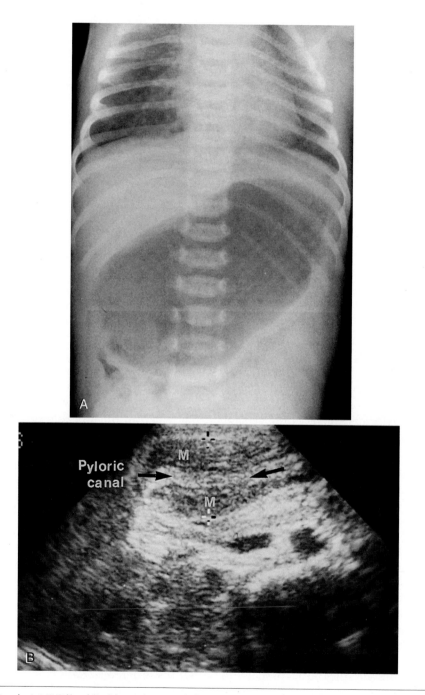

FIGURE 9–19. Pyloric stenosis. *A,* A KUB film of the abdomen shows a markedly dilated, gas-filled stomach. *B,* A transverse ultrasound study of the upper abdomen shows the thickened pyloric muscle (M) on both sides of the pyloric canal.

unused during fetal life (Fig. 9–20). Hirschsprung's disease is due to the absence of neural cells in the distal segment of the colon; these children present in the first 6 weeks of life with

obstruction or constipation. The disorder should be suspected in any infant who fails to pass meconium in the first 24 hours of life. In about 75 per cent of patients the abnormal segment is

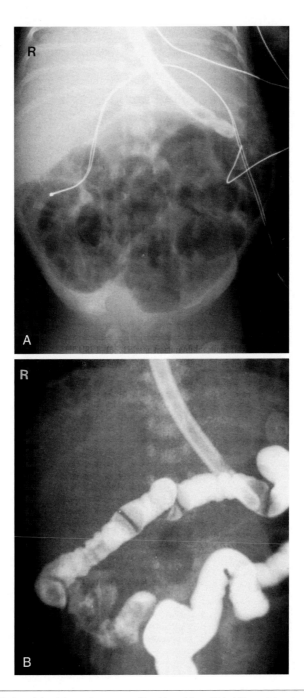

FIGURE 9–20. Meconium ileus. *A,* An AP view of the abdomen demonstrates dilated bowel. In a child of this age it is not possible to differentiate the colon from the small bowel. There is, however, no gas seen within the rectum. *B,* A Gastrografin enema has been performed, and the colon is noted to be very small (a microcolon). There are intraluminal defects seen in the colon at the level of the ileocecal valve, because there is usually obstruction at this level resulting from the thick tenacious meconium adhering to small bowel.

restricted to the rectosigmoid colon. On a barium enema, a narrowed segment may be identified (Fig. 9–21).

Intussusception is invagination of a segment of bowel into more distal bowel and usually occurs with ileum telescoping into colon. Forty per cent of patients present between 3 and 18 months of age, most with pain and vomiting. A lesser number have an associated abdominal mass or rectal bleeding. Intussusception is rarely seen in neonates. Clinically the children have an acute onset of colicky pain, and they may cry, draw up their knees, and vomit. Sometimes a sausage-shaped mass can be felt in the upper abdomen. Radiographically, plain films are often normal. If the intussusception has occurred within 24 hours prior to patient presentation, there is a good chance that a radiologist can reduce it with a water-soluble contrast enema. Currently, however, most radiologists prefer to reduce intussusception simply utilizing air (Fig. 9–22). If this fails, surgery is necessary. Reduction by a radiologist should not be at-

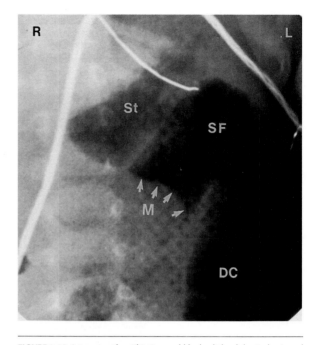

FIGURE 9–22. Intussusception. This 3-year-old had colicky abdominal pain and rectal bleeding. There is invagination of a segment of bowel into more distal bowel. Ileocolic and ileoileocolic intussusceptions represent 90% of occurrences. Here, a film has been obtained while the radiologist is reducing the intussusception with air. Air is seen in the distal colon and the splenic flexure, and the mass representing the leading portion of the intussuscepted segment is clearly identified.

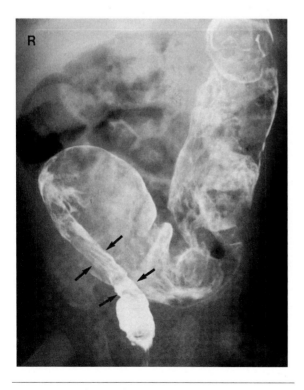

FIGURE 9–21. Hirschsprung's disease. This abnormality is due to an absence of myenteric plexus cells in the distal colon. A barium enema demonstrates a narrowed segment in the rectum and a markedly dilated sigmoid and descending colon.

tempted if there are clinical signs of peritonitis or shock. Other relatively common lesions to bear in mind when it looks as though there is a proximal bowel obstruction in a child 6 to 30 months of age are an incarcerated inguinal hernia and appendicitis.

Necrotizing Enterocolitis (NEC). This is the most common gastrointestinal emergency in premature infants. It usually develops within the first week after birth but can be seen up to 2 months after birth. Clinical signs are abdominal tenderness, rectal bleeding, and a septic shock–like appearance. The earliest radiographic sign is air within the wall of the bowel (pneumatosis) or a bubbly appearance of the bowel. Another early finding is small bowel dilatation due to an adynamic ileus (Fig. 9–23). Common complications and indications for surgery include free air within the peritoneal cavity, which indicates a bowel perforation. Gas in the portal vein may also be identified. In contrast with adults, in which this condition generally portends a fatal

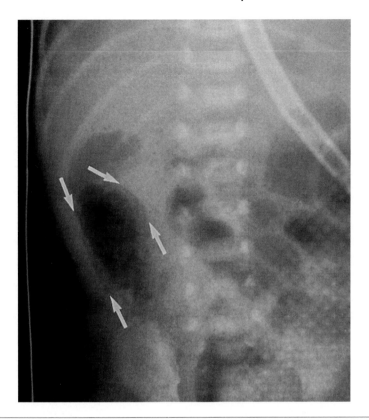

FIGURE 9–23. Necrotizing enterocolitis. This represents the most common gastrointestinal emergency in premature infants. A film of this 5-day-old infant shows abnormal collections of air within the bowel wall *(arrows)*.

outcome, the outcome in children with portal venous air is not as bad.

On a supine view, if there is a large amount of free air within the peritoneal cavity, the air will outline the falciform ligament of the liver (the "football sign") (Fig. 9–24). This is a fairly subtle sign; a large amount of air may be present in the peritoneal cavity, and on a supine film you may easily overlook it. For this reason, a left lateral decubitus view, which will show air over the lateral margin of the liver, is often recommended.

Meckel's Diverticulum. This is a vestigial remnant of the omphalomesenteric duct, and it may contain gastric mucosa. Clinical signs are painless rectal bleeding and, occasionally, intestinal obstruction. Meckel's diverticulum follows what is known as the rule of 2's. It occurs in 2 per cent of the population; it usually presents before 2 years of age; and the diverticulum is usually located in the ilium within 2 feet of the ileocecal valve. If gastric mucosa is present in the diverticulum, there may be resultant ulceration and hemorrhage. In patients with rectal bleeding prior to 2 years of age, Meckel's diverticulum should be considered. The imaging study of choice is a nuclear medicine scan done with technetium pertechnetate. This concentrates in the normal and ectopic gastric mucosa and allows identification of Meckel's diverticulum (Fig. 9–25).

Neonatal Jaundice. In some very young infants (2 to 3 weeks old) there can be development of jaundice. The usual diagnostic dilemma is whether the infant has neonatal hepatitis or biliary atresia. The imaging test of choice is a nuclear medicine hepatobiliary scan. This involves giving a small amount of radioactive tracer that is concentrated by the liver and then excreted via the biliary system. If any excretion into the

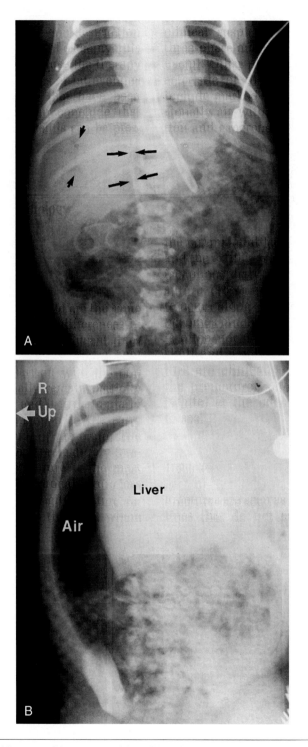

FIGURE 9–24. Complications of necrotizing enterocolitis. *A,* A supine abdominal film of the abdomen demonstrates diffuse mottled air throughout the bowel wall and shows air within the portal venous system *(short arrows)* as well. There is outlining of the falciform ligament by free air *(long arrows)* anteriorly in the peritoneal cavity. To the uninitiated, the amount of free air is difficult to appreciate. *B,* A left lateral decubitus view obtained in the same patient immediately afterward demonstrates a very large amount of free air overlying the surface of the liver.

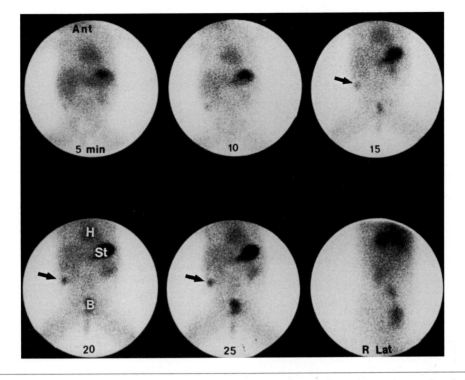

FIGURE 9-25. Meckel's diverticulum. In this 2-year-old child who had unexplained rectal bleeding, a nuclear medicine study was performed utilizing radioactive material that concentrates in gastric mucosa (technetium-99m pertechnetate). Sequential 5-minute images of the abdomen are obtained. On the 20-minute image, the heart, stomach, and bladder are clearly seen as well as an ectopic focus of activity *(arrow)* representing a Meckel's diverticulum.

small bowel is detected on the images, biliary atresia is excluded. Occasionally in patients with severe hepatitis, follow-up images are needed at 24 hours post injection to be certain of the diagnosis.

Abdominal Masses. Abdominal masses in children are usually initially worked up by clinical examination and a plain film of the abdomen. The differential diagnosis of an abdominal mass varies with the child's age. A mass in the abdomen of a child of any age most likely arises from the kidneys. In a neonate, 55 per cent of masses are renal in origin (hydronephrosis or multicystic dysplastic kidney), and the remainder are usually gastrointestinal duplications, cysts, and hemangioendotheliomas of the liver.

If a mass appears to be in the flank in an older infant or child, Wilms' tumor, neuroblastoma, and hydronephrosis account for about 80 per cent of the lesions. Other possibilities include abcesses, cysts, and hepatoblastomas. Neuroblastomas have calcification approximately 90 per cent of the time (Fig. 9–26) and

are usually seen in patients under the age of 2 years. They present as masses external to the kidney and tend to displace the kidney rather than deform it. Since neuroblastomas arise from neural tissue, they are also relatively common in the region of the adrenal glands, along the sympathetic chain, and in the posterior mediastinum (Fig. 9–27). Wilms' tumor begins within the kidney, and on an intravenous pyelogram it will be seen as a mass within the kidney, deforming the normal collecting system (Fig. 9–28). Wilms' tumors are bilateral 10 per cent of the time and are rarely calcified. The average age of presentation is 2 to 3 years, which is older than the usual age for neuroblastomas.

Urinary Abnormalities. There are two relatively common urinary problems in children—hydronephrosis and ureterovesicular reflux. The most common cause of hydronephrosis in a child is an obstruction at the junction of the lower portion of the renal pelvis and the upper ureter (UPJ). The entity is bilateral in 20 per cent of cases. The initial imaging test of choice is an

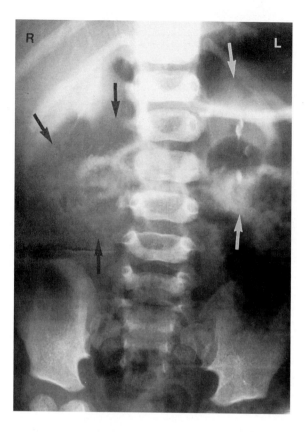

FIGURE 9–26. Retroperitoneal neuroblastoma. On this intravenous pyelogram, the left kidney appears to be functioning well *(white arrows)*. On the right, no functional kidney is identified, but there are multiple scattered tiny amorphous calcifications, which are often seen with this tumor.

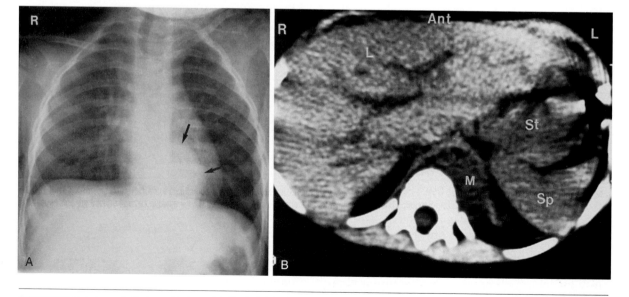

FIGURE 9–27. Posterior mediastinal neuroblastoma. *A,* A PA view of the chest demonstrates a rounded retrocardiac mass *(arrows)*. *B,* On a transverse CT scan, the liver, spleen, and stomach are seen, but there is also a mass (M) in the left paraspinous region.

intravenous pyelogram. Although the dilated collecting system can be visualized with ultrasound, there is usually not enough anatomic detail of the ureter and there is no information about renal function. Postoperative follow-up functional studies in these children are usually done with a nuclear medicine Lasix renogram, since the radiation dose is lower and there is no risk of a contrast reaction. If only information about the degree of dilatation of the collecting system is desired, ultrasound is the test of choice.

Ureterovesicular reflux is due to maldevelopment of the flap valve that is created as the ureter crosses obliquely through the bladder wall. Less commonly, it can be due to ectopic insertion of a ureter when there is ureteral duplication or to a ureterocele. On a contrast study, any visible reflux of urine from the bladder into a ureter is abnormal. If severe, it is surgically repaired because of the increased risk of infection. The most common imaging method is a cystogram. The patient is catheterized, contrast is put into the bladder, and the radiologist looks for contrast in the ureters. This involves a relatively high radiation dose to the child's gonads, but the anatomic resolution is good. If repeated evaluations of reflux are necessary, a nuclear medicine cystogram can provide good quantitative information with a much lower dose.

Multicystic dysplastic kidney is a unilateral process resulting from a severe UPJ obstruction in utero. As a result, there is no functional renal parenchyma, and the kidney is represented by a large number of noncommunicating cysts. Calcification may be present. There are absent or only very small renal vessels. A retrograde pyelogram shows a blind-ending ureter. Surgery is not immediately necessary. There is another congenital condition called multilocular cystic nephroma, which has large cystic areas. Calcifications in this entity are rare.

Neonatal or infantile polycystic disease does not present with a dominant abdominal mass. Each has ectasia of renal tubules, but there are no obvious cysts that are visible by imaging methods. Ultrasound is the test of choice in

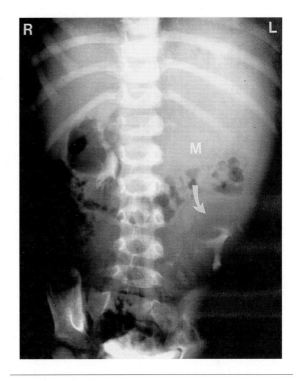

FIGURE 9–28. Wilms' tumor. On this intravenous pyelogram, the collecting system of the right kidney is identified along the lateral border of L1, L2, and L3. The collecting system of the left kidney has been displaced inferiorly by a mass (M), and the collecting system has been distorted, suggesting that the mass is intrarenal in origin. This is a common way of differentiating an intraparenchymal Wilms' tumor from an extrarenal neuroblastoma.

the neonatal form, most tubules are ectatic, and death usually occurs in months or years. There is little associated hepatic fibrosis. In the infantile form, about 20 per cent of the tubules are ectatic, and symptoms do not appear for 3 to 6 months. There is moderate hepatic fibrosis. In the juvenile form, fewer tubules are ectatic, and symptoms appear at 1 to 5 years of age. The liver fibrosis is severe in this form, and death results from portal hypertension.

General Suggested Readings

Silverman F, Kuhn J: Caffey's Pediatric X-Ray Diagnosis, 9th ed. St. Louis, CV Mosby, 1993.
Swischuk L: Emergency Imaging of the Acutely Ill or Injured Child, 3rd ed. Baltimore, Williams & Wilkins, 1994.

Appendix 1
Typical Price Range of Some Imaging Procedures*

Diagnostic Radiology

Chest	$30–130
Abdomen	30–130
Pelvis	30–140
Hand	24–104
Ankle	24–110
Barium enema	90–300
Intravenous pyelogram	100–240
Mammogram	45–200

Computerized Tomography

Brain with contrast only	240–700
with and without contrast	290–950

Magnetic Resonance Scan

Brain with contrast	525–1600
with and without contrast	880–1700

Nuclear Medicine

Bone scan	190–460
Myocardial perfusion	455–710

Ultrasound

Fetal	120–500
Right upper quadrant	70–300

*Price includes hospital and physician charges. Lower end of range is the fee paid by Medicare, and the upper end is the total fee charged (as compared with paid). Many contracted imaging services offer 20 to 40 per cent discounts on charged fees.

Appendix 2
Radiation Doses From Various Examinations*

Examination	Effective Dose (mrem)	Gonadal Dose (mrem)
Extremities	1	<1
Skull	22	<1
Chest (two views)	10	1
KUB (abdomen, one view)	60	97/221†
Lumbar spine	130	218/721
CT (head and body)	110	—
Barium enema	410	175/900
Hip and pelvis	50	210/600
Nuclear Medicine		
Bone scan	440	320/440
Lung scan	150	228/30
Cardiac (thallium)	710	1900/560
Hepatobiliary	370	19/50
All Ultrasound	None	None
All Magnetic Resonance Scans	None	None

*The effective dose from natural background radiation in the United States is 300 mrem per year.

†Refers to male/female. Gonadal dose in the female approximates dose to the fetus in a pregnant female.

Index

Page numbers in *italics* refer to illustrations; page numbers followed by t refer to tables.